ADVANCE PRAISE FOR *LAY THEM TO REST*

"Part murder mystery, part master class in forensics, Laurah Norton's *Lay Them to Rest* leads readers through a twisty personal investigation complete with a startling reckoning. Norton seamlessly transplants her passion for justice from her fantastic podcast to the narrative page—a must-read for true crime fanatics."

—**Kate Winkler Dawson**, author of *American Sherlock: Murder, Forensics, and the Birth of American CSI*

"Laurah Norton's *Lay Them to Rest* is a beautifully woven mystery that captivates the reader from the first page as they root for her to solve the case. Norton's expertise and her dedication to the victim shine through. This book and Norton's work [are] the good in true crime that everyone should pay attention to."

—**Sarah Turney**, victim advocate and CEO of Voices for Justice Media

"Rarely do readers of true crime get something as fresh and engaging as Laurah Norton's *Lay Them to Rest*. Norton's passion and empathy shine in this candid and personal account of her work with unidentified persons. Her admiration of those who share her passion gives an intimate look behind the scenes of complex investigations. She effortlessly guides readers—with the help of industry experts—without losing focus on the people at the heart of the case. *Lay Them to* Rest leaves a lasting impression even after [turning] the final page."

—**Kristen Seavey**, victim advocate and creator of the *Murder, She Told* podcast

"In *Lay Them to Rest*, Laurah Norton not only gives a master class on ethical research and reporting but a humanizing and empathetic look at some of the most marginalized and overlooked victims: the nameless. *Lay Them To Rest* gives readers an unwaveringly honest look at what true crime actually is and entails; Laurah's journey is equal parts obsessive and compassionate, exhilarating and patient, driven and human. I've never seen a more honest and comprehensive look at an investigation, which never shies away from juggling advocacy, working with law enforcement, and managing personal attachments. Every consumer of true crime media should be required to read this work."

—**Josh Hallmark**, creator of the *True Crime Bullsh*** podcast

"Laurah Norton pulls back the curtain on forensic science and allows readers easy access and understanding of the important work being done in this field."

—**Nina Innsted**, missing persons advocate and host of the *Already Gone, They Walk Among America*, and *Up and Vanished: The Trials of Ryan Duke* podcasts

"In *Lay Them to Rest* Laurah Norton immerses readers in a captivating exploration of true crime's true essence: the victims. Laurah takes us on a gripping journey as she illuminates the mystery surrounding 'Ina Jane Doe,' delving into the relentless and collaborative efforts of agencies, forensic scientists, and experts to unveil her identity, honor her story, and provide the closure she deserves."

—**Melissa Rice**, cocreator of *Moms and Mysteries* and board member of The Bridegan Foundation

"Laurah Norton's beautiful and compelling narrative brings the reader along as the team cracks a cold case, all while [presenting] a hard look at the science—and art—of how they do it. With deep research and surprising moments of humor, this book has a place on the shelf of everyone who has ever wondered what it takes to solve a mystery."

—**Charlie Worroll**, creator of *Crimelines* and cocreator of the *Crimelines and Consequences* podcast

"Laurah Norton takes us behind the scenes as she helps to solve a cold case in real time, skillfully breaking down layers of complexity in a way everyday readers can understand. A gripping must-read for anyone interested in true crime."

—**Kristi Lee**, creator of the *Canadian True Crime* podcast

LAY THEM
TO REST

LAY THEM TO REST

On *the* Road
with the
Cold Case
Investigators
Who Identify
the Nameless

LAURAH NORTON

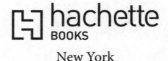

New York

Hachette Books
Hachette Book Group
1290 Avenue of the Americas
New York, NY 10104
HachetteBooks.com
Twitter.com/HachetteBooks
Instagram.com/HachetteBooks

First Edition: October 2023

Published by Hachette Books, an imprint of Hachette Book Group, Inc. The Hachette Books name and logo are trademarks of the Hachette Book Group.

The Hachette Speakers Bureau provides a wide range of authors for speaking events. To find out more, visit hachettespeakersbureau.com or email HachetteSpeakers@hbgusa.com.

Books by Hachette Books may be purchased in bulk for business, educational, or promotional use. For information, please contact your local bookseller or email the Hachette Book Group Special Markets Department at Special.Markets@hbgusa.com.

The publisher is not responsible for websites (or their content) that are not owned by the publisher.

Print book interior design by Amy Quinn

Library of Congress Cataloging-in-Publication Data

Name: Norton, Laurah, author.
Title: Lay them to rest: on the road with the cold case investigators who
    identify the nameless / Laurah Norton.
Description: First edition. | New York: Hachette Books, [2023] | Includes
    bibliographical references and index.
Identifiers: LCCN 2023013020 | ISBN 9780306828805 (hardcover) |
    ISBN 9780306828812 (trade paperback) | ISBN 9780306828829 (ebook)
Subjects: LCSH: Cold cases (Criminal investigation) | Murder victims—Identification. |
    Dead—Identification. | Forensic anthropology. | Forensic sciences.
Classification: LCC HV8073 .N635 2023 | DDC 363.25—dc23/eng/20230629
LC record available at https://lccn.loc.gov/2023013020

ISBNs: 9780306828805 (hardcover); 9780306828829 (ebook)

Printed in the United States of America

LSC-C

Printing 1, 2023

For my father.
And for every person yet to be identified—for the families waiting for them.

CONTENTS

Author's Note   ix
Prologue: What Came Before   xi

CHAPTER ONE
The Case: The Woman in the Woods   1

CHAPTER TWO
The Method: John and Jane Doe   19

CHAPTER THREE
The Case: Assembly   39

CHAPTER FOUR
The Method: Forensic Anthropology   61

CHAPTER FIVE
The Case: Ina, Illinois   71

CHAPTER SIX
The Method: Skeletal Analysis   91

CHAPTER SEVEN
The Case: New Hampshire   115

CHAPTER EIGHT
The Method: Dental Comparisons
and Odontology   149

CHAPTER NINE
The Case: A Trip to the Dentist   163

CHAPTER TEN
The Method: Forensic Art   177

CHAPTER ELEVEN
The Case: The Reconstruction   195

CHAPTER TWELVE
The Method: DNA Analysis and
Investigative Genetic Genealogy   207

CHAPTER THIRTEEN
The Case: Astrea   227

CHAPTER FOURTEEN
The Case: Redgrave Research   237

CHAPTER FIFTEEN
The Answer: Susan Minard Lund   253

CHAPTER SIXTEEN
The Announcement   269

Epilogue: What Comes After   *289*
Acknowledgments   *299*
Notes   *301*
Index   *311*

AUTHOR'S NOTE

The vast majority of conversations and all interviews included in this book were recorded so they could be reproduced in print. When that was not possible, the author worked with the subjects to reproduce the dialogue from our shared memory, text messages, and email. Some conversations and scenes have been condensed for length and clarity.

PROLOGUE
WHAT CAME BEFORE

At the risk of sounding like an absolute twenty-first-century cliché . . . it all started with a podcast.

I've been interested in unsolved cases, real or fictional, for as long as I can remember—detective novels, unexplained events, *Unsolved Mysteries*—but if you'd asked me back in school what I'd be writing about now, I never could've guessed where I've ended up: researching and writing about the unidentified dead, often called John and Jane Does. Burying myself in old articles, police reports, and transcripts of blurry taped interviews, or poring over maps of highways and parks and forests that had been bulldozed into subdivisions . . . it's hardly a choice that comes up in the guidance counselor's office, is it?

I'd studied fiction and creative writing in college and grad school, but after I graduated, I realized I was more interested in nonfiction—seeking out real stories, with real people, that hadn't been explored. I ended up in a full-time non-tenure-track job in the English department of a large university in Atlanta. Gradually, life settled in around me; I got married, and as my thirties hit, I had my son. I taught fiction, and wrote it, sometimes, but was hungry for other stories. Literature paid the bills, though.

But then, in the long sleepless nights of his newborn era, I started listening to podcasts.

For hours upon hours, I'd pace back and forth in the rickety little hallway of our first home, bouncing my restless baby, *Serial* in my ears. When

I finished that gateway series, I downloaded everything "true crime" I could find. I got an Audible subscription so I could listen to Ann Rule's books. Then there were the web forums. That's when I discovered that all the cases I'd obsessed over, watching reruns of *Unsolved Mysteries*? So many were still unsolved. *Why?* I needed to know. *What had been missed?* I dug through Google Scholar and the university archives while the laundry ran. I became an expert at scrolling Reddit with one hand. The other was full of baby.

Fully immersed in this world, I stumbled across a particular podcast in 2016 that changed everything—not the show itself, so much as the story. Although, it's a very good podcast. The host, Robin Warder, had been asked to cover a case that was almost totally unknown to anyone, one that had taken place in Georgia—just two hours away from Atlanta. And that was strange to me, because by this point I had begun to follow just about every cold case in the Southeastern United States. And this one, which I'd never even heard about before, concerned the disappearance of fifteen-year-old twins, Jeannette and Dannette Millbrook.

The twins were last seen on March 18, 1990, in Augusta, Georgia. Their case had somehow been closed about a year after they were reported missing by their mother, right after they would have turned seventeen. The case closure meant they were removed from the NCMEC—the National Center for Missing and Exploited Children—database. But the twins hadn't returned home. In fact, they'd never even been located. I decided to search for more information, but there was almost *nothing* out there. After a lot of searching, I discovered another podcast had been contacted by the same advocate who tipped off Robin Warder. Between the two, I discovered that in 2013 the twins were relisted in the NCMEC database, and on the Charley Project, an online collection of more than fourteen thousand "cold cases," mainly in the United States. A few articles had been written when their case was reopened in 2013, but other than that, I couldn't find much more information. Who, and what, had failed?

I brought up one of those articles—about the case reopening for Jeannette and Dannette Millbrook, back in 2013—in a composition class, interested to hear what my students might think. We discussed how little news coverage existed, and why their case had been closed when they were still missing. My students had a good discussion that day, and I kept thinking about the news photo of their mother and their younger sister, holding framed pictures of the twins: frozen in time at fifteen years old, in blurry yearbook shots. Later, I'd find out that these were some of the only remaining photos of them. The twins' mother had given the rest over to law enforcement. They weren't returned.

Around the same time, it just so happened that I'd gotten a small grant to design a podcasting class for the university. I was teaching myself to use the audio equipment I'd purchased for the task. But before I instructed my students in narrative podcasting, I needed to do a test run for myself. I'd originally planned on making something that would never leave the confines of my hard drive. *Writing Flash Fiction. Writing Even More Flash Fiction.* Something exciting like that.

But maybe, just maybe . . . I could do something useful while I learned.

———•———

Later that spring, my college friend Brooke and I met up for a playdate, and as we watched our boys fall over in a pit of plastic balls, I told her the story of the missing twins. Brooke was a licensed professional counselor and understood a lot; I enjoyed talking through cases from podcasts with her. She asked interesting questions about people that I'd never think of: the *whys* of who they were, not just the *hows* of what they did. Now that I was thinking of starting one of my own, I realized I couldn't do it without her. I wanted to take a dive into the twins' case, with fresh eyes, and I hoped she'd be willing to use her expertise to work directly with the family, doing interviews—if they were interested and gave us permission to cover the case. Meanwhile, I'd do the research and write the scripts. After we'd finished, we'd work with the twins' family to review and approve it all, and in return, they'd have a media source for the story that was complete.

Brooke, wincing as my toddler nailed her smaller toddler in the face with a red ball, agreed.

After flipping through a few websites on the history of the American Southeast, we decided to call our show *The Fall Line*. The metaphor worked on a few different levels: the geographical divide across Georgia, our home state, and the crack that seemed to widen and swallow up the cases that didn't hold enough public interest to stay afloat.

That was the start. We had no idea what we were doing on the audio front, but we found a lot on everything else. And, to our surprise, people listened. We raised money for a reward. A billboard. The twins' family gave national interviews. And then, there were many more cases—suggestions flooding our new Gmail. Before I knew it, I had two full-time jobs: English professor and researcher of cases with scant media footprints. I learned to file FOIA (Freedom of Information Act) requests for more details on missing-persons cases and cold cases. I started visiting police departments and sheriff's offices and medical examiners. We searched county and state databases for the missing and murdered who'd had no media coverage, often reaching out directly to families. Soon, they started coming to us.

Fortunately, I didn't teach on Fridays. We'd go do interviews then, or after classes, or weekends. My husband worked six days a week, so childcare was tricky to arrange. But we managed. We drove down tire-rutted roads in remote Southern towns to interview the families of victims whose stories the media hadn't bothered to cover, and we set up recording equipment on kitchen counters or back porches. We listened to mothers and fathers, sisters and brothers, friends and teachers talk about the day their loved ones were found in ditches or along dirt roads or disappeared right off the front porch. There was no end to it. So many people had been seeking news coverage that never came.

With so many families seeking publicity for their own loved ones' cases, it took us a while to come across John and Jane Does, which are what law enforcement calls victims whose remains have been found but remain unidentified. Still, when you're researching missing-persons cases, it's inevitable that you also begin to learn the ins and outs of the databases that catalog the dead—both the identified and the unidentified. Often, it comes down to a matching game—linking up reports of missing individuals with reports of found remains, cross-checking for specific details that can help identify the decedent. A unique tattoo. A special necklace. A scar. A healed broken bone. It took a little doing, but soon I understood how to use keyword searches on sites like the National Missing and Unidentified Persons System (NamUs), and the Doe Network. The latter was designed by passionate volunteers who'd solved some of the first amateur sleuth identification cases. In addition to searching for key identification details, I also learned how to check for exclusions—that's when a missing person had been ruled in or out as a match for a decedent, based on things like dental records or fingerprints or DNA.

We didn't cover an unidentified persons case on *The Fall Line* until 2018. I knew the background information for this particular victim would be scarce, at least until the advent of message boards; after all, news media couldn't do much, narratively speaking, with an unknown person whose body had been found. There was no family to interview. No trail to chase. There were a few Doe cases that had caught the public's attention over the years, but they generally reflected the same characteristics of the most famous missing persons and unsolved murders that were tied to identities: in general, young white children and young white women. And even those few were, at best, regional.

This had been the thing that bothered me most from day one: Doe cases got the least coverage, even though they were the ones that needed it *most*. So, I filed a fresh batch of FOIAs on the unidentified dead, the ones whose case numbers I'd been tracking in NamUs and whose nicknames were set to Google Alerts: Julie Doe. Dennis Doe. Christmas Doe. When I got the very first file, I knew—*these* were the cases I needed to write about, above all. There was no one out there advocating for them. No family holding a memorial for Jane Doe 1980. Or if there were, it was under a different name. But maybe their attention could be attracted and connected to the unidentified. After all, if you can construct a story with the pieces that death has left behind, someone might recognize the life that preceded them.

As helpful as my own curiosity was, I also knew that in order to really understand the reports I was receiving with these cases—descriptions of bones, ancestry estimations, entomology reports, forensic reconstructions, email communications regarding DNA and isotopic testing and soil and all the languages of science—I needed to speak to experts who could help me translate these findings and reveal how this new information could be used to help solve these cold cases. What evidence needed to be reanalyzed? What new methods should be applied? What signs should we be looking for to signal that something crucial had been missed, or could be done again, or tried now, with new technology?

That's how I met Dr. Amy Michael. At the time, she was a lecturer at the University of New Hampshire, in the anthropology department. Now, she's an assistant professor with her own lab, the Forensic Anthropology Identification and Recovery (FAIR) Lab. We were introduced by mutual colleagues who thought she might help me sort through some of the more confounding FOIAs I'd received on a few cold unidentified decedents (UID) cases. As luck would have it, she *was* able to help and, in the process, became one of my best friends. It's not often I find another professor who shares my affinity for loud music and cult horror classics. Before Amy, I'd spent most of my time in academia feeling like I was visiting alien landscapes, populated by a species utterly unknowable but subsisting on the same diet of textbooks.

Amy helped me make sense of so much. She showed me how to interpret the previously impenetrable language of medical examiners and forensic anthropology reports. She assigned me reading—whole textbooks sometimes, but also articles and case studies on specific foundational topics. I began to recognize a thorough skeletal analysis when I saw one. Amy also taught me that her field, biological anthropology, and its application to forensic science, was far from static.

Anthropologists continually refine and redefine and reform their opinions, and that has a lot of implications for these kinds of criminal investigations. For example, if a skeleton was recovered and examined in 1986 but not identified, it should be regularly revisited. That was Amy's view, at least, and one she was pushing to make a norm. New technology might be able to reveal new clues about who this person was. Mistakes could be caught—or not even mistakes, necessarily. Perhaps we can gain new understanding or reinterpretation on an unidentified person's ancestry, their age, their sex characteristics. Getting new eyes trained by new mentors on new methods could be the difference between an identification that finally brings worried families some peace and an everlasting cold case.

It didn't take long for Amy to become a permanent fixture in my life. She's a regular guest on the podcast. I virtually visit her classes and teach FOIA best practices or lecture on ethical true crime. She realized my research skills could help with the cases in her lab, and the interviews I'd become used to doing with families could add much to post-case study. We knew we wanted to work together more permanently. I wanted to help, somehow, with the actual identification process, to make a difference in these cold cases I kept coming across. And in late 2020, we found our chance: to work on and fund the identification of a woman then known only as Ina Jane Doe.

———————

Ina Jane Doe, called "Ina" after a nearby town, was found in Wayne Fitzgerrell State Park in Jefferson County, Illinois, in January 1993. Ina had been decapitated by her killer; only her head and several attached vertebrae were recovered at the crime scene. Authorities had done their best to identify her—they'd commissioned forensic art, completed an exhaustive search of the forest, reached out across state lines for more information, and conducted a thorough investigation—but despite their efforts, the killer's attempt to disguise her identity was successful.

All law enforcement knew was that she was a presumed white female, assumed to be somewhere between thirty and fifty years old, with red hair. The anthropologist who first examined Ina Jane Doe described her as having skeletal asymmetry and a possible neck condition called torticollis, or wry neck syndrome. Both aspects were reflected in the forensic art produced in her case. Those theories, and the artistic choices, were the initial reason why Amy wanted to approach the sheriff's office to offer skeletal reanalysis.

And that's where we began. Amy had been on the receiving end of casework for years—in addition to teaching anthropology classes at the university, she was also working on forensic cases for the state police in New Hampshire. But this was a little different. This case ultimately rested in our hands. We would be the ones to secure a lab for the extraction and—if that was successful—the sequencing. A kit would need to be prepared for upload to a public genealogy website. And then would come the final bit of connective tissue: investigative genetic genealogy. It was going to take a lot of time, money, and effort to do our due diligence, and even after all that, nothing was guaranteed.

In the last few years, dozens of John and Jane Does have been identified in the United States alone. That includes some of the highest-profile and longest-running cold cases—the Boy in the Box. Lyle Stevik. Delta Dawn. Baby Horry. Orange Socks. The Somerton Man. The Lady of the Dunes. A litany of nicknames every web sleuth, forensic anthropologist, investigative genetic genealogist, and crime researcher knows—we talk about them in shorthand. *Delta is solved. They ID'd Lyle.* We know that Doe cases once thought impossible to solve now have a real chance at closure.

With each passing year—each month—the tools of identification are refined, reworked, sometimes revolutionized. The headlines can feel like magic: "After 30 Years, Identified." "Unknown Woman Finally Has a Name." "Mysterious 'John Doe' IDed as Local Man."

But for every case that gets solved, there are still *so* many more that desperately need a second—or a third—look.

Many people are called to the cases of the unidentified: scientists of every discipline, artists, researchers, writers, genealogists, investigators, even podcasters. Perhaps we're driven by the same paradox: Does are found and lost in the same moment, caught between mystery and resolution. A body is discovered; a crime is revealed. Sometimes a killer is even caught. But the victim is still nameless. A family out there, somewhere, still waits for answers. There's a feeling that you get sometimes at night— no matter what your religious beliefs might be—that they all rest uneasy, living and dead.

If you do this work—amateur, professional, it seems to make no difference—that can weigh heavily on you. So, you stay up too late, scrolling web page after web page, trying to match John and Jane Does against the thousands of missing-persons cases listed in NamUs. You scour archived newspapers and web forums looking for names of those who never made it into the system in the first place—who were never officially reported missing but found all the same. They became the bags of bones along highways. At borders. Under bridges. Across state lines, on the routes that truckers favor. You don't always get the answers you're seeking, but sometimes you realize you need to take a step back so you can move on to the next search and work on how to address the most ignored or underfunded cases: decedents at the Southern border; the unidentified, unhoused, stolen ancestral remains lying in museum collections; the unmarked graves of Native children at residential schools; boxes of bones sitting on university shelves. It just never ends.

Ultimately, all we want to do is to be able to lay them to rest. Maybe that means we can help close a case—though it might not always mean closure for the loved ones who've been wondering what happened for all those years. More often, it's the beginning of another mystery, another unspooling, the threads of a second investigation into a murder. Sometimes, an identification in and of itself can answer many questions at once. But in others? There might be nothing, a dead end. Or something else opens up altogether: a vast warren of possibilities, twisting in against one another, recasting old suspicions that once lay dormant, bringing new ones to light.

Unless an identification is tied to an accidental or natural death, or suicide, there's always an "*and then.*"

But that takes different expertise.

It's difficult to get a precise count, but there are approximately forty thousand unidentified decedents in the United States. That statistic has been used since 2007 when the Department of Justice's Nancy Ritter published an article covering the scope of our national problem with cold Doe cases—something she called "the silent mass disaster."[1] The figure is still used today, though some argue it could be closer to sixty thousand.[2]

After all, this reported number does not account for the cases that have not been entered into systems. And there's always the question of where the money is going to come from, since funding for new DNA testing and genetic genealogy isn't built into many departmental budgets. The official funding for Doe identification—which in turn solves at least some missing-persons cases—will never be high enough to meet the need. Lab costs *alone* for DNA testing can run several thousand dollars per case; running several together, in batches, can save money, but it's still an expensive business and it's never guaranteed, especially in cases where the DNA has been mishandled or has degraded over time. DNA testing might be revolutionary, but it is not a panacea.

And what about cases where samples have never been taken in the first place? Exhumations can be costly. And then there are the cases where there are no bodies to test. The remains have been cremated beyond salvaging. Or they've been lost somewhere along the way: in a move from one office to another, in a flood, in a fire, due to bad recordkeeping by a cemetery. Fortunately, because DNA isn't the only tool in our arsenal, other forms of identification can and will continue to help us identify Does. Forensic reconstruction; dental comparisons and odontological study; study of identifying details of the body, like medical implants or fingerprints; skeletal analysis—these methods are not static. Advances in each aspect of possible human identification are vital in the common goal: resolution of cases. I've spent more than a year following experts who want to solve more cases faster and better. I recognize the scope of what they're facing, but more than anything I'm full of hope that they'll close more cases each year. That there will be fewer unidentified dead ignored and forgotten.

Those stories are just waiting to be told. But to tell them well, you have to unravel the forensic web—why some victims are identified, and some aren't, and how that's changing with every advance. There are many experts who have recognized the gaps and are working to build bridges and address the faults. To appreciate what they do, it helps to separate the science, strand by strand, method by method. Because it's those steps that make the magic headlines appear and create the satisfying endings.

That's the story of Ina Jane Doe: not just her death or the discovery of her remains in a lonely corner of a rural state park. It really comes down to the science behind every attempt to connect her to the woman she'd been in life, and to the people who never stopped looking for her.

CHAPTER ONE

THE CASE: THE WOMAN IN THE WOODS

January 27, 1993—Wayne Fitzgerrell State Park near Ina, Illinois

I
t was January in Jefferson County, Illinois, and two local girls—ages
ten and twelve—decided to go on a walk. Or maybe it was a run;
news reports varied. It was late afternoon on a Wednesday, but the
day reached fifty-five degrees and managed clear skies, which wasn't too
bad, especially for winter in the Midwest. It was as good a time as any
to tromp through the state park that stretched across two local counties, Jefferson and Franklin, and wrapped around Rend Lake. The state
recreation area covered more than three thousand acres,[1] and most of
it seemed to touch the water in one way or another. The northernmost
edge of the property cut between Jefferson and Franklin, a boundary
line that began beneath the lake. That edge of the park was close to the
town of Ina, Illinois—a tiny place that nevertheless had made headlines
just a few years before when an entire family, the Dardeens, had been
murdered nearby.

The far shore of Wayne Fitzgerrell Park cut a ragged curve, creating
peninsulas as it wound down toward its southernmost tip, culminating in
a point out into the water. Illinois Route 154 bisected the southern point
of the park, near the town of Whittington; that's where the more formal

1

entrance to the recreation area was, and where campers would pull in, during the various seasons, with RVs and trucks. Inside, they'd be able to peruse a picnic area, a horse barn, a boat launch, and the newly built Rend Lake Resort,[2] which drew in guests from all over, but especially neighboring Missouri and Kentucky, and of course, Illinois. Hunters came when the season called for it, to stalk game or shoot fowl from land or boats. During the summers, families could prop their feet up and cast a lazy line from the docks built onto little cabins along the lake.

Of course, in the middle of winter, the sunshine-fueled activities that often populated the area with tourists had mostly come to a pause. But locals still enjoyed the park's natural beauty, and security still did multiple rounds of the property each day from their vehicles. Park logs from late January 1993 showed no sign of suspicious or unusual activity.

The girls were exploring the park on foot when they noticed something red tangled up in the briars and brush. It sat at the base of a tree, on the right-hand side of the access road to the park's primitive campground. Perhaps they imagined it was an assortment of autumn leaves that had been spared during winter's erratic snowfalls. Or maybe they suspected right away, even if they didn't want to.

Upon closer inspection, the girls must have realized the red coloring they'd spotted from afar was hair. Not a wig, or a discarded doll, or mannequin. This was human hair attached to a very human head, lying in the underbrush, with no body in sight. It was close to dusk. But they must have seen enough. And the girls must have run to find help.

Fortunately, they didn't have far to go; an official record with the Illinois State Police was opened just thirty minutes later, at 5:20 p.m. That's when the Illinois Division of Criminal Investigation, in Marion, Illinois, contacted Special Agent Charles Parker, who would become the initial reporting agent on the case. Special Agent Parker was informed that there had been the decapitated head of a presumed white female discovered at the north end of Wayne Fitzgerrell State Park. A number of officers were already on scene.

The park wasn't busy that Wednesday; it was late January, after all. Winter vacation was over, and with deer season just finished, there were only a few guests registered to camp overnight.[3] There wouldn't have been many who saw the law-enforcement vehicles gathering at dusk, strung along the primitive campground road. There were cars from multiple agencies and both neighboring counties—Jefferson and Franklin. Officials knew they'd have to determine where on the county line the crime scene sat, though both agreed to assist with any search. Troopers. State police. Sheriff's deputies. Blue-and-red lights casting color and shadow across trees set back from the road, dense in some spots, scattered in others, and mostly bare of leaves.

Thick brush crisscrossed the roots, and a steady ribbon of yellow winter grass separated the road from the woods. Under the glow of all that light, officers stepped forward to take a closer look at what the girls had seen: the decapitated head of a woman, whom the pathologist would initially estimate to have been between her late twenties and late thirties at the time of her death. She appeared to be white. Her head had been severed just below the fourth cervical vertebra. There were no other immediate signs of her remains in the area.

Law enforcement's first impression that night was chilling: The officers suspected that whoever had dismembered this woman could have thrown her head from the driver's side window of a vehicle, into the brush. Who knows where the crime itself may have occurred. There must be a thousand places where the evidence of murder—and certainly, it must have been murder, to commit such violence after the fact—could have been secreted away forever.

But then again, she hadn't been hidden.

Assuming the perpetrator deposited her remains from a car, it wouldn't have taken much longer to tuck her remains deeper into the woods, or to drive just a little farther down the road to the lake. But instead, she'd been left just a little way off the road. It seemed that she hadn't been placed there so much as she might have been thrown. Maybe from a moving vehicle. Had the killer been frightened or forced away from the original drop-off spot he had in mind? Or had they really been that bold, or callous, or careless?

She was found at the north end of the park, closer to the town of Ina than to the town of Whittington, on the south end. Consequently, it was determined that the county line fell through the primitive campground, and the crime scene lay on the Jefferson County side of the divide, meaning it was Jefferson County's case to handle, along with the Illinois State Police.[4] Many agencies would be there, to help, into that first night and the coming days. But the woman would be forever associated primarily with Jefferson County and the little town near the north end of the park. In months, or maybe years, without a name to call her, she would become Ina Jane Doe.

Her case began officially with a State Police Case Action Report. The file would eventually stretch four hundred pages long, give or take, and contain photos, reports, VICAP printouts, phone notations, leads, test results, forensic reconstructions, records of evidence transfer between the coroner, the pathologist, a forensic odontologist, the lab, a forensic anthropologist . . . but the earliest was a slightly faded copy of a case report written by a member of the Illinois State Police. It was typed up afterward, from notes taken at the scene later that night. Twilight had set in by then. The woman's red hair must have looked a different shade to the agent who was gathering as much information as quickly as he could before he lost all the light. Perhaps that's why he described the victim as brunette. There are always inaccuracies.

This initial report was just a page or so of typed text, prepared a week after the first trip to the crime scene. It was soon accompanied by long lists of items collected at the scene, which were carefully bagged and placed in filters. Bag 1. Bag 2. Who had custody of Bag 7; what it contained. Where it would be taken. The language of investigation has always been to the point and detached. It has to be; the steps must be easy to retrace, again and again, by all the investigators who may follow.

———•———

From the case file of "Ina Jane Doe," Freedom of Information Act fulfillment, excerpt:

CASE NUMBER 93PO723. JANUARY 27, 1993. REPORTING AGENT, S/A C.P. [ILLEGIBLE WORD]: JANE DOE

[. . .] At approximately 6:00 PM on 01/27/1993, the reporting agent (R/A) arrived at the Primitive Camp area in the Wayne Fitzgerrell State Park north of Illinois Rt. 154 [. . .] The R/A's attention was directed to a thicket on the north side of the Primitive Camp Area Road. The R/A observed the decapitated head of a white female lying on the right side.

The decapitated head had brown hair which was partly entangled in briars [. . .] Crime Scene Technician (CST) O. photographed the scene, took measurements, and processed the scene for evidence. At approximately 7:00 PM, Dr. G., Jefferson County Coroner, arrived at the scene. CST O. also examined the scene and took photographs, and at approximately 8:05 PM, the decapitated head was placed in a plastic bag and removed from the scene by Capt. A.

At approximately 8:55 pm [. . .] the R/A, Capt. A, and CST O. met with Dr. G. and Dr. K. Dr. K x-rayed the plastic bag containing the decapitated head. An examination of the teeth revealed that a three-part root canal had been performed on the first molar of the lower left side, and the second molar on the lower left side had a filling. There was also a filling in the first molar on the lower right side, and there were no wisdom teeth present. It was also determined that the head had been severed at the fourth cervical vertebrae [. . .]

Attached to this report is a copy of a map depicting the area with an 'X' marking the approximate location of the decapitated head.

The X was tiny, placed at the edge of a line that looked just like all the others. Following the thick black line of the map, the scene of discovery was 2.2 miles northwest of the park's main entrance, and then another 1.2 miles north up the primitive campground road.

Though the search began at that spot on the night of the twenty-seventh, they'd have to return in the morning. And then again. Then they'd fan out, on foot, with dogs, and then to search by air.

[. . .] At approximately 8:00 AM, on 01/28/93, the reporting agent (R/A) met with personnel from The Illinois State Police, Division of Criminal Investigation (ISP/DCI), and Division of State Troopers (DST), the Jefferson County Sheriff's Department, the Franklin County Sheriff's Department, and the Department of Conservation. Following the meeting, a foot and aerial search was conducted of the area where the decapitated head was found. The search included both sides of the access roads and the parking areas.

———•———

The language of a police file can seem disconcerting at first when it is viewed by outsiders. After all, it isn't a suspense novel laid out with perfect detail so real that you feel like you're standing in the cold woods yourself. In fact, you can forget there was a "there" at all. Or a woman. Because, for the context of that document, she'd been reduced to a part of what had once been whole: *the head.*

But when you take a step back, the rest of it shifts back into focus. You remember that *the head*—the person—lived through thousands of moments of life. That crown in her tooth had likely come with an afternoon numbed by Novocain, a thick, cotton-y feeling in the mouth, and then an aching jaw for a day. Her hair—naturally reddish, it would turn out, once examined in the light—wasn't touched by gray. Then again, redheads generally don't go gray early. And she was so much more than just her appearance. Was she a mother, a sister, a classmate, a friend? Had she made plans the day she died—to cook a meal, to pick up children from school, to finish a shift at work? All the clues they might have used, to make educated guesses about who she was and the life she left behind, had been carefully removed. She could have been anyone.

She was certainly *someone*, and that didn't end the moment she died. But one thing you pick up when you follow the medical examiners, the anthropologists, and the rest of the specialists investigating the murders and identities of the dead is that the most decent of these professionals treat human remains with incredible respect. The best of them also want to solve their deaths and reunite victims with their identities. But they also distance themselves. It's often necessary.

Perhaps, when they stop to think too long about the woman behind the decapitated head, found by the girls in the park, it's harder to see the big picture. But maybe she's always there, in the background, driving the case. I've read enough files and can sense when that urgency is there, under the antiseptic language.

Don't get me wrong; there are definitely law-enforcement officers who *don't* care much about cases, especially cold ones. That is a truth you learn quickly. And when you try to help families gain attention for missing loved ones, it becomes depressingly clear: Some cases only get a cursory examination. And there will always be families that know damned well that their loved ones' files were lost, or thin, and will never be touched again, and they can't even get a phone call returned. And too often, there's nothing they can do about it.

But then there are those four-hundred-page files. Perhaps they begin with a report that might feel cold. Perhaps focusing on a decapitated head, in language that feels a million miles away from the horror of the moment. Underneath that, though, you'll see the willingness to try out an array of methods, spend money on reconstruction, on testing, on anything, to get a person identified. *The head* is the language of the paperwork, not the heart. The memory of a slackened face against the dried grass, the decomposition. The knowledge that one person could and would decapitate another with a few clean strokes. But lying beneath all that are pages and pages of attempts at something resembling resolution, the undercurrent of every hour spent on a case that ultimately leads you right back to where you started.

In 1993, newspapers reported that Ina Jane Doe's head was estimated to have lain in the park for two or three days, but the pathologist's report amended that to four to five days, with an outside range of two weeks.[5] The weather was cold but not consistently below freezing; records indicated highs in the mid-fifties and lows in the thirties on the twenty-seventh.[6] The week or so before had featured days both cooler and warmer, with some evenings reaching freezing temperatures.

According to the pathologist who first examined her remains, there were no signs of animal predation or insect activity; that notation seems to indicate a PMI, or postmortem interval—time elapsed since death—on the shorter range of the scale. Even in winter, if Ina Jane Doe's remains had rested along the side of the road for weeks, some scavenging would be expected. It was a small mercy that the head was still intact; her features were fairly recognizable, though the pathologist was uncertain of her eye color. He thought they had been dark—probably hazel or brown. A red-headed white female with hair that touched her shoulders, and, maybe, dark eyes. She was perhaps twenty-five or thirty, or so said the very earliest reports.[7]

That age estimate was later amended to thirty to fifty after all the experts had contributed their opinions. A wide range is normal, especially when a person is an adult and found in a state of decomposition or partial or full skeletonization. Without postcrania—that is, the rest of the skeleton below the skull—to examine, age-range estimations can be even broader.

All examiners noted that Ina Jane Doe had extensive dental work at some point in her life—including a rather unique crown and filling that might be used to identify her.[8] But there was also significant decay affecting a number of her teeth. That's a somewhat unusual combination: painstaking (and often expensive) dental restoration alongside advanced dental deterioration could signal some kind of change or shift in her life, whether it be physiological, environmental, or economic. That, too, could be a thread that might lead to her identification.

Her manner of death was listed as homicide. The effort made to hide her identity made it impossible to definitively rule on cause of death, though notations of her injuries were made and a suggestion was offered. The coroner carefully stored what had been recovered of Ina's remains for two days in his freezer. Meanwhile, the local forensic tech helped officers from every department in the area search the rest of the park. That tech brought back samples in bags and vials—leaves, a tiny fleck of red material that had clung to the forest floor—and carefully entered them into the system. Long red hair from a comb used to examine Ina was bagged and marked. Once the pathologist took samples of blood and tissue, those specimens were labeled, too, and delivered to the lab for analysis.

In those first few days, records traced the path of each item and aspect of the case, from a single filter of dirt to the victim herself, to follow the chain of custody. The pathologist learned as much as they could during their initial inspection, and then sent Ina to be carefully examined by an anthropologist. But they could have learned so much more if the killer hadn't dismembered her or they'd been able to find the rest of her body. In all likelihood, that had been the point. It was still in the early days of forensic DNA swabbing, but in 1993 they could check for fingerprints, swab for semen, and test blood type. No samples were submitted for DNA processing.

Back then, few departments had easy access to that kind of technology and testing, let alone the budget. The United States' first criminal case had successfully been won, at least partially, thanks to DNA evidence, in 1987.[9] But DNA collection was still not the norm, and this kind of evidence works best when you have something to compare it with. It would be another year before the 1994 DNA Identification Act, which established the National DNA Index System. The NDIS created a database and federal oversight of that system, where local and federal law enforcement could upload different DNA profiles of samples taken from various crime scenes, which would eventually become an element of the FBI's CODIS—the Combined DNA Index System.

If Ina had been found years later, they might have been able to find remnants of the perpetrator's DNA on her. But even so, if that person wasn't in the system, there still wouldn't be a match. The same could be said for her own DNA sample. Most departments wouldn't see the true possibilities of investigative genetic genealogy until 2018 when scientists and genealogists used it to throw the door wide open for cases that had long gone cold, ranging from long-standing Doe cases to infamous serial perpetrators like the Golden State Killer, Joseph DeAngelo.

But in 1993, choices were limited. Illinois authorities could, and would, complete and submit a Violent Criminal Apprehension Program (VICAP) report for Ina. VICAP, developed and implemented in the mid-1980s, creates a repository for analysts who can then potentially connect crimes that might not otherwise be linked; for example, an investigator might notice a pattern in line with a case they're working on, based on demographics, location, signature, or method.[10] Illinois authorities would also begin their attempts to match Ina to a missing-persons report from another state, even as her remains made their way to a forensic anthropologist for further study.

Despite their efforts, investigators faced a number of challenges. First, the "crime scene" was not, in the literal sense, the scene of the crime but rather the point of discovery. What's more, the majority of her skeleton was still missing, and law enforcement had no way of knowing if the murderer had further scattered her remains. The rest of her body could be anywhere, even in the nearby lake—the search of which would be an enormous undertaking, beyond the resources of a small department. It stretched thirteen miles long and three miles wide and had depths of up to thirty-five feet, though it averaged closer to ten.[11]

But she could have been taken anywhere else, too. She had not been a large woman in life. Stature was incredibly difficult to estimate, given the evidence, but no one thought she would have been over five foot five or so. On the park's grounds alone, there would have been a hundred places to obscure the rest of her, especially if the killer had continued the ugly work he'd begun: dismembering and scattering her remains. There was no guarantee the rest of her body would be recovered, which in turn decreased the amount of information the investigators could feasibly glean about her life and her death. In hiding what was left of the victim,

Ina's killer had essentially forced investigators to work in reverse: Take this awful crime and turn it back into a person.

Jefferson County authorities had perhaps more experience with homicide than outsiders might've expected. Another similarly rural county might be looking at their first violent death in decades, had girls from their own town come upon a woman's remains in the woods. But Ina's murder wasn't the sheriff's department's first shocking case over the past decade—not by a long shot.

Jefferson County was and is a comparatively sparse county: By 1990, there were only thirty-seven thousand residents, with fewer than five hundred living in Ina.[12] But the 1980s had been hard on the town and the region. A ten-year-old girl was raped and murdered. A double poisoning was plotted by a reverend and his lover, each set on freedom from their respective spouses without the bother of divorce. A teenager had killed each member of his family, one by one, over in Mount Vernon.

And Jefferson County was the same department that in 1987 handled the gruesome Dardeen family homicides. Three-year-old Peter Dardeen was found beaten to death. So was his mother, Elaine, who'd been seven months pregnant with his baby sister. Elaine had gone into early labor during the attack, and the newborn baby was beaten to death, too. Elaine was also genitally mutilated after death. All three victims were discovered together, in Elaine and her husband Keith's bed. The apparent murder weapon was Peter's baseball bat.

Keith Dardeen became suspect number one—he was missing, as was his car. What's more, he hadn't reported to work at the Rend Lake water treatment plant. But a day later, authorities discovered Keith's body in a nearby wheat field. Unlike the rest of his family, he'd been shot. And investigators discovered that Keith had also been subjected to extreme postmortem mutilation: His penis was sliced off and inserted into his mouth.[13]

No one understood why such terrible brutality had befallen the Dardeens: They had no secrets, no enemies. Eventually, Jefferson County authorities began to look further afield. Two serial killers were considered as possible suspects—one based on profile, and the other, a confession.

The first was Ángel Maturino Reséndiz; known as the "Railroad Killer," he hopped rides across the country and killed in at least three states, including Illinois. After his 1999 arrest, Reséndiz was seriously considered as a suspect for the Dardeen murders.[14] Aspects of the killings matched his patterns—and Ina is a railway town—but authorities were never able to link him to the area at the right time.[15]

Then there was Tommy Lynn Sells, the so-called "Coast to Coast Killer." He rode the railways, too. He'd been convicted of the murder of a teenager, Kaylene Jo "Katy" Harris, in 2000. Sometime in the early '00s, Tommy Lynn Sells began to talk—a lot. He confessed to the Dardeen family slayings and many other murders across the United States. And on the surface, he seemed to know some unreleased details of the Dardeen case—he was able to describe items in their home, for instance. But he took that confession back, along with others, sometime before his execution in 2014. When asked about the details, Tommy showed little compunction in explaining his technique. He repeated back details investigators had unknowingly dropped, and he took a guess at what decor a house in the 1980s might have.[16]

He was never prosecuted for the Dardeen murders. And in the years since, no one else has been either. Their families have no answers.

On the surface, Ina Jane Doe's murder may not seem very similar to the Dardeen family killings as she was a single victim. Though dismemberment was a key feature in both cases, she was likely decapitated to obscure her identity, with the killer intending to dispose of her remains across several separate locations. Plus, she was purposefully removed from the scene of her murder, and her cause of death could only be guessed. Although mutilation was also a feature of the Dardeen murders, and Keith was moved from the family home and from the apparent scene of his death—likely his own car—there were no efforts made to obscure his identity or those of his wife and children. Keith's and Elaine's bodies also showed signs of violent overkill; with Ina Jane Doe, that determination couldn't be fully made without postcrania, but what the pathologist gleaned from her limited autopsy didn't show signs of that kind of rage.

And yet, like the Dardeens, the motive for her murder was unknown. And her case, grisly and tragic as it was, had landed in the tiny town of Ina, so small in the early 1990s that it was described by KMOV News as having "one stop light [. . .] at the intersection of Main and Third streets."[17] There wasn't room for much more; the village proper is only about two and a half square miles in total. Back then, there was a Baptist church. A barbecue joint. An antiques store.

And nearby, the beautiful state park that attracted a steady stream of visitors, both locals and tourists. The Dardeens lived on the outskirts of town, much like the park sat on the edge between counties. It was rural but not inaccessible. Anyone might pull off the highway, circle around that lonely lakeside road at the park, or to that mobile home where the family had lived, and then be gone as quickly as they'd arrived, crossing over either county line. Then? Maybe on to Indiana, or Michigan, or even Kentucky, Missouri, or Tennessee. In Ina Jane Doe's case, that might include as many stops along the way as were necessary to fully dispose of her body.

The Dardeens could have been killed by a stranger, though that was always less likely than the perpetrator having some kind of connection. But they at least lived in the area and had ties to the community. Jefferson County authorities were sure that Ina Jane Doe, on the other hand, didn't live in the immediate area. There were no missing-persons reports that came close to matching her description, and no one had come forward with any information that tied her to Ina or the surrounding towns.

It followed, then, that the killer wouldn't be, either.

Travel far enough, and the story wouldn't cross the pages of the right local paper. If luck fell on the side of the murderer, national broadcasts would stay silent—the thread between missing and found neatly snipped. In 1993, that message would be easily lost across a few state lines. And the way the media wrote headlines—like "Decapitated Head Discovered" or "Woman's Head Found"—a family might fail to recognize a missing mother, or sister, or daughter in those words. They might not even want to. It would take digging down into the details to get to the few characteristics they might recognize.

As the search for Ina Jane Doe's identity, and her killer, continued over the early months of 1993, Southern Illinois authorities kept watch, on the lookout for similar cases. And it wouldn't be long before another woman was found, in a park, in Illinois. Four months after Ina Jane Doe's remains were discovered, another victim was found just outside Litchfield. That's a town about a hundred miles north of Ina, up I-57.

At first, the case seemed an eerie match for Ina Jane Doe. The remains of a presumed white female, somewhere between thirty and forty years old, had been found in a park. She'd been decapitated, and her head not found at the scene.[18]

In this instance, a fire had been set where her body lay. The killer had been there at some point, lurking among the rest of the park's visitors, but had gone unnoticed; it wasn't until flames consumed a pile of brush that the crime attracted attention at all. According to the *Pantagraph*, an Illinois newspaper, the fire was blazing so bright and so hot that the men who stamped it out didn't know, at first, what lay beneath the brush. When they finally saw a shape, outlined in ash, some onlookers thought they'd come upon a burnt mannequin. It must have been agonizing, that slow dawning, that in the soot and dirt, they'd come upon the remains of a human being.

The victim's autopsy report revealed more information—such as the fact that she had given birth and had a serious uterine tumor "that probably would have forced her to seek medical attention"[19]—but did not help to establish her cause of death. She was estimated to be approximately the same stature as Ina—about five foot four to five foot six. Though initially thought to be white, her race was updated in news reporting, and articles began to describe her as "a light-skinned Black woman." That's why the use of "presumed" is often useful when investigators are first describing the components of a case; what appears to be true may be reassessed, and then either confirmed or corrected.[20]

Also like Ina, authorities suspected that the unknown woman had been killed elsewhere and brought to the campground, and that, per the *St. Louis Post-Dispatch*, "burning was incidental to the crime—an effort to hide her identity, and not part of some kind of ritual."[21] What was most interesting, though, was revealed in the next line of the same article—that the local authorities noted, "the crime does not appear to be similar to any other recorded by the FBI, which has used the files in its VICAP program to aid in the investigation."[22]

Strangely enough, there's no reference in this article made to the head of a woman being found in another park—also by Illinois State Police, just two hours south, and a few months earlier. At the time the article was printed—August 1993—Ina Jane Doe's death had been under investigation for seven months. The Litchfield Jane Doe had been found in May. News media didn't connect the two stories, but there are records in Jefferson County and Illinois State records that confirm they did get word of the case—dot-matrix-like printouts that came, with bullets of information, like telegrams.

Eventually, further details would be released to the press. From the case file of "Ina Jane Doe," Freedom of Information Act fulfillment, excerpt:

. . . On May 8, 1993, at approximately 10:40 p.m., an unidentified white female body was recovered from a fire in a wooded area 200 yards from the water at Lake Lou Yaeger, Litchfield, Illinois. The decapitated body was burned [. . .] and [was] transported to the site in a U-HAUL brand box and remnants of black garbage bags were attached to the victim's limbs.

Authorities are looking for a late 1970's or early 80's Ford cargo-type van, dull orange/red/rust in color, similar in style to the one shown above. The sited van observed leaving the scene where the body was located had no ladders or spare tire on the back doors. The back door glasses possibly had dark windows. AFIS suitable fingerprints of Jane Doe were searched in numerous AFIS databases as well as FBI criminal and civil fingerprint files with negative results.

Unlike Ina Jane Doe, the Litchfield Jane Doe would be identified in a little over a year. Every detail counts, and in her case, there was a lot more to go on: the van, the bags, the specifics of the victim's health condition. But those weren't the key to her identification. In fact, state police sorted through the missing-persons cases of over five hundred white females and had no luck. It was only a year into the investigation, when they expanded their search to include missing Black women, that they landed on a report concerning Lynn Matchem-Thomas, who the *Chicago Tribune* described as "a 35-year-old clerical worker from St. Louis reported missing May 6, 1993—two days before the headless body was found."

She was separated from her husband, Curtis, but he'd been the one—along with her mother—to report her missing. He was a mental-health counselor whose home had been searched the day his wife went missing. But not his entire home. He hadn't allowed Missouri police into the basement. Curtis Thomas would eventually be charged and convicted of Lynn's murder—something that didn't surprise investigators once she'd been identified. They'd been expecting a close tie to the victim; as the lead detective told the *Tribune*: "The more trouble they go to, the closer the relationship."

Would that be the case for Ina Jane Doe as well? Who had driven down that primitive campground road in late January? Had it been their last stop, or their first? There were no clear signs of the killer left to trace—no clear description of a van to follow, or a suspicious person to track down. Just a report that a girl on her way to the local college had seen a vehicle parked near the primitive campground, on the side of the road, a few days before Ina was found. But she was hazy on the details. That wouldn't be enough. So, for investigators who longed to close the case, their only hope was working backward, from the victim's remains to her identity, and hope that clues would light up a path to her murderer, piece by piece, as evidence fell into place.

But the puzzle of Ina Jane Doe's identity didn't form a clear picture of the crime that had taken her life. Despite a forensic anthropologist's examination and two artist's renderings, no one recognized the woman in the woods, and that seemed strange based on the image both the drawing and sculpture conjured. They were similar reconstructions, though they were created by different artists: a page boyish haircut; distinctive, almost jagged teeth; dark eyes; and a face that seemed affected by some mild paralysis and/or the pull of muscles caused by torticollis. Those images, one in black-and-white, and one sculpted, in color, should have stoked the memories of someone.

That's what had always bothered me: If those representations were accurate, her people, if she had them, would have known her on sight. Either she had none, or, for close to thirty years, everyone had been pointed in the wrong direction. And that meant that Ina Jane Doe hadn't had a chance. Not really. No matter how much work had gone into her case, it was all headed off, in every direction, except toward the truth.

CHAPTER TWO

THE METHOD: JOHN AND JANE DOE

Doe. That's a word I've typed a thousand times over the past six years. With the right turn of phrase, it can feel like a true name, an invocation, meant to call forth the person who is waiting there, just under the surface, to be reunified with their identity: *Ina Jane Doe. Julie Doe. Dennis Doe.*

But really, we all know *Doe* is a taciturn kind of communication: *We cannot identify this person. This mystery remains unsolved.*

The unidentified dead are often named after counties where they are discovered but not always. It's not a uniform rule. That "Ina" also sounds like a person's name, and not a place designation, was more chance than design. When there are too many victims from a county, or city, years and months are assigned: Los Angeles County John Doe 1980. Los Angeles County John Doe 1999.

Some decedents are known by what was printed on a piece of false identification, or as a name they gave out, eventually determined as an alias: *Sebastian Pasqual*, in Florida. *Pablo Hernandez Cruz*, in West Virginia. *Lyle Stevik*, in Washington. When the DNA Doe Project, a nonprofit that works on unidentified-decedent identification, takes on a case that doesn't have a well-known associated name, they try to choose one that will stick in the minds of people who encounter it. *Slaughter Creek Jane Doe*, for instance, is more memorable than *Travis County Jane Doe*.

When they're raising funds to help law enforcement cover the cost of testing, anything that attracts the public can help.

John Doe, Jane Doe. Those placeholders are meant to be temporary. But we all know that sometimes they become permanent. Their cases wait under the "Cold Case" tab on local law-enforcement websites and in state bureau databases for more information to be revealed. And it makes sense; identification, in past decades, could be incredibly difficult. Even now, it still can be. There are many cases older than Ina Jane Doe's that are still unsolved. Finding information on just how many, and what the demographics of the cases can tell us, though, is tricky. But there is a lot to say on other topics: who become and remain unidentified, the methods by which Does are reunited with their names, and why this great new tool, investigative genetic genealogy, hasn't wiped the cold-case slate clean.

———•———

Who are the unidentified dead? There are all kinds of deaths that end with a Doe decedent; it's not nearly as uncommon as you might think. Despite the landscape created by true-crime podcasts and television shows, the unidentified deceased aren't all homicide victims. It's just that those deaths are the ones that make the news. A study published in 2008 collected data on 10,748 unidentified decedents recorded as such between 1973 and 2004. That is a huge number as far as research into Doe cases goes. It's difficult to find and track the unidentified dead.

Researchers found that 82.7 percent of these deaths were due to injuries. When I read *injury,* I thought accident—but no; that phrase included any mortal wound. Among injury deaths counted in the study, 31.8 percent were officially classified as homicides.[1] It was a lower number than I expected, but that's perhaps the prejudice of a crime researcher talking. The world is not as dangerous as the media tells us it is—though that is certainly scaled, demographically, to who you are. For instance, the same study noted that though female-labeled Doe victims are more likely to have been murdered, they are less likely to remain Does; in 2009, males made up 80 percent of the overall recorded UID number in the United States. The researchers also discovered that Black Does, men and women, are more likely to remain unidentified than white decedents.

There's a clear connection between missing people and unidentified people, and those 2008 findings correlate with what we know today. The Black and Missing Foundation pointed out in late 2022, "40% of the missing-persons reported in 2021 were persons of color."[2] And though Black women made up only 13 percent of the population in 2020, "a third of the almost 300,000 U.S. girls and women reported missing in 2020 were Black."[3] That seems to line up with the findings of the 2008 study: Regarding prevalence among the unidentified, when race was recorded, "the Black male rate was 1.9 times the white male rate, while the Black female rate was 2.4 times the white female rate." When I checked National Missing and Unidentified Persons System (NamUs) in late 2022, cases tagged as "Black" made up roughly 22 percent of the total female-identified cases in the system.

That's never going to be a precise count due to a number of factors: uncertain information about the deceased, how case information is entered by law enforcement, and how racial categories are assessed and assigned—and even the actual number of deceased in the United States versus what's represented in the database. In 2022, NamUs listed approximately fourteen thousand unidentified decedents—a number far below the estimated forty thousand in the United States. I've yet to find an update on that figure from 2007, besides one estimate that it could be as high as sixty thousand; forty thousand is still used by both governmental, nonprofit, and university publications, and was referenced in a report on the crisis of missing and murdered Indigenous women and girls as recently as 2022. Anecdotally, many professionals have told me that the people who they see as long-term unidentified in their offices, making up that 40,000+, are the people who are given less attention in life: people who are unhoused, who have lived in various systems—foster, penitentiary—people who are living on the margins due to a confluence of factors that might include age, income, citizenship status, substance dependence, illness, and more. Anyone can go missing and become unidentified. But there are people whose disappearances are never actually reported—the "un-missing," as a forensic anthropologist once described to me—who likely make the numbers harder to calculate.

We go back to NamUs's numbers and reports because it is *the* official, national system devoted to missing and unidentified persons. Its purpose is, per the National Institute of Justice, to serve as a "national information clearinghouse and resource center for missing, unidentified, and unclaimed person cases throughout the United States."[4] An entry for a Doe case in NamUs might include as little as a short description and a contact number, and as much as a detailed write-up, full dental records, case photos, information as to DNA availability, and more. What can be accessed depends on the authorization of the user (general public or authorized by law enforcement) and what is uploaded. If I'm logged in, I can see basic case details and contacts, forensic art, and clothing items, if those photos are provided; very rarely I might see a postmortem photo used for identification. If Amy logs in, she can view all the other, reserved info that is limited to medicolegal officials: possible dental charts, fingerprints, and more.

The concept itself is relatively new; NamUs was launched in 2007 and is still in the process of ongoing evolution. As of 2021, its operations were transferred from the University of North Texas Health Science Centers, where the work was funded by ongoing government grants with oversight from the NIJ, to the North Carolina–based Research Triangle Institute (RTI), a nonprofit contracted by the NIJ.[5]

NamUs can also offer services to other official departments within the government, such as the storage of dental records, fingerprint search and storage, collaboration with the FBI on latent fingerprints and palm prints submitted via NGI (Next Generation Identification), forensic anthropological skeletal analysis, DNA extraction, and via contract, sequencing, and now, genetic genealogy. The NamUs "clearinghouse" concept hasn't been fully perfected; it can take months or sometimes years to wait for test results, due to backlogs. There are *so many* cases. But it's undoubtedly a vital resource, and it has the potential to be an incredible one. Dedicated scientists and experts are working hard to make it so.

But here's the kicker: NamUs use—whether that be for missing, unidentified, or unclaimed persons—is not compulsory in all states. There are law-enforcement agencies across the country that have never entered a single case into the system and perhaps have never consulted it in regard to their own cases. Without consulting NamUs and logging in with official credentials, professionals miss out on the information that the general public can't see, like fingerprints or dental records, additional photos, plus other case information they can quickly access to rule in or rule out a match.

My friend Todd Matthews knows a lot about NamUs. He should; after all, he helped create it. He's also one of the founders of the Doe Network, a website database that preceded NamUs by almost a decade. He has a passion for data and for sharing it with as many people as possible: That's how cases get solved. And Todd wants law enforcement, medicolegal professionals, and the public to use NamUs thoroughly and well.

Todd was actually tapped to help create the official NamUs site because of his success as a civilian database-organizer. The volunteer-run Doe Network helped the government realize that such a project was not only possible but an important tool in resolving cases. Todd is perhaps one of the most famous civilians in true crime; he's the man popularly considered to be the world's first web sleuth—he famously used 1990s internet technology to identify "Tent Girl," a Jane Doe victim in Kentucky, as Barbara Ann Hackman Taylor. Todd recognized how digital communication could help solve cases, and as soon as it was technologically feasible, he worked with other passionate cold-case enthusiasts to begin the Doe Network in 1999. What began as a listing of cases has become an extensive, searchable database.

Each Doe Network entry contains information garnered from police reports, newspapers, and other publications, and as much identifying information as possible: clothing, photographs, forensic art. Case circumstances are described as are all details of the decedent: whether DNA is available, or fingerprints, or dental information. At the bottom of the page for a decedent, like Ina Jane Doe, you'd find plenty of additional information, too: contacts for police or medical examiners, links to other websites where information is listed, and a note as to when the page had been updated. It's not fancy, but the pages are comprehensive: Everything is contained in one place, easy to read and understand. Even if you're not familiar with an indexed database, you'll find what you need.

That functionality was certainly a big reason the Doe Network appealed to the law enforcement who checked it, before NamUs was established. It's why Todd kept it up, even after he began work at NamUs, and throughout his tenure, until January 2020. Todd told me, "Actually someone at the Department of Justice said, 'Why does the Doe Network still exist?' And I said, 'Well, because there's still very much of a need, and that was why you called me.' It's a different thing. Doe Network is very different in the way that I operate it. We used anecdotal data, newspaper articles."

That part is important, at least to me: One of the biggest missing pieces in many police files are relevant news articles about the crime. It's rare that I find them included, and they can offer important details that the rest of the files don't. Todd explained, "There were a lot of things in Doe Network I could show, like the cause and manner of death if it was in a newspaper article. There was no category in NamUs to say the cause and manner of death, so it is very limited in its ability to share certain data. Even if it was public knowledge, there was no way for it to be 'the source of cause and manner of death was this and this.'"

With the Doe Network, its success has always been based on the passion of its volunteers, who are willing to put the time into keeping the database up-to-date. But for the government-funded NamUs, things are more complicated. Todd has pointed out time and again that NamUs is as useful as its participants make it. Like the National Crime Information Center (NCIC) and VICAP—both federal databases that store essential information—it is an active database *dependent* on participation to truly function at its best. When a NamUs profile is up-to-date and filled out as completely as possible, it's an incredible resource. The search engine function has helped me sort through cases in a dozen different ways that aren't possible anywhere else; as long as the information is *there*, it is exactly what we need to research cases and find patterns or compare missing-persons to decedents.

Regardless of what database you're using, it can often feel like we don't have much information on Doe cases, but compared with many countries, there's a wealth of it. Our freedom of information laws and public access are practically transparent compared with, say, those of the UK or Australia. Plus, we aren't limited to official federal, state, county, and city databases; all the information that is released through those channels and the press allows for Doe Network to exist. It also fuels other essential Doe research sites, like Charley Project, the most comprehensive citizen-run database for cold cases, and Unidentified Wiki, an online encyclopedia of unidentified decedents. In Doe cases, this web of volunteer websites is vital for research.

Because of the relative difficulty of solving Doe cases—which are often double layered, the search to find both an identity and the person who killed the unknown decedent—every scrap of evidence is precious. The tags in clothing. Jewelry. The constellation of moles and scars and tattoos that make up our skin. Shoes. A fresh haircut. Invisible evidence caught beneath fingernails, between the treads of sneakers, the folds of cuffs, the most minute traces that might now be collected in an M-Vac machine. The medical information meticulously etched into a set of dentures. The serial numbers assigned to breast implants. The particularities of a dental crown. The blood sample, smeared on a card and stored in an evidence folder, however degraded, might produce *just enough* usable DNA. The more I've spoken to experts through the last few years, the more amazing it's all become—just how unique the sources might be for information that cracks a case.

Television and books and even podcasts have created a mantra in the past five years: *DNA is king.* That's the story, right? The inevitable social-media comments on any case, whether it's an article share or an awareness post of a NamUs profile, often come down to the same singularity: *Is there DNA? Why haven't they done the DNA? DNA could solve this. It says there's DNA available; this should be solved.* DNA science is certainly amazing, and it has incredible potential to solve cases. In fact, when I began researching unidentified-persons cases, I assumed that they were all solved by DNA; I saw those headlines popping up in the news in what seemed like an endless stream.

Nowadays, there is rapid DNA testing available that would have changed the landscape of a mass disaster like 9/11, where forensic anthropologists and odontologists worked side by side to identify the dead. For example, new technology like the ANDE machine was developed for improving efficiency on field operations, so that STR DNA testing can be done, in the best conditions, in under two hours.[6] STR profiles are the sort you've heard about on TV for years, that are stored in CODIS— useful if a close relative, or the victim or suspect is available for testing. A SNP profile is developed differently and is the kind of test you take if you want to get your ancestry done on 23andMe or another private database. That kind of DNA profile can find relatives very far removed from the original source. The ANDE machine is an amazing advancement for forensic science, because traditional testing takes weeks. But it's an expensive one, too. When I interviewed a representative from a medical examiner's office in Tennessee in early 2022, they mentioned they had the only ANDE in the state at the time. Cost and availability are serious considerations in cold cases, whether they involve a state-of-the-art machine or classic testing. If it wasn't, the case log would be clear.

That said, DNA testing has become much more affordable than it once was, and that should continue. And DNA matches aren't the only piece of the identification puzzle. Experts have a lot of tools at hand. There are numerous other paths to human identification: dental comparisons; skeletal analysis; X-ray comparison; the use of visual identification and photos; medical implant serial-number matching; fingerprint comparison; the juxtaposition of tattoos, identifying marks, or even old injuries (like broken bones) that can be found in a missing-person's medical records. Each method has helped close cases. Some, like dental comparison, fingerprint comparison, and skeletal analysis, have been the workhorses of identification for years.

We spend a lot of time, as a culture, discussing the most prevalent methods—art, dental identification, skeletal analysis, DNA comparison—but it's worth taking time to mention a few other ways the dead are reunited with their identities. Tattoos and identifying features, like birthmarks, are clear examples. When Ina Jane Doe was discovered, her most minute features were inventoried and described in detail before her autopsy, down to a mole located within the curve of her right ear.

In the perfect circumstances, it could have been enough to identify her—if only the right person had seen the description or remembered that small detail. We never know what people will remember, though; that's the trouble. Humans are so apt to fixate. But on what? Our minds play tricks. Maybe you never told them about that wrist you broke back in middle school. Maybe even you forgot about the hairline fracture.

But methods of bodily comparison exist that can supersede the need for memory, which is fallible and so dependent on chance. And that is lucky. After all, what do your friends and family remember about you, really? If they had to write down a list of your identifying features, what would they miss? What have you forgotten to tell them?

———⋅———

Luckily, many methods don't rely on our memories: They exist in records. Although it has limited scope in unidentified decedent cases, fingerprinting remains a powerful tool—it's just a matter of the right circumstances, and the databases that might include the decedent. For cases of skeletal remains, or partial remains with no hands, like Ina Jane Doe, prints of any kind are not going to be of use, unless there is a crime scene that retains a perpetrator's prints.

But it's a method that the public is familiar with; in fact, many of us have already been fingerprinted. And it's not limited to those who have been arrested or had prints required for work; if you grew up in the 1980s or 1990s, for example, there were fingerprinting drives at elementary schools, libraries, and even grocery stores. It was the height of the *stranger-danger* era, when missing children's photos ran on the backs of milk cartons. I have vague memories of lining up in the elementary school cafeteria in the 1980s to have my fingers rolled across an ink pad; in the auditorium I'd watched McGruff the Crime Dog, in all his threadbare-mascot-costume glory, tell us to "take a bite out of crime" and stay away from anyone offering us candy or a look at cute kittens from a windowless van.

I certainly wasn't the only one getting fingerprinted. An October 1983 article in *Education Week* reported that "in recent months, the parents of thousands of schoolchildren nationwide have agreed to permit them to be fingerprinted so that the identifying prints could be used in the event the children disappear."[7] It was not a coincidence that, per the reporter, it was around the same time that the TV special *Adam* aired to 38 million viewers on NBC. *Adam* dramatized the kidnapping and murder of Adam Walsh, the son of John Walsh, best known as the activist and host of shows like *America's Most Wanted* and *On the Hunt with John Walsh*. At the end of the program, missing children's photos were featured to help raise awareness. Apparently, this led to "thousands of calls" to NBC. Most were tips.

Ironically, for all the popularity of fingerprinting children in the late twentieth century, there was no unified effort to gather the data into a system where their prints might be referenced. All that talk of initiatives and legislation and child safety-kits that pervaded 1980s and early '90s media, the hope that these prints, collected in childhood, would revolutionize case closure? It never really materialized. Plus, even then, there were privacy concerns. Parents had to sign permission forms, and the fear of a database being constructed of the prints was discussed by legislators. Per *Education Week*, the child-fingerprinting initiatives were intended to help parents catalog information they could keep as part of their family records.[8]

Unless a family managed to hang on to that card for years, it could do little in a missing-persons case or help to identify a Doe decedent. I don't think that my mother could produce my card now, several decades and three states later. Would Ina Jane Doe have been too old to have been included in the initiative? Maybe.

And in the United States, we don't maintain the fingerprints of average citizens. There's no general database that can be analyzed with the same tools employed in what is popularly known as an Automated Fingerprint Identification System (AFIS). AFIS is the general name for any fingerprinting system in which a print can be run and matched by various points. The national database was long known as Integrated Automated Fingerprint Identification System (IAFIS). In 2011, the FBI shifted the official terminology for IAFIS to Advanced Fingerprint Identification Technology (AFIT) to reflect the enhanced capability of the system; the AFIT system falls under its Next Generation Identification (NGI) initiative.[9]

It's a dizzying array of ever-shifting initials, but the takeaway is this: Their databases are now tracking more than just fingerprints. When TV detectives say they're going to *run the prints*, AFIT is the system they're referencing. But they can run a lot more, now. There's a lot happening according to their website: development in ridge technology, the use of palm prints, mobile fingerprint technology, and even eye scans—and those are just the major bullet points.

Most pertinent to unidentified persons cases within the NGI is a specific service aimed at helping to resolve Doe cases. Practically speaking, the "advanced search algorithms" expand the government's ability to compare an unidentified person's prints against any civilian whose prints are retained by the FBI because they're federal or civilian employees or have been "submitted by state, local, and tribal agencies."[10] In terms of the pool of identification, the NGI estimated that in 2021, the total number of prints in the system—offender, latent, and civil—amounted to roughly 162 million. The Department of Defense maintains its own, separate record of military fingerprints and other data, and began a digitized database in 2009.[11]

In totality, that may seem like a *lot* of records, but many unidentified decedents, even those found immediately after death, or early enough in the decomposition process to have printable fingers, still don't come up with a match. AFIS systems have definitely solved unidentified persons cases; it's a matter of the right records passing into the right system at the right time, so they can be matched.

For instance, a fingerprint match that came from improved systems and communication solved a twenty-seven-year-old cold case in 2017—one that had been featured on *Unsolved Mysteries* back in 1995. The unidentified decedent's manner of death, and the details investigators released about her made it seem as if she should have been almost immediately recognized. Late on the evening of April 1, 1990, a young woman tried to cross—or perhaps simply stepped into traffic along—the Pacific Coast Highway in Huntington Beach, California. Reports have differed. What was consistent among them was the description of what came next: She was struck and killed, and when police recovered her body, she was still recognizable.

The *LA Times* carefully described her clothing and added in a particularly unique detail that anyone who knew her surely would have recognized: "she had a strand of hair wrapped around her finger like a ring, and a lock of hair in her pocket."[12] The hair seemed to be her own; she was brunette. She appeared to be white and young; she was estimated to be somewhere between eighteen and thirty. Per the *Times*, the Orange County Sheriff's Office wasn't able to release a photo of her face to the media—there had been too much damage done in her fatal accident—but a forensic sketch was done. Eventually, the National Center for Missing and Exploited Children provided updated, colorized art as well.

Officers did receive some leads on the case after it was announced to the public, as people in the community reported interactions with the decedent; Unidentified Wiki gathered considerable details on her case, and there were reports that she spent time hitchhiking in the area before her death. Some of the alleged details she shared with acquaintances were that her name was Andrea and she "came from a prominent family" who had adopted her and were based in Virginia. Some said she mentioned a search for her biological parents. Some suspected she was a teenager, though she claimed to be twenty-six.[13] Even with all this information, investigators still couldn't find a missing-persons report that matched.

As the years passed, and new investigators and coroners inherited the case, the unidentified woman's details were reviewed again. In 2016, a new supervising coroner named Kelly Keyes reached out to Virginia officials about a missing woman named "Andrea," and the results were much the same: no hits.[14] But the game changer came just a year later when the FBI partnered with NamUs to "to examine fingerprints from the database against those from unsolved cases."[15]

Of course, the unidentified woman's fingerprints had been run before, back in 1990, but the FBI's databases had continued to expand significantly in the years since, and, most importantly, older records had been scanned in. And in the end, that's what finally helped solve the 1990 Pacific Highway case, officially identifying the victim as Andrea Kuiper. In 1987, at just twenty-three years old, she'd been an employee of the Department of Agriculture, and the fingerprints she'd submitted as part of her application had finally been digitized. Many wondered why the case hadn't been solved sooner, but upon a closer look, investigators realized that her parents had not reported her missing—which is why there had never been a record of her disappearance to begin with.

Families have complex reasons for that choice, and though Andrea's loved ones didn't provide much detail regarding their decision to refrain from filing, they did cite her bipolar diagnosis as a complicating factor in their intermittent communication with their daughter at the time of her disappearance. They also told reporters that they'd gotten an update from a friend of Andrea's that she was doing all right just a few months before the April 1st accident on the Pacific Highway. They held out hope that Andrea would eventually get back in contact. As the *LA Times* reported, all the family has ever wanted was to "see Andrea driving up to their Virginia home in a car full of beautiful children and say, 'Hi, it's me.'"[16]

———•———

Unique physical characteristics can be key in identification, too, though they can also spark misidentifications, or even complex theories that ultimately lead to dead ends; perhaps that's because of our need to create cause where there is only suggestion. And what we consider to be defining, individual features—well, those characteristics can turn out to be disappointingly commonplace, or at least less unique than we'd hoped.

That's been clearly illustrated in the recently solved case of "The Somerton Man," one of the longest-running and most famous Doe cases in modern memory. On December 1, 1948, on Somerton Beach, just a little outside Adelaide, Australia, a man dressed in a full suit was discovered by a crowd of summer revelers—it was the hot season in the Southern Hemisphere, after all. That made the man's outfit, from his dress shoes to the collar of his shirt, so absolutely out of place that they would have drawn attention on their own, but that wasn't the only strange thing about him. It was his absolute stillness and the burnt-out cigarette that had tumbled from his mouth and onto his collar that concerned the beachgoers.[17]

Two things were immediately apparent: The man was out of place, and he was dead. Some locals claimed to have seen him on the shore the night before, sitting sprawled out on the sand, in front of the ocean; they'd just assumed he was drunk. At least one had seen him raise a cigarette to his mouth with an unsteady hand. Now, though, it was clear he'd been in some kind of distress. Initially, investigators at the Adelaide hospital considered the possibility that the unknown man might have passed away from heart failure. But there were other considerations . . . and a handful of complications.

For starters, the man found on Somerton Beach had died without any kind of identification on his person. On a beach, that wouldn't be unheard of, *but* he'd been dressed in a suit. His cause of death remained unclear, though investigators suspected poisoning. What's more, that suit had the labels carefully removed. All investigators had to go on were the contents of his pockets, a suitcase they later tracked down at the train station, which contained a confusing mismatch of items—some of which were clothing items that suggested he might have traveled to, or from, the United States. They studied the man's body for clues; as *Smithsonian* noted in 2011, "The dead man's calf muscles were high and very well developed; although in his late 40s, he had the legs of an athlete. His toes, meanwhile, were oddly wedge-shaped." Based on that information, the theory that the deceased might be a ballet dancer was posed. It would be only one of many possibilities offered over the coming decades, and hardly the most outlandish.

During a later, careful examination of the Somerton Man's clothing, an expert discovered a new clue in one of his pockets: a rolled-up scrap of paper printed with two words: *Tamám Shud*. The English translation of the phrase is, depending on who you ask, "it is ended," or "ended," or "finished." That scrap would later be matched to a book of Persian poetry, *Rubáiyát of Omar Khayyám*. For a long time, investigators couldn't find the specific copy of the book from which the scrap might have been torn; though I assumed there could not have been that many copies floating around, ABC Australia noted that it was actually fairly popular among Australian military during and after World War II. But eventually, two men came forward and said they'd found a copy in their car that matched the torn scrap. Each assumed it had belonged to the other; when they saw a news story about the unsolved case, they realized the strange book they'd discovered in the back of their car might have been placed there, perhaps by way of an open door or window.[18] By whom, they weren't sure; maybe it had been tossed in by the Somerton Man himself. Maybe his killer if there was one. Perhaps an entirely unrelated person. But authorities were pretty sure it *was* the right book; the missing scrap from its page perfectly lined up with the paper found in the deceased's pocket.

The book contained other information, too, including what authorities thought might be a peculiar kind of handwritten code—a string of letters that, despite their best efforts, and an invitation to code breakers around the world, no one has been able to solve. There was also a phone number. The mystery surrounding the "code" has long fascinated true-crime enthusiasts who have posited that the Somerton Man was a spy, and that perhaps he died as a result of espionage—i.e., poisoning.

The phone number written in the book led to an Australian woman. Her backstory seemed, to some, to support the mystery military theory as she had at least vague connections to the military. The woman—who was for decades known only by pseudonyms in the media, and later by a nickname, "Jestyn"—told investigators she had indeed given a copy of the *Rubáiyát* to a man. She'd gifted the book to Alfred "Alf" Boxall, who was an Army lieutenant in the Australian military. Investigators thought that was a lead . . . until they found Alf Boxall, very much alive, with his copy of the book intact. How "Jestyn"—whose real name was Jessica Harkness Thomson—came to have her number written in that copy of the *Rubáiyát* has never been fully established.[19] But the military role of Alf Boxall felt like a strong clue to any number of citizen detectives. Perhaps there was a military-intelligence angle hiding under the surface?

The prevailing theory of many web sleuths was that Jessica had actually given away two copies, including one to the Somerton Man, and that this unknown man had come to Adelaide to visit her, though Jessica never confirmed that. She died in the late '00s without ever establishing any connection to the unidentified man. But rumors persisted, and not just because espionage is tantalizing. Why? Well, Jessica had a son in 1947, and some researchers theorized her child was fathered by the Somerton Man—despite the fact she was married to another. It may seem a little far-fetched, but believe it or not, that theory was based not only on wishful thinking but on "identifying" features.

That child had two very distinct physical characteristics that occur in only a small percentage of the European-descended population. Specifically, he had uniquely shaped ears: "his upper ear hollow (the cymba) was much larger than his lower ear hollow (the cavum)." But that's not all. The child also was missing his lateral incisors. He'd been born without them, in fact, which shifted his teeth so that his canines sat directly next to his central incisors. Notably, as can be seen on postmortem photos, the Somerton Man displayed both these features.[20] The fact that her son, Robin Thomson, became an accomplished ballet dancer in his adulthood? That only strengthened the physical connections that enthusiasts drew.

There were also professional researchers interested in the case, and the possible connection between Jessica and Robin Thomson and the Somerton Man. A professor from the University of Adelaide, Dr. Derek Abbott, began arguing for an exhumation of the Somerton Man on the grounds of promising leads such as these. Abbott became interested in the case in 2009, and he'd pursued his own inquiries, including the genealogical lines of the Thomson family, for years. It was only in 2021 that the approval was finally granted. As government officials commenced testing,

Abbott and American investigative genetic genealogist Dr. Colleen Fitzpatrick had begun their own research. They didn't have access to the Somerton Man's remains, but they had something else: hair. Per *Smithsonian* magazine, they'd collected samples from the plaster death mask made before the deceased was buried. It was enough for a successful DNA profile, and they began the work of tracing family lines.

Per *Smithsonian*, Drs. Abbott and Fitzpatrick reached a conclusion before the Australian government. In the late summer of 2022, they had an announcement: They had identified the Somerton Man. Though the Australian government did not officially endorse this ID, there was plenty of supporting research for their candidate . . . one that would disappoint every internet sleuth with an espionage pet theory.

DNA testing ruled out a familial connection to the Thomsons. The Somerton Man was identified as Charles "Carl" Webb, an Australian citizen—not a spy, but an instrument maker and electrical engineer—one who inherited some American-made clothing from a family member. Why did he have that scrap of paper? No one has solved that bit of the puzzle, although Webb did have a fondness for poetry. The mysterious "code" in the book? Dr. Abbott has told Australian news outlets that Webb liked the horse races; he theorizes the deceased was keeping tracking of horses he'd bet on, by first initial. As for Jessica's phone number? No answer there, either. Researchers are still working on that. But they've certainly disproved something that once seemed practically indisputable: the familial connection of Webb to Thomson. Yes, Webb and Robin Thomson shared a dental characteristic and the unusual ear features found in 1 percent of the population. But ultimately that information meant exactly *nothing* for the case.[21]

All this to say: the study of physical features can certainly be helpful in identification—after all, the FBI regularly checks ear shape and size when they're comparing photos—but if we concentrate too much on similarities that we believe to be indisputable "proof," then we can head down the wrong path.

Still, tools in the non-DNA arsenal *are* important, provided they can be used in a concrete way to do a true comparison between an unidentified person and a missing individual. Medical implants and devices have the powerful potential to identify Does, but it's not a cut-and-dried, A-to-B process. Currently, medical devices—which might be anything from a cochlear implant, breast implants, or pacemaker to a steel rod in the arm or leg—are marked with serial numbers that can, ideally, be traced to a manufacturer, a doctor, and a patient. There are certainly cases where IDs have been confirmed by medical implants or devices—when an identity was suspected but not 100 percent known—and some where a completely unidentified Doe was connected to their name by an implant or a steel pin. But for some cases, particularly older ones, devices and implants can lead to a frustrating dead end. The trail takes us somewhere but not far enough.

As of 2022, breast implants are the most common cosmetic medical implant on the market.[22] Though breast augmentation has been a common procedure for decades, implant serial numbers have only been required since the 1990s,[23] which means that while some implants prior to that time had tracking methods or even a version of serial numbers, that information wouldn't necessarily lead to a single patient.

Examples that come to mind include decedents like a woman nicknamed Julie Doe, whose body was recovered in Florida in 1988. Though her 250cc breast implants could be identified by brand, and as having been discontinued in 1983—thus likely not implanted after 1984—that's as far as investigators could track them.[24] If they'd known in 1988 that Julie's implants had been part of gender-affirming surgery, it's possible that detectives could have done more—for starters, they could've narrowed down the hospitals if she'd had surgery in the United States—but the fact that Julie was trans wasn't discovered until 2015 when DNA testing was performed.

Now there's a barcode system that should, in practice, connect each implant to its owner. The serial-number requirement was used in 2009 to confirm the identity of homicide victim Jasmine Fiore.[25] Her case was well-publicized because of her modeling career, and because her husband,

Ryan Jenkins, had appeared on the VH1 reality dating show *Megan Wants a Millionaire*. Jenkins was the primary suspect in Fiore's death. Her body was discovered mutilated and placed in a suitcase that was tossed in a Los Angeles–area dumpster. Someone—presumably Jenkins— had "removed her fingers and teeth [. . .] to prevent identification." Her face had been mutilated postmortem, and without the serial numbers on her medical implants, it could have taken longer to positively identify Fiore.

Success stories involving medical devices reach far beyond the United States. According to the British Transport Police, a medical implant was used to identify a victim of the King's Cross Underground station fire of 1987. Thirty-one people died in that blaze, and all but one were identified by 1988. The final victim, known as Body 115—a presumed white male between the ages of forty and sixty, and around five foot two—long remained a mystery. Investigators had considered a missing man, Alexander Fallon, as a possible match for the final victim, but Body 115's estimated height and age weren't a match for Fallon's; his family reported him as seventy-three years old and five foot six.

As authorities continued to study Body 115's case, they made sure to record the particulars: a set of full dentures, signs of "heart and lung disease," and an unusual piece of medical hardware in place. Per the Transport Police, they found "a clip found in the brain, used in a right frontal/temporal craniotomy. The clip used had been preserved and was identified as a Sugita No. 5 clip manufactured in Japan between 1977 and 1982." There were "no more than 300" of that particular clip imported into the UK within the possible timeframe. And there was more—the area of the surgery itself was unusual. "About a third of craniotomies [were] carried out on the left-hand side [. . .] that would leave only 200 on the right. Only 100 would appear on the right side of a male." Police found evidence of exactly such a surgery in a photo of Fallon—and then located the surgeon who had operated on him. Body 115 was thus formally identified as Alexander Fallon, a widower from Scotland who had moved to London in 1974 after the death of his wife. He had unstable housing after that point, keeping in contact with his daughters by letter until 1987.[26]

There are so many other case solves that don't make the news, mostly because the decedents don't become long-term unidentified Does; a medical examiner or anthropologist matches up an X-ray to a medical record, and spots that injury, the fused spine. Research is able to trace a knee replacement straight to the doctor who completed the surgery. It happens more often than you'd think.

For the longest-standing cold cases, DNA will likely be the key to solving them, but there's no harm—and much to be gained—from using more immediate methods. There's a reason Dr. Amy Michael suggests cold cases be reviewed every five years. Maybe a missing person's fingerprints have finally made it into the right database. Perhaps someone will spot the details of a surgery that were missed before, leading to a match. Skeletal-analysis methods are continually refined, and databases grow. A case review, by fresh eyes, can be a powerful tool in a world of stretched budgets and uneven case funding. By any number of means, John Doe and Jane Doe can be reconnected to the identity they held in life.

CHAPTER THREE

THE CASE: ASSEMBLY

May 2021—Atlanta, GA

I had been dreaming all week.

That was unusual. Normally, I slept hard and deeply, and didn't dream at all. Nighttime, after my son was in bed, and my husband had drifted off beside him after telling him "just one more story"—that was when I did my best work. The house was peaceful; it hummed with fans, air conditioning, and the sounds of crickets from the swath of deep woods that sidled up to our fence. In that quiet time, no one needed me. I could finish a podcast script or research past midnight without interruption.

I might spend a few hours digging through census records, or trying to match an earring found in the desert to a missing girl, or reviewing the accounting of each bone recovered from a crime scene—contemplating all the while whether the missing pieces fit, like a puzzle, with another case. Maybe there were transcripts of an interview with a murderer to read, or an autopsy to study, with each organ described like a piece of awful produce plucked from a garden: *Glistening. Smooth. Shiny.*

It could be a shock to the system, to move from that to my real life. Another reason why night was easier: I could shift from death reports and blurry scans of police files to the solitary rituals of tooth brushing and lunch packing, and not have to pretend that everything was fine. I'd have some time before I needed to quietly wake my husband, still asleep in my son's little bed. Some things were easier to forget than others.

I once spent three days trying to understand how poorly mixed concrete might have affected the decomposition of an unidentified child's body. She'd been put into a suitcase filled with it, and then inside an old TV cabinet, a revenant of the 1970s or early '80s. More concrete had been added, and she'd been left in a forest in South Georgia. Maybe her killer, or killers, had planned to sink her in a body of water. But that hadn't happened. And when a logger had come upon the cabinet, sitting off the highway in the woods, he tipped it over, and some of the concrete broke, exposing the toddler's little tomb.

I wanted to understand whether the wet concrete poured into the suitcase might have affected various estimations at autopsy. There were a few studies available, but nothing that really helped me understand if the PMI, the postmortem interval, suggested by the medical examiner in this case was perhaps longer than she'd actually been dead. Based on the way the concrete shattered, I suspected it had been improperly mixed. Perhaps that could throw off an estimation of how the heat of the setting concrete might have sped up decomposition, if at all. The medical examiner thought she'd died in November. But I wondered if decomposition had been hastened by that concrete. Maybe she'd died closer to Christmas. That's when she was found—and why she was called "Christmas Doe." She had on a red-and-white outfit, with matching bow clips in her braids. Had she been dressed for an occasion? Pictures? It was July when I was researching her case, and I felt sick at the smell of the hot asphalt all that summer.

But still, I didn't dream. Not often. My friends told me they did when they were deep into research or writing about terrible things. I could usually leave work behind.

That week in May 2021, though, things had shifted.

Since February, a drive folder labeled "Ina Jane Doe" had sat patiently in an open tab on my laptop. I returned there every day to reorganize, relabel, and slowly fill it with piecemeal news clippings I hoped might help form a picture. Or maybe pictures—intertwining stories of missing women who could be Ina Jane Doe. With so few base details, we had dozens upon dozens of possibilities. It wasn't a perfect game of match; many of the missing aren't actually reported as such. You could search forever and not find the right listing. But you have to check. And so I did, along with Amy's students, setting our parameters a little wider than NamUs had—at least to begin with.

Age range, somewhere between twenty-five and fifty-five. Presumed white. Presumed female. Sometimes I limited to red hair, sometimes not. I scrolled through face after face, captured in black-and-white or faded color. There were school photos, wedding photos, cropped candid photos taken at barbecues and parties and beaches, stern driver's license shots, mugshots, photos taken from old student IDs. Auburn, orange, strawberry, ginger, red brown. Brown eyes. Hazel. Color unlisted.

But I could stop and start the work, and not get too lost in it. Until May. That's when Amy got the go-ahead to take on Ina's case, and I suddenly had free time. I'd just begun a year of unpaid leave from my university to concentrate on the cold-case work that had slowly consumed my life. Travel time had always been scarce, something to fit in on the weekend when I'd drive two states over to interview a family, or a medical examiner, or visit a closed-down state hospital. But now, I finally had more uninterrupted time to devote to Ina's case. For months, Amy and I had been planning, and emailing, and requesting records, and saving money, and when we'd finally decided to see Ina's case through, that past winter, we'd all begun working ahead, hoping Amy would get the approval for the skeletal reanalysis. Jefferson County had agreed, and we'd be heading to Illinois in June.

We texted almost every night. That spring, it was mostly logistics:

What did Jefferson say?

No mailing. They don't want to risk it.

Will you fly?

I'll drive and meet you at STL. You can fly in and meet Audrey
and Kyana there.

If an Illinois sheriff's office was surprised that a New Hampshire–based
biological anthropologist had contacted them and offered to do a skeletal
reanalysis of their 1993 unidentified Jane Doe case, they hadn't said so.
They'd also been fine with Amy's mention of bringing along a colleague,
an academic and writer from Georgia with experience in researching cold
cases. She didn't mention my true-crime podcast as a credential. That was
a wise decision. People could be funny about that.

With a date finally in place, I felt like I had catching up to do—but
on what, I wasn't sure. The problem with unidentified-persons research
is that there is no precise beginning or end. And that meant staying up
late and reading every archived message board. Of course, you start with
the case itself. On the actual crime, on the victim we knew as Ina, there
wasn't much. There was, however, plenty of discussion in the forums, on
Reddit, and Websleuths, and Facebook, and in a few more far-flung corners. But that primarily came down to the art that had been commissioned for her in the early 1990s. It had created quite a stir.

The original anthropological analysis of Ina inspired two separate artist's renditions, a drawing and a forensic sculpture. Each showed a woman
with marked torticollis and distinct facial asymmetry that looked in the
artists' imagining like a kind of partial paralysis. Ina was pictured with
her mouth positioned askew, and her cheek and chin sagging to one side.
In the clay reconstruction, Ina Jane Doe was also shown as having very
distinctly crooked front teeth, with one broken off at a jagged point—
something that Amy had noted when we discussed the case. Both artists
had presented Ina with a mid-length bob and dark eyes, and maybe somewhere in her forties. I could recognize the connection between the art and
the descriptions in the report, but for some reason, when I read the blurry,
digitized news articles late at night, describing Ina, and where she'd been
found in the park . . . I couldn't see anything of her in them. Which was

silly. There wasn't any real physical detail. But it wasn't how she took form in my mind's eye—a hazy picture, but a woman with long hair, a little older than me, maybe someone I might see when I visited my parents in the mountains, shopping at the Ingles. I'm not sure why I associated her with the country, and not the city. Maybe it was the forest.

Though very similar to each other, the forensic renderings were memorable and distinct in their own right. Both were shared, often: the drawing and a photo of the bust. And because of Ina Jane Doe's possible torticollis, which the report suggested might have been congenital or acquired—if she had it at all—theories developed based on those characteristics alone. Some thought that Ina Jane Doe might have been injured in a car wreck. Others proposed that she'd had neck issues or facial asymmetry for most or all of her life. Some wondered if she'd had a disability that rendered her vulnerable to a caregiver who could have injured her. Either way, those characteristics became important to those combing the missing-persons databases and news archives.

When I talked to Amy about it, however, she wasn't convinced by the online discussion. She pointed out what I'd sensed from the photo that accompanied the journal article, published by the first anthropologist to study the case: Ina's skeletal asymmetry seemed mild. Her vertebrae weren't shown along with the journal article, so Amy couldn't comment on possible torticollis. But if Ina truly had such unique physical features . . . I just couldn't shake the feeling that someone should have recognized her, in nearly thirty years. Her family would know her. Her friends, her neighbors. They'd see something in that art, in the brilliant red of her hair, and call Jefferson County. But from what the soon-retiring detective captain relayed to Amy, that call never came. No one saw their sister, or mother, or daughter looking back from the newspaper or flyer or screen. And that was why Amy wanted the reanalysis. It was time to try something else.

Nothing is static, she typed. *Not even bones.*

It was in the middle of this whole process that the dreams started up.

Every morning, my phone shrilled at 5:30, when I was supposed to get up early enough to drink coffee in peace—and some days I woke with a start, remembering the woods. Mostly the trees—big, towering things, with arching branches that crisscrossed overhead into a dark canopy. It made a green ceiling over everything, but I knew it was winter in the dream. On the ground were dead leaves and red hair, in little piles all over the forest floor, like tiny fires half hidden in the brush. I knew that if I disturbed one, there would be . . . something underneath. But I always woke up before I found out just what.

Maybe it was that I would see her, her real face, and know her when I did.

It wasn't a real place, that forest I visited in my dreams. I hadn't been to the scene yet. I hadn't even seen precise photos. Google Earth and images of the park were the best I could do. My brain was filling in the rest with a kind of fairy-tale forest. I wasn't sure who I was supposed to be in the dream, or what I was supposed to do. Was I finding her there for the first time? Sometimes there were faces hidden in the branches, and a road curling like a pencil shaving toward a bare clearing.

I decided I shouldn't clip digital newspaper articles right before bed. It was better to stop by midafternoon and answer emails about podcast ads for things like shampoo and food-subscription boxes until I could trick myself out of it. Feel less haunted.

Everything I found that directly covered Ina Jane's case was already nesting in a neat little Google Drive folder; there were a half-dozen articles or so. But it didn't even begin to start answering our questions. Had other partial human remains been found along Illinois roads? What about Indiana, Kentucky, Ohio, Tennessee? The answer was, unfortunately, of course there had; there is nothing quite so singularly macabre as trying to come up for every possible synonym for dismemberment you can think of and running it through a newspaper archive. *Partial remains recovered. Human torso. Decapitated body. Woman's leg. Hands found.* It went on and on, and just when you thought you'd exhausted every possible combination, another police officer's unique description would appear, culled from a report, and spark another hour of searching.

And even then—I knew I was still just at the tip of the iceberg. One thing I'd learned early on in podcasting: Don't ever assume you have everything just because you've exhausted the available sources. There's always another case, just a rephrased search term or archived article or retired journalist away. You don't know until you stumble on that lucky bit of information in the strangest of places. There might be a gem among the paranoid comments on an old blog post. Or maybe it's in person, a casual aside from a waitress at a roadside restaurant when you finally make it to the little town to do the interview. There's always something more lurking close by, waiting to be found.

In the final week before we had to start packing for our trip to Illinois, I worked in my bedroom hunched over or sprawled across my bed, fan blowing, TV playing endless loops of trashy reality TV. It was my necessary research background; something about tables being flipped over in fancy restaurants and people marrying each other at first sight provided balance to, well, everything else. Luckily for me, my son was enrolled in a neighborhood art camp, and though he managed to turn every single assignment into a hellish Minecraft landscape that we duly displayed on the refrigerator, it still allowed me a good five hours of precious, uninterrupted research time. Amy was prepping on her side, too, going over the anthropologist's published paper about the case, and reviewing everything else she could find on the possible skeletal features that had been mentioned—features that Ina Jane Doe might or might not have. She wanted to work as quickly as possible; Ina's case had been cold for a very long time, but there still might be family members and loved ones waiting for answers.

When Amy was in the lab at school, we couldn't talk; she had terrible reception. It was a big, echo-y space, full of microscopes and sinks and wide black counters designed for her students' work. But when she worked from home, we were in near-constant communication. There were plenty of logistics to discuss. When I thought about it, I could imagine her setup. After all, I'd already been to her house in New Hampshire, a white-painted New Englander full of curiosities: delicate birds' bones she'd found on hikes, antique books and vintage art, and an elderly black pug named Lucy who would be your friend for life if you had any beef jerky in your possession. I always had a lot of that because I ate keto and was visiting a vegan. Subsequently, Lucy and I had an understanding.

When Amy was home, Lucy was with her, tucked in on the big wraparound couch with a pile of blankets because they never had to deal with real heat in New Hampshire. Some iteration of *90 Day Fiancé* or a Netflix dating show would be playing on the television. That was clear because she'd feed me commentary about whatever couple was behaving terribly until I gave up and turned on my TV so we were watching the episode together. We talked about almost everything. I didn't mention the dreams—it felt unprofessional, even when I was only speaking with a friend. Cases were supposed to stay in their own little category and be put away when we stopped working. Everyone knew that wasn't possible, but the pretense was kept up. Otherwise, you couldn't move in the world.

But even so, our text threads were very strange:

What was that NamUs Profile?

I left the Post-It in my office.

Why is she putting up with him he is a giant asshole

They are going to get divorced in the finale.

Did you see that dental chart?

No let me check

Do you follow Darcey on IG?

Yes. Do you have field pants?

. . . what are field pants

Pants you wear in the field. To go out in the field.

English departments don't have "fields"

To an exhumation or on a dig. OK you obviously don't, you need to buy field pants. Go to the thrift store. Don't spend more than five bucks.

I still don't know what they are???

I was eventually told to purchase sturdy fatigue-style pants that I could wear out in the woods or in various conditions that would protect my legs—basically, clothes I wouldn't mind throwing away. We might not need them but better to be prepared. We planned to circle back through to Missouri to visit one of Amy's friends, an anthropologist at a school southeast of St. Louis, after we finished work in Illinois. Since we were going to be so close, she wanted Amy to consult on a case. Amy wasn't sure what we might be in for there, or in the state park near Ina. As the writer in this relationship, I couldn't imagine that I'd be doing anything that required disposable trousers, but I still put them on my list.

In the meantime, we had some last-minute work to finish on possible perpetrators. That was basic background research. It wasn't something we could devote a lot of time to just yet; without Ina Jane Doe's identity, we didn't know anything about the most likely suspects in her life. But it was good practice to do research of similar crimes that occurred in the same general area, around the same time period; you never know what notes can come in handy months down the road. More than once, I've gotten a case file and seen a name in it that I'd found weeks before, in a newspaper article, mentioned in relation to another crime.

Amy didn't often mention serial killers, and neither did I. That was a sore subject for both of us, probably because people wanted to talk about them, with too much excitement, all the time.

In the vast majority of cases, serial murder is the exception, not the rule. But mention a cold case anywhere, and the worst of them are summoned like Bloody Mary at the bathroom mirror: *Bundy. Ridgway. Keyes.*

Even someone like Samuel Little. We'd covered the most prolific serial killer in the United States on my podcast back in 2019, and I *still* got emails from people wondering if I thought he might be connected to this case or that. Little had confessed to ninety-three murders—a horrific number—but that was also less than the total number of people murdered in Atlanta in 2020. Some of those 157 people were killed by strangers, sure, but many weren't. The odds said that Ina was more likely to know her killer than not. Efforts to move her from the crime scene, to hide her identity, supported that theory—but didn't prove it. There were always those who broke the mold in the worst ways possible. She also died in 1993, the edge of what crime historian Harold Schechter termed "the golden age of serial murder." That period, the thirty-year stretch from 1970 to 1999, accounted for the active years of roughly 88 percent of the known serial killers in the United States.[1]

Even with all we knew about the ordinary versus the extraordinary, Amy and I had briefly discussed the possibility of serial killer Gary Hilton, also called the National Forest (sometimes National Park) serial killer, being involved. As far as I knew, he'd still been living in Georgia in 1993—and law enforcement hadn't tied him to a crime until the mid-'00s—but he was suspected in a number of murders dating back to the 1990s. And there were a few similarities that gave us pause. Hilton dismembered his victims and left their remains in parks. Some he knew, but in the suspected cases, there were victims to whom he had no obvious ties.

In 1995, Hilton had heavily influenced the direction of a movie, *Deadly Run*, which served as an eerie foreshadowing of one of his later murders—and his future victim disposal sites. In the movie, a take on the "most dangerous game," a killer drops a woman off in the woods and hunts her. Rather than ending as a classic slasher movie night—with her ultimate "final girl" survival—the killer decapitates her. Horrifically, Hilton's 2008 murder of Meredith Emerson, in Georgia, bore similarities to the film. And southern Illinois wasn't so far from some of Hilton's later stomping grounds.

Meanwhile, a number of message-board posters online had posed a possible connection between Ina Jane Doe and the "Redhead Murders."

These were a series of killings that had similarities but had not been defin-itively linked, and occurred between 1983 and 1985,[2] though some believe the murders occurred from 1978 to 1992.[3] Reddish-haired women were found strangled, some wrapped in blankets, and bound with duct tape, disposed of off the highways of Tennessee and Kentucky and surrounding states. Illinois wasn't far off. January 27, 1993, might be considered part of that extended timeline. Ina obviously fit the redhead component of the victimology, and we knew that NamUs and every other public source we had access to described her as redheaded, except for two early articles, which described her hair as brown. We weren't so sure about the shade of red just yet; we'd know more when we got access to Jefferson County's file and photographs if there were any. Either way, Ina Jane Doe fit the rough victim profile that investigators had used as part of the system for identi-fying possible murders in this series.

But like so many theories involving serial murder, the seams had to stretch to make the known information fit Ina Jane Doe's death: the year, the manner in which she was found (farther off a highway), and in the Midwest. She had not been left whole. The other women hadn't had their identities obscured via dismemberment.

It was natural that serial killers would be the focus of online ama-teur researchers, especially when digging through Doe cases: There are often no other immediate trails to follow. The victims' backstories are obscured. There's an urge to play connect the dots with virtual red string across the digital landscape of known entities. Still, cold cases are not neat packages. All roads don't lead due north to the infamous.

Ultimately, Amy and I didn't consider it very likely that she was one of the victims from the Redhead Murders. I did make note of Gary Hilton and asked Kyana, Amy's lab manager, to gather up a few articles about him, for background's sake, but it wasn't a lead we would spend real time on—not unless other clear connections made themselves known. At the end of the day, the possible is not the probable. The probability is that a killer knows their victim, and that this relationship holds the key to the crime. But that's the trouble when you don't have a name—there's no last action to study. Even if we had one, we'd still be at a disadvantage: all those digital footprints that we take for granted that we can step backward in, like magic, to find out every swipe and click that can count up the moments and motions of a day? There were prototypes in 1993. But nothing like what we have today. We'd essentially be searching in the dark.

And so, the four of us—two professors from opposite ends of the East Coast and a couple of Amy's University of New Hampshire undergrads, Kyana and Audrey, who'd managed to get travel approval—prepared ourselves for the trip to Illinois.

I imagined the two of them already owned field pants.

I wanted to see everything that we could, but especially the park, which had some areas that were more "rustic" than others. We knew that Ina Jane Doe's remains had been found in the area known as the "primitive campground," but what that really meant, practically speaking, we weren't sure. The online maps and brochures didn't tell us much. You can study all the information you want until your eyes blur—but going to the location in person is always better. You can see, immediately, all the mistakes you've made as you've assumed. What constitutes "a small outcropping of trees," really? A hundred Reddit threads could be closed with a walk around a state park, or with an in-person trip to a lonely, rural highway, and a few minutes with a measuring tape. Of course, that's not feasible for most people. Not even for researchers and writers who have to construct scenes as if we've crunched across gravel ourselves, gazing into the dense forests described in case reports.

I've always preferred to go in person when I can, and not just to get the lay of the land. I traveled for the podcast with my co-host, Brooke, as much as possible, and we felt the interviews always turned out better when we could meet people face-to-face. Law enforcement could get a feel for us. Families were more comfortable in their homes or favorite coffee shops or some neutral location where they could see who we were and ask us questions, too. They weren't speaking into the void and hoping their story would come out all right.

There was another, practical reason to go in person, too: Jefferson County was not willing to mail Ina's remains to us—and we didn't expect them to. With only her skull left to analyze, chances at testing were limited, and ties between the victim in life and in death were finite. After we'd established contact with law enforcement, Amy discovered that Ina's four cervical vertebrae—still attached when her remains were discovered—were not readily available. Not lost, probably. But they weren't stored with her skull, or in the cold-storage room at the justice complex. There had been a burst pipe in the building, and a major move had to happen because of it. It was possible that Ina's verts had been maintained in their own evidence container and had been separated during the rush to preserve property into another area of the building, or moved to the coroner's storage facility.

I'd seen similar problems a dozen times in similar long-running investigations. I knew of one case where the search for a victim's hands had been going on for years. In that instance, authorities knew they were in storage—that wasn't the issue—but "storage" meant one of several enormous warehouses holding tens of thousands of items. Records, inconveniently, had not been digitized.

In that particular case, DNA testing could not proceed. Luckily, though, Jefferson County had what they needed for DNA extraction. Ina's skull was intact, which meant she had both her cranium and her mandible—her jaw, with nearly all her teeth in place. Her molars and portions of the cranium were both strong candidates for DNA testing.

It felt strange to discuss a person like an item to be sampled—like volcanic rock or soil or something that hadn't done the same things we all do: Checked the mail after work. Sunk her teeth into an apple. Drank cold water on a hot day. Watched a bad movie. Submerged herself into a warm bath. But when we become unidentified, the scientific is the only way back to the specific.

The local department was also sorting through their cold storage for other conserved evidence. If her hair had been preserved, it could be tested as well. And there likely would be other evidence in storage that would be valuable in her homicide investigation—once her identity was established.

In any case, since Amy had family she'd planned to visit in Illinois and that colleague, Jen Bengtson, in Missouri, who needed help with another case, driving seemed the logical choice for her. She would personally retrieve Ina's remains and deliver them to her secure lab on the University of New Hampshire's campus. Those two bits—the visit to the sheriff and case consulting—are how her students, anthropology majors and star lab assistants, had gotten university approval to join in for field experience.

The plan was this: The four of us would meet in St. Louis. There was a real airport there, big enough for direct flights—and I'd be coming from Atlanta, so that was a plus. The two University of New Hampshire students, Kyana and Audrey, were headed in on flights from New England. They'd both taken time out of their summer breaks for this "field experience." It would be something to add to their CVs, but they were two of Amy's best students. Really, they just wanted to learn. I was still a professor then, too, and had been talking to Kyana about research methods. The students had already helped me understand some of the anthropological terms we were tossing around via email. That was the kind of learning environment I had always liked best: taking turns as teacher and pupil.

Amy decided to leave a few days earlier, driving her ten-year-old Toyota RAV4 all the way from New Hampshire. She didn't know what kind of storage container Jefferson County was working with, and she'd need to plan ahead for delicate packing.

And then there was the issue of getting through airport security. It can be done, but she didn't want to gamble. On the possible loss or damage of or to the victim, that is. She wasn't worried about the TSA on her own account; after all, biological anthropologists are generally made of pretty stern stuff. But she was trained to handle bones with respect, and precision, and care. And there was so little left of Ina Jane Doe. We needed to do whatever we could to protect her.

Detective Captain Scott Burge, who'd agreed to let us work with Jefferson County, was pleased with this plan. Captain Burge was the third lead detective to handle Ina's case, and he'd put in plenty of hours trying to identify her. It was an investigation that had stayed with him for a long time. He was set to retire in the fall, and the captain wanted to know her name and see her murderer caught. By now, the department had been on the hunt for twenty-nine years. He was open to suggestions.

It was clear in many ways that both departments involved in the case, the Jefferson County Sheriff's Office and the Illinois State Police, had taken Ina Jane Doe's death and her identification seriously. You might think that would be a given. But I've covered enough under-investigated cases on the podcast to know that isn't always true. And in unidentified-persons investigations in particular, the on-the-ground work could be thin. Fortunately, JCSO and ISP were serious and methodical about her investigation; I gleaned that from the scattered regional newspaper coverage and the measured public statements of officials. It was also clear when Amy spoke to Detective Captain Scott Burge about Ina Jane Doe. He told her he'd spent months organizing the files on Ina Jane Doe's case—that's *files*, plural—and how his small department followed up on all the various leads, hoping they might discover her identity. He was receptive to Amy's position on skeletal reanalysis. He also understood how radically investigative genetic genealogy had changed the landscape, and he was willing to let us do our work to help in the case.

People often make the mistake of thinking rural departments won't have forward-thinking investigators. That's not necessarily the case. I've visited tiny offices in my home state of Georgia where everyone's up-to-date on the latest DNA technology and that have sent detectives to trainings at Quantico. What's more, at least in my experience, smaller departments with a lot of homicide experience are willing to listen. Jefferson County was certainly open to seeing what we could discover.

But what would that be? Best-case scenario, our team would identify Ina Jane Doe, and her family and loved ones would know what had happened to her. Law enforcement could then use that information to pursue her homicide case; we hoped they would. Cold cases were worked in the spare hours, and there were no devoted squads or task forces in such small towns.

Of course, we would need a team to manage anything. That would be simple enough; no action-adventure assembly montage necessary. Amy was the bone expert, and I was handy for fiddling with pieces of old paper, but the lab work and genealogy required outside help. We decided to consult another anthropologist, an anatomist, and investigative genetic genealogists, and to contract a lab. If Jefferson County agreed, we'd ask an artist to update the forensic art as well. We knew who we wanted to use, and we hoped that by the time Detective Captain Burge was ready to retire, the case would be close to solved. Nothing would move *quickly*— the testing, the paperwork, the bureaucratic steps, the little pieces that needed to be in place for everything to follow the proper procedure— those could be maddening. By fall, though, the process would at least be well underway.

But to get in motion . . . I had to get in motion. I'd put off travel plans until a week out. I could blame that on the lack of sleep, but it had been that way since I was old enough to go leave the house and reasonably be expected to return. I'd always arrive late, with no gas in my car, and missing at least one essential item—usually my suitcase, or homework, or passport, or wallet. My first and best portable CD-Walkman was lost somewhere in England after my semester abroad there in the early '00s, a Social Distortion album still stuck inside. I hoped some angry teen would unearth it from an alley or back room of a dive bar and treat it like the holy relic it was.

So, in keeping with that tradition, I booked a last-minute ticket to St. Louis via the Delta app, guaranteed inconvenient departure time. According to Amy's itinerary, we'd be traveling around the Midwest for at least five days, so I filled a suitcase we'd bought for a family trip (translation: big enough for three people) with what seemed like the proper amount of random black clothing and the prescribed "field pants." Those ended up being a pair of old gray fatigues I'd dug up from my house show days, which had since been sitting in the back of my closet. I was saving all the band T-shirts for my son. He told me that my music was "terrible," but at barely seven, he still had time to develop taste.

I packed all my various cords and recording equipment, too. My husband had neatly zip-tied them into little bundles that I would, *through absolutely no fault of my own*, manage to somehow unwind and tangle before I made it back to Atlanta. I always carried those with me through security because my Zoom H4n Pro digital recorder seemed to strike every TSA agent as a possible explosive. I was tired of having my clothes and moisturizer and tampons rifled through every time I took a flight. I couldn't leave without the stuff, though. I wanted to record what we were doing in the field: What we saw at Wayne Fitzgerrell State Park when we walked the primitive campground. My thoughts on the files. Amy's initial, informal skeletal analysis. Recording everything and then having it transcribed meant I had an accurate version of what we actually did and said, not just how we remembered it.

Those are always two very different things, aren't they?

The last tasks involved double-checking that our babysitter would be available and writing a list of what was in the freezer for my husband. He was excellent in many things, but planning dinner was not one of them. Without serving suggestions, they'd be eating corn dogs for every meal. That went straight on the fridge, with double magnets for safety.

The night before that first flight, I sat at the little oak-wood table in our kitchen, stuffing a few protein bars into the side pocket of my messenger bag while my son dribbled blue kinetic sand onto an old baking sheet. He was fresh from a swim lesson, and his dark blond hair was still damp against his cheeks. I paused and brushed it back from his eyes.

"You remember I'm going out of town, right? With Dr. Amy?"

He didn't look up. Sand formed into little spheres under his fingers, and he lined them up, one by one, against the edge of the pan. They looked like tiny blue snowballs, ready to be pelted at some imaginary target.

"You're going to go find someone."

"Pretty close, bud. Trying to find out more about someone." I put my bag down on the floor and gave his shoulder a squeeze.

After the times he'd talked at school about my work, we told him a little but not too much. My son knew about the stacks of folders and the long interviews we did upstairs, and the times his mom and his "Auntie Brooke" were gone, off to "go and talk to families." But when he'd gone to kindergarten and promised his computer teacher that I'd find his "missing people"? I couldn't live up to that. Not then. A podcast was something but not enough. That was around the time Amy and I had started making our plans to close cases.

At seven a.m. the next morning, I headed to the Hartsfield-Jackson Atlanta International Airport in an Uber that met me at the bottom of our steep driveway. Our metro Atlanta neighborhood was still quiet, except for the distant sound of recycling trucks trundling down the streets. I always took rideshare; getting dropped off by my husband meant missing two exits, being dropped off at the wrong terminal, and then racing through TSA and jogging across the United States' busiest airport to catch my flight. With that as the alternative, I'd rather pay $50 to be driven there two hours ahead of schedule. When it comes to Atlanta air travel, you want to be bored and early.

It was a silent drive, which I always appreciated; the young woman who picked me up was wearing a single earbud and gold-and-black sunglasses, and the only word she said besides "Hello" was "Delta?" In Atlanta, that was always a good guess.

There wasn't much I liked about planes, except that it was a good time to work uninterrupted—as long as I sat next to someone who wanted to ignore me as much as I wanted to ignore them. But my 9:30 flight to St. Louis was so short that I'd barely gotten a few pages of a podcast script edited and a free bag of almonds eaten before the captain announced our descent. I hadn't even had time to go over my Ina notes again. I sighed. I wanted to be as prepped as possible before we arrived at the sheriff's office. That meant I'd have to do that in Amy's car, on the drive to Jefferson County.

After crawling up into the overhead bin to rescue an elderly woman's hopelessly wedged overnight bag, I was safely deboarded and on my way to meet Kyana and Audrey, Amy's students, at baggage claim. The Lambert Airport seemed tiny in comparison to Atlanta's, but to be fair, Hartsfield-Jackson is bigger than some towns. It was a short walk to the main entrance, where luggage could be fetched and rides caught. I'd talked to Kyana before—we'd been working on research together for a while by that point—but we hadn't actually convened in person. I was pretty sure both Kyana and Audrey had been in the class of Amy's I'd visited—digitally, of course—to lecture on filing FOIA requests.

I had just wrestled my enormous suitcase off the carousel and managed to get upright as Kyana and Audrey rounded the corner, fresh from their flights. I recognized them almost immediately from the digital-class visit—varying shades of blond hair, and each dressed appropriately for the heat in rugged shorts and tank tops. Both carried backpacks that could be tossed in the back of a truck or in a ditch at a dig site and were definitely full of appropriate field clothing.

"Professor Norton?" Kyana asked, but it was a formality. The airport wasn't teeming with other women who were dressed head-to-toe in black in the middle of summer.

As we headed upstairs, I found my sunglasses buried somewhere in my bag. Sunlight streaming in from the big, paneled windows promised a very bright day outside the airport.

"Yeah, but call me Laurah. Amy goes by her first name, right?"

They agreed that she did. I don't stand on ceremony with my students, let alone other people's. Besides, I had a terminal degree, an MFA, and not a doctorate, and no one was quite sure what to call me. It was better to get to first names before we devolved into *Mrs.* territory.

We walked the short stretch toward the main entrance and exit together, Kyana and Audrey slowing down a bit to keep pace with me. They were polite and a little shy, which was absolutely appropriate, considering they were meeting a sweaty semi-stranger technically old enough to have given birth to them, although their packing skills were a good indication that they had been raised by more responsible people.

We made our way outside to wait for Amy. She was on the last leg of her trip from New Hampshire and had called to say she'd be there within ten minutes. So, we parked ourselves by what seemed to be the smoking section—that was a blast from the past—to wait at the curb for a dusty RAV4. The ground beneath our feet was littered with blue surgical masks and cigarette butts, and the air felt thick as anything. The hair twisted back against the nape of my neck was already beginning to curl. Unfortunately, St. Louis was as hot as Atlanta and just as humid; there was no escape from the summer. The tornado shelters I'd seen at the airport had been a fun new addition, though.

We broke out the snacks, munching on granola bars and trail mix and sipping from enormous metal water bottles when we ran out of conversational topics. I didn't want to ask them embarrassing, old-person questions about finals or their plans for graduate school. I was almost at the point of asking what podcasts they listened to when the RAV4 pulled up just a hair too tightly to the curb. I noticed because I was sitting on my suitcase right at the lip of the concrete, and the car door nearly skimmed my knee.

The passenger's side window rolled down, revealing dark brown, chin-length hair and oversized sunglasses.

"Sorry, sorry, sorry. Traffic." She wrinkled her nose and gave me a look. "Christ, that's a giant suitcase."

Amy was late, but Amy was always late. Not on purpose. She just seemed to exist in some slightly different space-time continuum, operating twenty minutes behind everyone else. I was also always late, and when we were together, it somehow multiplied, putting us roughly an hour behind schedule.

Amy hopped out to help me, since I was still scrambling. Like most of the times I'd seen her, she was dressed in chunky shoes—for the added height—and jeans and a white graphic tee of some variety. This time it was *Exonerate the West Memphis 3*. She would button up a blouse over it before we arrived at the sheriff's office, to cover her tattoos and the slogan. I had my cover-the-tattoo-and-T-shirt blouse shoved in my purse. Along with my natural-born Southern accent and a few extra pens, it was essential administrative travel gear.

I settled in the front seat and plucked a few errant Post-it notes from my jeans. Post-its and a complex system of phone alarms were Amy's system of life organization. Chimes would ring every fifteen minutes or so—I don't know how she knew what designated where she was meant to be—and mysterious messages like *CORONER* were stuck all over her desk at work. And now, to me.

Amy cranked the engine and a blast of blessedly cool air hit me right in the face. In the back seat, Audrey and Kyana made responsible seatbelt-clicking noises. Amy frowned into the rearview mirror, checking for traffic behind us, and then shifted the Toyota over two lanes, merging out into the main highway. The flat Missouri pavement stretched out before us like a perfect, smooth sheet of metal, coasting all the way to the horizon without interruption.

"Time to go pick up Ina," she said, her foot on the gas.

CHAPTER FOUR

THE METHOD: FORENSIC ANTHROPOLOGY

Amy has told me a dozen times: Maybe the work of a forensic anthropologist can seem exciting, and seductively simple, if you watch a lot of crime procedural television. But television lies. An unusually stylish scientist swoops into the children's playground or jobsite or groundbreaking ceremony where a skeleton has been unearthed, glances down, and announces that *this is a crime scene.* Next thing you know, they're in the lab, rattling off a list of discoveries so specific that the human skeleton seems as traversable as a Monday-morning crossword. But it's often a lot more complicated than that.

First off, Amy always says, it's a recovery scene. Why does everyone think crime scene and recovery scene are synonymous? And how do they know it's not a historical set of remains?

It's hard out there for the practical forensic anthropologist.

The truth is, when it comes to the discovery of human bones, the difference between historic and forensic skeletal remains was a confusing concept for me to parse. There's whether a possible crime has been committed *and* the age of the remains in question. And that's where a forensic anthropologist comes in.

Spending time with Amy, I saw both kinds of cases. If a construction crew comes upon skeletal remains while working, law enforcement is called, and the state archaeologist or local anthropologists will help them make an initial assessment. It's often obvious—like when a forgotten cemetery has accidentally been disturbed, or a cranium with a bullet hole is discovered, hidden away in a chimney. But sometimes things aren't so simple. Maybe weather or environment or both have made contemporary bones look older. Or maybe "historic" discoveries also uncover evidence of foul play.

I stumbled on an article in *Smithsonian*, published back in 2009, that perfectly illustrates the layered work of a forensic anthropologist: studying human remains within different layers of context—some cultural, some scientific—and making judgments that are informed by time, place, and environment. This story concerned an archaeological project that had uncovered a clandestine grave, dating back to the seventeenth century. Archaeologists were exploring forgotten settlements in Anne Arundel County, Maryland, when they dug up a human skull where one should not have been: in the cellar of a colonial home. They called in forensic anthropologists from the Smithsonian, who located a buried hearth just underneath it.

There, "underneath a layer of fireplace ash, bottle and ceramic fragments, and animal bones," were the remains of a presumed adolescent male with evidence of healed antemortem fractures as well as more recent injuries.[1] According to *Smithsonian*, "the boy's right wrist was fractured in a way that suggested he used his arm to block a strong blow shortly before his death. That injury, along with the awkward burial, points to a violent end." There'd been a law against private burials of indentured servants enacted in the area around the time that this unknown teen would have likely been buried. It had been a measure meant to staunch some of the abuse of servants. In this case, however, the landowners had kept their ugly secrets very close to home.[2]

Clandestine graves, or burials, are exactly what they sound like: hidden. Much of the current literature associated with clandestine burial covers their role in massive human-rights crises across the globe. But there are also many examples that exist on a smaller scale, and forensic anthropologists can be called in to explore clandestine graves. Some of my friends who practice forensic anthropology have backgrounds in bioarchaeology, which calls for the careful excavation of ancient bones; the approach is very similar—except for the knowledge that a crime most likely occurred. In both cases, the bones are often scattered, and there's reconstructing and *siding* to be done—that's determining which side a portion of bone belongs on, like: *Is this patella from the right knee or the left?* They'll also identify fragments of other materials that tend to get mixed in with the remains, like chips of rock, and then further examine what they've gathered to be sure it's human. It's laborious, tedious work—not exactly the *Bones*-style Dr. Temperance Brennan examinations that sent a generation of students into forensic anthropology classes.

Not that my friends have minded the influx of students; Amy has always said that anything that gets them into the chairs to learn about skeletal biology is fine with her. But she could do without reporters asking her things like "Tell me, how do the bones speak to you?"

It's a strange way to dance around the work of forensic anthropology. Ina Jane Doe's cranium and mandible don't speak. She did when she was alive. But her skeletal remains aren't a romantic symbol. They are evidence that she was murdered, and that, until we find out what happened to her and who is responsible, her killer is getting away with the crime.

Forensic anthropologists examine the deceased for evidence of trauma, both antemortem and *perimortem*—meaning that it happened at or around the time of death—to help them both identify the victim and learn more about what happened in the hours or moments before they died. How many injuries did this body sustain? Sometimes, skeletal damage can illustrate that: a bullet hole through a rib, or damage to the bones of a cranium. But the expert must also sort out postmortem damage, too.

When skeletal remains are exposed to the elements, and to animal scavenging, all kinds of damage can occur. Ina Jane Doe herself had a broken tooth, but did that breakage happen during the attack that ended her life, or after her death? That was just one of the things Amy planned to take a closer look at later down the line, with the help of her friend Dr. Samantha Blatt, from Idaho State University. Though there is an entire field of forensic science called forensic odontology, anthropologists also weigh in on teeth; after all, they are hard tissues that stay preserved after death. In Ina's case, determining when her tooth was broken, and how, could be an important detail in either her identification or in the criminal investigation later on. But it could also be impossible to tell for sure.

One of the reasons we sought out Ina's case was because she was a victim who had not had a skeletal reanalysis. Any case that hadn't been reviewed in the last decade, that hadn't attracted funding, was a good candidate for the work Amy and I wanted to do. I thought about the process as akin to digitization: If it was vital to digitize records to bring them into the modern age, then why not apply new anthropological learning to old cases? An anthropologist's review was one of the most accessible things a department could seek out, but Amy told me that a reanalysis was highly unusual. Once a report is in the file, it's considered finished. What could a new set of anthropologists, nearly thirty years after an initial examination, find in Ina? For her?

———◆———

Technically, "forensic anthropologist" is a title. My understanding is that many biological anthropologists—like Amy—*practice* forensic anthropology, because the term "forensic" simply means "relating to or denoting the application of scientific methods and techniques to the investigation of crime."[3] It's been explained to me that, if we are being very formal, to call oneself a forensic anthropologist, one would need to have earned board certification in the field: a D-ABFA (Diplomate of the American Board of Forensic Anthropology). But in the interest of simplicity, I'll use the term "forensic anthropology" to encompass the practice by both board-certified and non-board-certified biological anthropologists. Otherwise, things are going to get *very* wordy.

Now a term I'm more familiar with, from college: *anthropology*: "the study of the human race, especially of its origins, development, customs, and beliefs."[4] In cultural anthropology, of course, that connection seems clear, but I hadn't gathered how important understanding the living is to the work of understanding the dead—not until I began to spend time with experts. I am a creative writer, and not a scientist. But I like learning and hope that by explaining some of the basics I've picked up by tagging along, you'll get a glimpse into their world, too. There's far more nuance and complexity involved in each discipline than could be fully understood in a year or two of study; that becomes clear every time Amy tells me I have mixed up the word *patella* with *parietal*. But the essence of the discipline? I think that can be captured pretty clearly, even by nonexperts, if you listen to these scientists talk passionately about their work.

Most people I've met in the anthropological space understand the dead because they care about the living—and know that none of us, when we die, exist as a set of bones, devoid of context. How we identify in life can be key to identifying us in death. Understanding a place, like the population of a city, or region, will inform the work of identifying its dead. That can mean the ancient residents or the current ones. Biological anthropologists who practice forensic anthropology emerge from a decade-plus of higher education ready to work on both current and cold cases. If they go into academia, forensic anthropologists take on casework between teaching and their own research, and likely too many faculty meetings. Forensic anthropologists also go on to work at the offices of medical examiners, with governmental agencies, like the Defense POW/MIA Accounting Agency (DPAA), in a full-time position with a law-enforcement agency, or with institutions like the Smithsonian.

Most that I've personally met are professors who also consult for local law enforcement—be that state bureaus, police or sheriffs, or the like. Amy might be called to the scene of recovery by the New Hampshire State Police or have remains shipped to her lab. They could come from any number of agencies. In other areas, a forensic anthropologist might come in to consult at the medical examiner or go out in the field.

In general, they consult on a wide array of cases, and what they take on depends on their full-time job. The work might include ongoing forensic cases, excavating mass graves, "legacy" skeletal remains that almost certainly need to be repatriated, unidentified persons, and the examination of historical remains that are unearthed or otherwise discovered. When the call comes, it could be anything; an anthropologist might be asked to examine skeletal remains discovered at the site of an obvious homicide or tasked with the reanalysis of a long-standing Doe case, or even sent mummified remains or bones seized or acquired by an agency. The possibilities are nearly endless.

And then there are the cases that . . . just sort of *show up*. Maybe someone stops by the university with a cranium they found in their uncle's attic after his funeral. Perhaps a clerk at an insurance firm began to worry about the strange carved bone someone unearthed in a storage closet. Believe me, it happens more often than you'd imagine. Maybe these folks call the police, but if there's a forensic anthropologist in the area, those skeletal remains will likely—eventually—land in their lab. I've heard of people bringing in human remains to work or school, assuming they'd found their families' long-stored Halloween decorations. Imagine their surprise.

And what then? It can depend on results from the skeletal analysis that the anthropologist performs, and what the agency that has sent in the remains—or in the case of mysterious or suspicious skeletal remains, which agency has taken charge—decides to do about it. Is the case suspected to be criminal? The medical examiner's office or law enforcement may fund testing if needed. Does the anthropologist have lab funds that can be used? Maybe samples are taken for radiocarbon dating. That's a method that had long been used by scientists to study ancient organic matter, and to great effect. And in recent years, scientists recognized the ways carbon-14 dating could be utilized in more recent forensic cases involving human remains. The National Institute of Justice funded a study at Arizona State University focused on the atomic age as a flash point in our timeline—the before and after time stamp on our hard tissue, you might say. Time really is written on our bones, in its own fashion.

According to the NIJ's website on the study, "Before the nuclear age, the amount of radiocarbon in the environment varied little in the span of a century. In contrast, from 1955 to 1963, atmospheric radiocarbon levels almost doubled. Since then, they have been dropping back toward natural levels. Over the past six decades, the amount of radiocarbon in people or their remains depends heavily on when they were born or, more precisely, when their tissues were formed."[5] This "bomb carbon" is artificial radiocarbon, different from the natural levels measured in pre-nuclear-age matter. The NIJ's study noted that "for teeth formed after 1965, enamel radiocarbon content predicted year of birth within 1.5 years." The study mentioned that soft tissue is most ideal for estimating date of death as it reflects the current environment's level of radiocarbon. When nails were available, for instance, year of death was "accurate to within three years." For a forensic anthropologist, who deals in bones? Soft tissue isn't their realm. But the testing is still useful: It can tell a forensic anthropologist if bones are from an individual born post-1950, when that artificial radiocarbon raised the levels.

The ability to perform this testing was a huge breakthrough, because estimating even the rough age of a fully skeletonized body can be difficult, especially if it was in an environment that might discolor or weather bone so that it appeared older than it actually was. The reverse was true as well—a bone might be extremely well-preserved but turn out to be hundreds of years old. Amy's friend Dr. Samantha Blatt had run into that situation before, in her Idaho lab. There are other signs that help determine how old bones are—one I always think of is dental work, the development of which has progressed in an orderly manner—but this testing has helped sort more modern cases from older remains that sometimes arrive at the lab.

It's always possible that historic remains might be accidentally unearthed right where they were initially laid to rest, but older bones are also likely to arrive on an anthropologist's desk as part of collections that had previously belonged to someone. Often, these collections were well-known to everyone and had been cataloged and studied by generations of students. But other times, one or two sets of human remains might have been donated by an alumnus, decades back, and forgotten about, only to be uncovered during a renovation or move. Sometimes, the officials who passed remains onto anthropologists weren't quite sure who had brought them in the first place. Other times, an anthropologist would be sent remains that had been held in a private collection, or by an institution that discovered, quite literally, it had skeletons in the closet.

And that's hardly a thing of the past. Per NBC News, a professor at the University of North Dakota inadvertently discovered in a storage area "more than 70 samples of human remains, many of them in boxes with no identifying information [. . .] at the school's library [. . .] the recesses of the nearly 140-year-old campus." That was in late 2022. The professor was searching for Native religious items that had been on display until 1988. Instead, she found the remains of Indigenous individuals scattered in boxes like forgotten files.[6]

When such a discovery is made, those ancestral remains in question then frequently end up in the hands of modern anthropology professors, like Amy, or Sam, who are tasked with discovering their age, and in making ancestry estimations. That would guide next steps, which, depending on origin, might be laid out in law—such as the 1990 NAGPRA, or Native American Graves Protection and Repatriation Act.[7]

NAGPRA is limited in scope, with guidelines set for federal and tribal lands, and federally funded organizations. And despite the act being in place for decades, *ProPublica* reported in early 2023 that federally funded organizations still hold Indigenous ancestral remains and funerary cultural artifacts. The news outlet designed a database to catalog "the repatriation records of these hundreds of institutions."[8] For instance, at the time of *ProPublica*'s reporting, they noted that "the University of California, Berkeley still has the remains of at least 9,058 Native Americans that it has not made available for return; the Department of the Interior still has the remains of at least 2,970 Native Americans [. . .]."[9] This database will likely grow as more data comes in.

These ancestral remains have not been returned, by process, to a community that, per NAGPRA, has "a relationship of shared group identity which can be reasonably traced historically or prehistorically between a present-day Indian tribe or Native Hawaiian organization and an identifiable earlier group. [25 USC 3001 (2)] Cultural affiliation is established when the preponderance of the evidence—based on geographical, kinship, biological, archaeological, linguistic, folklore, oral tradition, historical evidence, or other information or expert opinion—reasonably leads to such a conclusion. [43 CFR 10.2 I]." This makes the process sound orderly. But it can be hard to establish those connections when a person's remains have been fully removed from their context, and stuck on a shelf, in a dusty box, in a museum's back room. According to *ProPublica*, NAGPRA has issued further regulations to address such issues, such as in 2010 when "a pathway for the return of remains and items whose cultural affiliation cannot be established." That's important, but it still hasn't solved the issue. *ProPublica* interviewed D. Rae Gould, "executive director of the Native American and Indigenous Studies Initiative at Brown University and a member of the Hassanamisco Band of Nipmucs of Massachusetts, [who] said it's common for institutions to say they can't figure out who they should return remains and items to." Gould said such institutions often "use arbitrary analysis they call science to say there's no cultural affiliation with modern day tribes." Basically, Gould points out that some institutions have used the supposed or actual age of remains to argue there's no way to determine cultural ties, and thus a path to repatriation, even though NAGPRA allows flexibility in interpretation.[10] And what about when it comes to private land and collections, and state or county-owned property? Laws vary by state.

When I spoke to several anthropologists about NAGPRA, they said that there are other issues that need to be addressed, ones that this new database hasn't captured: For instance, there isn't enough funding made available to cover the cost of repatriation. NAGPRA doesn't allocate those funds by default; either institutions or tribal governments are expected to absorb the cost of transport and burial or apply for grants via the secretary of the interior to offset the expense.[11] The application and dispersal process may delay repatriation as well. Additionally, there generally isn't permanently allocated funding in place to help cover the cost of examination at schools or institutes that hold ancestral remains. And very few universities have a dedicated director or coordinator to handle NAGPRA and examine the nuances of the laws and dedicate time to answer the more difficult questions: What if there are no communities who are ready to repatriate the ancestral remains? How could processes be improved and communities better served?

If it seems like a lot to take in, it is. I've been learning from foren-sic anthropologists like Amy and her friends for only a few years or so. Hanging out with them is a more accurate term for it, really, since there's a lot of bad television involved in our downtime, and eating junk food in hotel rooms, and for some reason, they really *love* going to oddity shops and cryptid museums and taking group photos in front of things like the World's Biggest Shoe—no idea why we had to see that, thinking back—but anyway, it's been enlightening. And for every bizarre misadventure or prediction about whether or not the relationships we saw on reality TV would combust, there were just as many moments that, large or small, changed my understanding of casework.

I've been to labs, exhumations, bone rooms. I've been in exam rooms, observing the experts take detailed notes and recordings; I've also joined in on official law-enforcement visits and evidence retrieval. I've attended conferences, served on panels, helped with presentations—even contrib-uted data to papers although my "data" isn't of the hard science sort. My family interviews have come in handy, though, afterward—particularly when a victim has been identified. They add context. Amy tells me that working with a writer creates an extended learning process after identifi-cation. Anthropologists want to understand people, after all. It's good to be helpful, in some small way.

What I've picked up, more than anything, is that the field of anthropol-ogy is dynamic, and holistic, and comparative. You'd think that there is only so much to learn about the skeletal system of the human body, and how to interpret it, and what we might take away from it; oh boy, is there a *lot* to discuss.

This is not an episode of *Bones*. Not unless Dr. Temperance Bren-nan is willing to spend an entire episode taking tiny measurements in a quiet lab, with the cliffhanger coming just before she begins to fill out her paperwork.

CHAPTER FIVE

THE CASE: INA, ILLINOIS

We made it into Mount Vernon, Illinois, in less than two hours. The trip felt like a parallel slide across a totally flat surface, a perfect line drawn from point A to point B. I was told we'd left Missouri at some point, but the road and fields, broken up by trees and barns, all blurred together for me. Amy had no trouble, but I'd never been good with geography. Later on, I wouldn't be able to tell the days of driving apart: leaves shifting in a rush over the car as we whizzed by, creating a fragment of shadow across the asphalt. Just little broken patterns, like spots on a map that had no key. That reminded me of rural Georgia. Or, at least, the faded red crosses painted across the tin roof of a shed did. So did the piles of moldering flowers and rain-beaten teddy bears at the edge of a splintered highway barrier. Someone had erected two white wooden crosses there, too; if there had been names or dates inscribed, the weather had carried them away.

Just a little ways from the sheriff's office, or where the Waze app promised it would be, we stopped at a gas station. We picked up snacks because that's what you do on a road trip, but our main goal was a quick freshen up—or a button-up, really. Amy and I needed to shimmy into our professional disguises, which we did with minimal contortion inside the car, in the back parking lot.

Besides a blouse, I always packed the same things in my extra-large handbag: laptop, copious pens, recording setup, batteries, and a spiral reporter's notebook. I couldn't read my own handwriting and preferred taking notes on my phone, but that made law enforcement nervous, especially when sensitive files were around. As a general rule, they didn't like the idea of unredacted reports ending up on a podcaster's Instagram feed. I had a portable wand scanner that I often carried for that very reason— another use for the batteries. It ate them up, and it was embarrassing to run out of juice halfway through a giant file and ask if the department had spares. They never did.

The wand scanner didn't make much sense when you really thought it through; those images could travel the web just as quickly from a laptop as an iPhone. It was just an extra, irritating step in my process, and I'd never know if I'd gotten the pages crooked until I was home. But if it made an office less jumpy, I was happy to oblige. Relationships took a long time to build, and I spent a considerable amount of time trying to get documents on victims who weren't covered by other media.

Visiting families was so different. They never cared what you looked like, or if you were just a podcaster. You could arrive at their house in a beaten-up car with one headlight, and with your audio gear packed in your kid's old diaper bag. They just wanted to know you were telling them the truth, and you'd do what you promised . . . put out an accurate account of their missing or murdered loved one's case. Because often, that hadn't happened. Whether it was due to lack of any coverage at all or the spread of misinformation, things had stalled. For the families we worked with, it was almost always the former. If the case was cold, and it always was by the time I met them, lots of things hadn't been happening for a long time. But for Doe cases, those families who were waiting? They were out of reach. So, the authorities were the first and the last line of contact for me. I learned to communicate in a different way.

Law enforcement had a different reaction to Amy and scientists in general. They needed *her*, and not the other way around. Still, Amy wanted to make a good impression. This case wasn't strictly within her purview as it wasn't a New Hampshire case. Moreover, we were forming a new relationship, and her approach was to present herself as neutrally as possible: the expert offering opinions devoid of the personality that spilled out of her when she wasn't taking charge of a thirty-year-old cold case. Except, maybe, for the small talk. Amy was also from rural Illinois, and she was able to speak like she was, which went a long way out here.

"Gum?" Amy offered around an enormous container of some kind of mint-blast cubes. We all took some. No one wanted to chance coffee or Dorito breath on a first meeting.

Otherwise, Kyana and Audrey looked perfectly presentable in their role as college students assisting and didn't require a wardrobe change. Neither needed a rundown on how to behave, either; medical examiners and other officials were a regular feature of Amy's lab back at school, and both had been out in the field. Amy believed in taking her students to experience as much as possible, like recoveries, or observations of exhumations. But this case still held something novel for them; they'd never gotten to work with out-of-state law enforcement before.

Honestly, before we rolled up, I didn't think there'd be much for them to see. Except for the station I'd seen in Beaufort County, South Carolina—which had been converted from an enormous 1990s-era dentist's office and felt like a set from *Saved by the Bell*—local police departments tended to have the same feel. Huge complexes like the APD in Atlanta were another matter, but the smaller outfits and rural ones—those tended to be pretty similar. Sometimes there'd be a justice center attached, and if that was the case, there might be a metal detector. This could often lead to problems whenever I arrived on the scene on behalf of the podcast; I'd have to field questions about my suitcase full of audio equipment if no one remembered to warn the front office about our plans to record.

Occasionally, the coroner would have offices right next door, or other municipal offices might be splitting space; I'd previously run into a mayor across the hall from a police chief in west Georgia. Once, I'd even visited a setup so small that there was a single, large courtroom that doubled as the conference room. We'd had to book an interview on the day that the judge wasn't hearing cases. The echoing of sound bouncing around the space had been impossible to scrub out of our tape.

As predicted, the Jefferson County Sheriff's Office was fairly nondescript: square, cement, a flagpole out front, and sporting a confusing arrangement of doors that made it unclear where we should park. Luckily, one of those doors opened as we were pulling up—not the one I would have picked, of course—and a man appeared. I assumed this was Detective Captain Scott Burge, our contact in Ina Jane Doe's case. I wasn't sure if Amy had texted ahead or if he just had an excellent sense of timing. Maybe they just had a great view of the parking lot. Burge was tall and middle-aged, and his neat gray hair and suit transmitted a clear message, at least to me: *law enforcement*. He shaded his eyes with a hand.

"Dr. Michael," he called, and waved over to us. I was still getting used to that: Everyone was happy to see anthropologists. Amy introduced me as a writer, which I was, and a professor, which was also true, and reminded the detective captain about her students and why they'd come along. Burge was fine with all of it since he was largely interested in getting us into the building and down to business. He was the third detective assigned to Ina's case, but he'd been with the sheriff's office for decades. He remembered when she'd been discovered, at the park. And with his retirement only a few months away, he likely didn't want to imagine a fourth, and fifth, and sixth to follow him.

We were ushered into the cool, beige interior of the department and were introduced to a few people—most importantly, Detective Captain Bobby Wallace. He worked in cybercrime, among other things, and would be taking over Ina's case when Captain Burge retired. He was a bit younger—maybe in his early forties, though it was hard to tell—and greeted us with just a hint of a drawl.

"Originally from Texas," he explained. He probably had to say that a lot in the Midwest.

After we shook hands, Wallace told me that he'd worked with some of the folks I knew over at the GBI, on some interstate cybercrime. Then, after he handed out his business cards to all four of us, he told us about a restaurant that we should definitely hit on our way out of town. It served something like two dozen kinds of lemonade.

"Every flavor you can think of," he opined. I could only think of about four, so I found this impressive.

Introductions made, Detective Captain Burge ushered the four of us into a back office. High shelves lined the walls, and a few nondescript desks sat on either side, creating a small pathway of open floor space. I wasn't sure if it was a work area with storage, or a storage area where people came to work. Whatever it was, it wasn't the evidence room; they had a separate, cold-climate area for physical items. Burge and the other detectives were still going through everything they'd collected for Ina's case, looking for any items that might be tested, like hair samples or blood cards.

On the desk closest to the door was a huge white binder and a cardboard box, fitted with a removable top—like the kind you might get from a fruit stand, or buy reams of paper in. This particular box, though, was designed specifically for its job: housing evidence. Indecipherable—to me—permanent marker ran along its sides and top, remnants of more than one recording system. I glanced back at Kyana and Audrey, who were hanging back a bit, making sure we didn't get too crowded in the small place. They'd worked with Amy in the lab long enough to realize what was in the box. Ina Jane Doe would be wrapped, carefully, and ready for transport.

Meanwhile, I realized Burge was speaking to Amy when he gestured toward the table. "You can copy the files and then bring them back on your way."

Amy blinked at me; she was not the file handler. Fair enough. I'd already filed the necessary forms online, anyway. I grabbed the three-ring binder and flipped through it while Amy filled out chain-of-custody paperwork at one of the desks. As cold-case files went, it was long. And as Doe files went, it was *extremely* long, in addition to being organized and detailed. Neat, creaseless paper, pristinely arranged into plastic sleeves? Files don't start out that way, especially when they've involved multiple agencies. Someone had taken a lot of time to put it together from many disparate records, from notes taken by phone to faxes and reports sent back and forth across the state. I remembered what Amy had told me: It had been Burge.

There were more binders, scattered in groups of two or three—and then a thick row, like a set of encyclopedias, just above our heads. "The Dardeen Case," Burge clarified, following my gaze.

Amy and Burge then returned to discussing the matter at hand: Ina Jane Doe—the care with which she would be transported to New Hampshire, and then the security of Amy's lab. Amy also explained the kinds of samples she would need to take for DNA extraction—a tooth, and any remnants of hair if Jefferson County found it. Ina would in fact remain almost completely intact, so that, hopefully, she could be returned to her loved ones once she was identified. The department would need to sign off on the testing, and Amy and I would pay whatever fee was needed.

After we were all in agreement, Burge carefully raised the lid off the box. Amy leaned in. She was examining how Ina's skull had been wrapped, in layers of protective paper, so we could be sure to rewrap her the same way and transport her with care.

Amy gingerly lifted Ina from the box. She'd told me that the first thing she taught new students in her lab was that the bones they handled didn't exist in a vacuum as objects devoid of connection. She wanted them to think hard about the *human* half of the equation when it came to remains, and act accordingly.

"Kyana, Audrey," she called. "Take a look. Tell me what you notice."

I knew less about human anatomy than anyone else in the room, but as I stepped aside to let the two students move forward, I noticed a few details. Ina's cranium and mandible had been cut during autopsy. I didn't always see the mandible cuts, or read about them in reports, but that might have been a requirement specific to her case—to what her killer had done to hide her identity. The horizontal and vertical marks were obvious, as was the glue that had been used to reconstruct her skull. That would have been for forensic art, maybe, so that the 3-D reconstruction of Ina could be made. Some artists worked on facsimiles, but others created their work directly on the bone, building up clay over carefully measured depth markers.

Amy had shifted into anthro mode. She held Ina's skull very gently, up at eye level, so she could follow the midline of the frontal bone and down to her teeth, forming an imaginary line in the air. She glanced at Kyana and Audrey. "What do you see?"

They were frowning down, too, and noted a few skeletal features that I knew I'd have to look up later. But one observation stood out: *mild asymmetry.*

"Might not have been noticeable in life at all?" I asked.

Amy had on her work face; I couldn't interpret her expression.

She finally said, "Might not have been. I need to do a full examination back at the lab."

That was what we'd been worried about from the start, the main reason why she'd wanted to do the skeletal reanalysis for Ina. The downside to forensic approximations was that the second word—approximation—was often skipped over. A viewer might treat a re-creation of the victim like photographic evidence, not a suggestion. And the current art for Ina Jane Doe showed marked asymmetry of the features. This meant that family and friends might have seen this representation of a face, meant to be hers, and not recognized her in it at all. After all, most families I'd met spent at least some time looking at Doe forensic reconstructions, even if they believed, or wanted to believe, their missing family member was alive.

Burge and I watched as Amy gently wrapped up Ina Jane Doe's skull and placed it back in the box. Kyana was tasked with carrying the evidence container to the car, and she held the corners of the thirty-year-old evidence box like it contained sweating dynamite. I could tell she wanted gloves. She was already a good scientist.

Everyone began to shift around in that "we're going to get going" way. I looked back up at those notebooks along the top of the ceiling, sitting in their rows. Besides the Dardeen case, there were at least a few other clusters.

I couldn't help but ask, "Do you have any other unidentified cases in the county?"

Burge was leaning against a desk, with one arm resting comfortably on top of the other. "There's two. A baby case. No body on that one. We do have an item of clothing that could be tested."

No body meant no skeletal reanalysis for Amy.

"And then there's the 1995 John Doe. Found him out in the woods in a sleeping bag."

Amy's eyebrows raised just a fraction. She was interested. "Is the decedent in NamUs? I don't remember that case."

The detective captain didn't think so.

So, it was unlikely anyone else even knew the case existed. Which meant that none of the people who spent time online looking for cases to match to missing persons would be including this decedent's profile.

I went for it.

"Could I take a look at the file? See if it's something we could maybe work on, too?" After all, we wanted to work on other cases that were unlikely to be solved just as much as Ina's. This fit the bill.

"Sure." Burge smiled, just a fraction. "You can make a copy while you're copying the other one. But you're gonna need to go up there and get it down." His eyes drifted to the shelf, high up against the ceiling.

I can't say I was surprised. After all, he was set to retire in September. Unnecessary climbing was no longer in his job description.

———•———

Ina safely secured, we headed down I-57 South. Kyana and Audrey discussed some of the stranger billboards we passed—possibly religious, but definitely threatening, like *HE IS HERE*—and I balanced both large binders on my lap.

"I think I left footprints on the paperwork on that desk," I whispered to Amy. She was wearing those huge sunglasses again, so I couldn't see her eyes; just a reflection of asphalt and blurred green.

"They'll never know it was you," she murmured.

They definitely would.

Hopefully, the documents hadn't been important. Size ten Converse prints might be difficult to explain to a judge. Maybe they'd been cross-word puzzles.

Ina Jane Doe's file was at least four hundred pages long, maybe more. There was the original anthropologist's report, the one that had served as a basis for the journal article we'd read, plus a pathologist's report, detailed field notes, records of who'd been at the park, jotted notations of tips and leads, NCIC printouts, missing-persons reports . . . we'd be reading for a while. From a brief glance, it seemed like the second binder, for the 1995 Doe, was half as thick. I hadn't had the chance to go through it all between standing on desks and filling out the proper forms. The decedent—he didn't have an official designation, but I supposed the Jefferson County John Doe was our working name—had been discovered just a few years after Ina. Luckily for him, it seemed that, with more physical evidence to go on, the sheriff's office and state police had been able to get further with their investigation.

I spotted an entomologist's report on the insects discovered in the sleeping bag. Then I noticed papers that indicated the victim's skeleton was sent to the Smithsonian for analysis. I paused.

"What would it mean for a department to send remains to the Smithsonian?"

Amy considered as she shifted into the right lane. "In the 1990s? Serious effort, that's what. Access to some of the best anthropologists."

I was interested to see what else Jefferson County had attempted in its investigation into John Doe's case.

"You want to take a look?" I asked the back seat passengers. They did indeed. After a few minutes of flipping, Kyana pulled out a copy of the Wayne Fitzgerrell Park map from 1993, which was one of the first pages in her binder, and scanned it with her phone. Smart. We might not have another way to find the paths in the park.

We reached our destination in less than thirty minutes. Amy and I were both eager to visit the park for ourselves; it had been a stop we considered absolutely necessary. Amy wanted a look at the terrain. We were a far ways off from January, but it still gave her a sense of place, some context for the scene of recovery. I wanted a sense of place, too: trees, the curve of roads, how far the lake stretched off into the horizon.

We pulled up to a heavy-hewn sign that directed us onto an asphalt road. According to Google, Wayne Fitzgerrell State Park had become Wayne Fitzgerrell State Recreation Center sometime in the 1990s, apparently to emphasize the park's focus on hunting and sport. Though you couldn't tell from the park's entrance, the land stretched back far and wide, with peninsulas created by the shoreline on three sides. Hunters came for deer and waterfowl as far as I could tell from their official website, and though the resort and conference center were closed, campers were still welcome. There was plenty of room for tents and RVs. Even so, the park wasn't busy that day, even in midsummer—maybe because it was still in the middle of the pandemic, or simply because it was a weekday. We didn't see any other cars on the interior road.

We stopped outside the main office, but it was locked, and Amy wasn't able to get an answer when she called the number. Personally, it reminded me a little too much of my unhappy stint at a 1989 4-H day camp. It had that main-lodge look. Instead, we pulled into the empty parking lot nearby, where a splintered wooden frame stood. Plexiglass protected a yellowing map. We'd seen several maps online and had a copy of law enforcement's version, but this one was stylized to suit its primary purpose: marking a spot for those already familiar with the terrain.

"We need to figure out where the primitive campground is," Amy told us. Kyanna pulled out the copy of the law-enforcement map so we could compare, and we crowded around the scratched glass to examine the display. It was old—pre-name-change—but it laid out the basics: what seemed to be a hotel, called Rend Lake Resort. The wide expanses of water. Different spots for camping, and spots along the shoreline with names like Shady Rest, Scout Point, and the County Line Picnic Area. A bike trail. Roads that neatly dissected the land. We found the primitive camping area marked at the extreme northern corner of the map. The county line itself seemed to float, suspended, in Rend Lake.

I took a few quick pictures of the map on my phone, but our movement disturbed the yellowjackets, or hornets, or something angry and winged that took up residence in the nooks and crannies of the wood. They buzzed out and circled Amy's head.

"Let's just try to find it," Amy said.

Kyana and Audrey were already halfway back to the car.

On our first drive through the park, we spotted the resort. It looked like a cross between a haunted mansion and an abandoned asylum. I'd seen an old article online about its construction; at one point, it had been something like a conference center crossed with a hotel. But that had all been shut down. Years later, the resort was beginning to fall into itself, though we could see through the open doors and windows that the rooms weren't empty.

Amy had eased her foot entirely off the gas.

"I want to go there. I know we can't, but I'm coming back sometime." A childhood spent in the rural Midwest had made Amy a connoisseur of weird old structures she had no business entering. It was either that or jumping off or onto things, Amy had told me once before, and she'd already broken her tailbone—her coccyx—jumping off a train trestle over a swimming hole located near a decrepit barn.

We kept following the main road, trying to match the lines of the various maps to the gravel and asphalt paths we spotted. Little roads split off like arteries, heading toward areas that—if our calculations were correct—would take us to ponds and horse stables and some kind of boat dock.

We thought we'd dead end eventually, but instead we hit the highway on the other side of the park, right out on the county line. There was a small back entrance to the park there, at the edge of Rend Lake. It was nondescript; if you didn't know it was part of the park, you might think you were turning onto a rural road. That meant we'd missed the turn-off to the primitive campground, somehow; it had to be very near this exit onto the highway. Amy swung her RAV4 around in a theoretically legal U-turn across the median.

"This is right off the highway, huh?" I hit Voice Memo on my phone. Otherwise, I might forget. "If you came in this way, at night, I bet no one would see you."

"In January? Probably not, unless there was security." Amy turned back onto a little entry road.

If Ina's killer *had* come into the park through this back entrance, there wouldn't have been a long ride through the property to reach the place where she'd been found. I'd wondered about that circuitous journey. But a simple turn, then another? It made sense.

Within a few minutes, we found what we thought was primitive campground road. Kyana matched our various maps as best she could: The sheriff's version showed both the primitive camp and the county line picnic area in similar arrangements, areas, and peninsulas, so it seemed like we could end up at either.

But as we pulled up at the top of a road closed off to through traffic by a thick chain, it seemed right. There wasn't any signage. Right now, we were technically going to follow the implied . . . suggestion, let's call it, by not *driving* down it. A walk was a different matter. The chain only extended the breadth of the road, anyway. Plenty of gravel on either side.

We had no idea how far it would be, so Amy passed around a bottle of sunscreen—it was at least ninety degrees that day—and we all grabbed our phones so we could record anything of note. We proceeded to walk down around a curve, not quite sure what we'd find, or how long we'd have to walk. I wondered if we'd know where exactly she'd been found. It all looked the same: clean asphalt, strips of grass, trees set back from the road in clumps that thinned and thickened, underbrush tangling up at the roots. Any one of them could have been the spot I'd seen in the file, marked with a spray-painted X.

Amy fell into step beside me but was quiet until I finished muttering voice memos into my phone. She'd made the executive decision to change into flip-flops for the walk, because she'd had on heels for our office visit. Later, at the hotel, she'd find a tick had wedged itself in between her toes.

"What do you think?" she asked.

"I can't decide if they came here because they knew this place, or if they got on the highway and just kept driving. If it was a random stop. Before I thought it was more likely the park was a destination. But if they came in the back way? Maybe not." I could feel sweat dripping down the back of my shirt. So much for escaping the Georgia summer.

"Could have been trying to find an easy access point to the lake. You'd see it, driving up that side."

That was an excellent point. And the lake would have been a logical goal, wouldn't it?

Amy took pictures of the trees and bushes. As we walked, I tried to place myself in the photos I'd reviewed: Which side of the road had the officers been on? *My right? So maybe the passenger's side of a car, coming down the road. The driver's side, returning?*

Kyana and Audrey reached the peninsula first. Their backs were silhouetted against the bright sunlight as I rounded the corner and saw Rend Lake, and what I guessed was the campground. It was roughly as the 1993 police report described it—but the few details there had been written up by people familiar with the terrain, and who'd no doubt had reason to visit Wayne Fitzgerrell on numerous occasions. We didn't see hookups that would make it easy to park a camper or enjoy any kind of modern convenience, that much was certain. But there was grass and shade and a swath of shimmering, gorgeous lake, and a looping curve that would send a car back the way it came.

"Easy access to the water," Amy noted. Mosquitos materialized around us as Kyana and Audrey moved in closer to the shore. Amy smacked her left arm, and I jumped. A little red welt was already forming.

"Wouldn't take long to park here," she said, gesturing, "and make it to the lake."

"So why didn't he?" We didn't know that Ina's killer was a he, of course. But it was a habit. "All this water, and a state park full of places where he could have hidden human remains, places where she might not have been discovered. And he leaves her on the edge of the woods?"

We walked around the edge of the road, tracing the path a vehicle would make if it had swung around and headed back down. We struggled to reconcile the killer's apparently conflicting choices: going to the effort of scattering her remains but leaving her in what amounted to plain sight. The dismemberment could have been purely logistical, for transport. But if that were the only reason in Ina's case, her whole body might well have been left in the same place: Plenty of other killers had done similar things. From what I'd read in the archives, the search of the park had been thorough, and they hadn't found any other remains. The lake hadn't been dragged, though.

I wandered into the brush while Amy contemplated the road and fended off bugs. Some of the trees and ground looked familiar, but that could be said about a dozen other trees. What I could tell, though, was how visible the crime scene would have been. If I could see the forest floor so well in June? January would have been even more bare, especially without snow as it had been when the girls had been out on their own walk and discovered Ina.

The girls were never named in the media. I was glad their privacy had been protected. But I wondered where they were, nearly three decades later. Had they had someone to talk to? Or were they expected to keep going on, like normal, after what they'd seen? Ina Jane Doe was a woman who had, in the newspapers, been reduced to *the decapitated head*. And those girls had been the ones who found her.

Amy called out. I was ankle-deep in the brush by then. "Do you think he was interrupted?"

Click. Memo. "Interrupted or spooked? Maybe. Campers or security? Or paranoia. Maybe something on the lake. Headlights on the road. Could have been out of his car, or maybe he never got out. Maybe he came back down the road, and thought he had to get rid of her in a different way than he'd planned. Quickly."

If the plan had been to sink Ina into the lake, there was no sign of anything that could have weighed her down—not found at the crime scene, at least. No cooler filled with rocks, or trash bag tied to a cement block. But the lake wasn't necessarily the goal. Making assumptions based on limited information was a bad way to do research. It made for a pretty good Reddit thread, maybe. But ultimately, it didn't help a family or identify a victim.

Click. "For all we know, the plan could have been to leave her somewhere else in the park. Or maybe he did. Maybe he did have time to sink remains in the lake, and then he was frightened, and hadn't planned on disposing of her head here at all. Maybe he did that so he wouldn't be caught with human remains."

Amy waved Kyana and Audrey over from their place out on the shore. "So whether the trip to the park was planned or spontaneous, we think that, maybe, something went wrong."

I stepped back out onto the path, and Amy frowned. "I think you were standing in poison ivy. Hope you're not allergic."

I was very allergic. But I'd worry about that later.

Click. "We know that coming up that back way, a turn into the park might be spontaneous. Or it could be a deliberate plan to cross county lines—maybe after crossing a state line, or two, or four—and a location chosen to confuse authorities. Took them a little while to figure out jurisdiction. And dismemberment, that was purposeful. And no one recognized her description. She didn't match any local missing persons. So, he brought her here from . . . somewhere. What went wrong was her being found, or found so quickly. But everything else seems to have gone his way. No one IDed her." I didn't bother to stop recording. I was interested to hear what they'd say.

Amy looked over at Kyana and Audrey. "So we're thinking she could have been placed at the edge of the woods. But what do you think about her being thrown from a car?"

"Driver's side?" I asked. They walked the short distance back and forth from the edge of the wood to the road, considering.

"Could make sense. Was the car moving, do you think?" Kyana's ponytail was clinging to the back of her neck. The perspiration had set in on all of us by then.

"No clue. I don't know that we'd figure that out. Positioning, maybe? But maybe not."

Research was like that. For every one small detail you were able to uncover, you had to widen the possibilities. From the little of the file I'd had time to read in the car, it said that there had been debris caught in Ina's hair—fragments from the forest floor, winter dry and brittle. Her head had been lying sideways in the brush; the placement of her remains didn't feel deliberate. If she'd been physically placed there by the killer, the scene wasn't staged. As far as I knew, anyway. That didn't make it any less awful to consider.

"Do we need to look at anything else?" Audrey and Kyana were checking the two maps.

"I don't think so." I leaned down and scratched my right ankle, then my left.

"Dude. Stop touching them." Amy stood over me, reflecting my sweaty face back at me in her sunglasses. "You're going to get that poison ivy all over." To Kyana and Audrey, she answered, "I'm good if Laurah is. We have a lot of scanning to do tonight."

"I think so?" I straightened and brushed off my hands. That was one of the places the poison ivy would show up in a few days—in thin lines across my palms. "But let's take more pictures on the way out." We took dozens of shots of the road, and the turn-off, and we paid attention to how long it took to reach the main entrance.

It felt like forever. The back way, that seemed right.

———•———

Amy had booked us two rooms at a hotel in a neighboring city that had a large, humid pool and a weirdly expansive breakfast bar; it took up half the lobby.

"Who needs this many waffles?" I asked no one. There were at least ten waffle makers.

"Slumber parties," Amy said. "Went to a bunch of them when I was a kid in Illinois. Hotel parties, big pool, big breakfast, all the rage."

She bounded up a set of interior stairs with her sensible luggage, AKA two tote bags. Audrey and Kyana followed suit because they had their backpacks. I looked for an elevator for a few minutes but only found a Skee-Ball machine and some kind of broken VR-simulator tucked in a back corner.

By the time I'd finally given up and dragged my suitcase up the stairs, they were on their second trip. It was absolutely necessary to bring everything from Jefferson County into the hotel room; Amy was the steward of record for both Ina Jane Doe and the files. The idea of leaving human remains in a parking lot, overnight, was unthinkable. Amy would keep that evidence box firmly within her sight until she was back in her secure lab at UNH. Her students were seeing, in practice, what she taught them in class: They weren't scientists who studied bone to understand bone. They studied to understand people. And they needed to remember.

The room stank like chlorine—probably because it sat on an inner balcony overlooking the enormous indoor pool—but there were two beds, cable, a shower, and a coffee maker. I had stayed in much worse places; my friends had played in bands that went on very short, very inexpensive tours. I tossed my purse on the bed and let my suitcase roll to a stop by a burnt-orange window curtain. "I'm going to start scanning this file. You can shower first."

Amy was already digging for her toiletries. We both had the same, strangely cheerful floral travel bag and we both hated it. But it had come as a free bonus with a subscription box that, yes, we both subscribed to, and you have to get full use out of free bonuses, even if they are grandmotherly.

She paused in front of the ill-lit vanity mirror and frowned. "Why didn't you tell me my eyebrows looked like this?"

"Because you didn't tell me mine looked like *this*." There had been a lot of sweating.

I heard the shower come on as I sat cross-legged on the bed with the heavy binder. One of my students had taught me that the iPhone Notes app could be used as a scanner, and it had changed my research life;

everything was sent straight to a dedicated Google Drive folder, just like that. Gen Z: truly magical.

I wasn't planning on reading through everything in the binder until later; there was no way to get it all finished before we had to return them. I'd be reading the scans for days, in the car, on the plane, when I got back to Atlanta. But I kept track, in a general way, as I flipped: Incident reports. NCIC report. VICAP entry. License plates—people who'd been camping that week in 1993. Security logs. How many times drivers had been through the primitive campground. Missing-persons leads that had been checked. Rule-outs based on dentals. Tips: A woman calling about a classmate she hadn't seen in years. A man who hadn't heard from his daughter. Ruled out. Ruled out.

Then there were the pictures. I'd seen the first three of the crime scene in the car. But then there was a single photo of Ina Jane Doe, taken as she'd been found. Long red hair, caught up in the brush. Her features slack. Her eyes looked brown, or hazel. The pathologist hadn't wanted to make a definite ruling on that. All the news articles said she could have been out there, in the park, for a week or more. I didn't think so, though.

I had seen the dead, in police records and in person, at medical examiners' offices back in Atlanta. But I hadn't documented an autopsy before. Those photos came next. Scanning them felt invasive, though I knew we needed them; the anatomist and the forensic artist we planned on consulting would need to see as much as they could to advise and re-create. Amy might spot something important. But after those pages, five or six in a row, I needed a break.

Online, there are true-crime fans of a certain stripe—or maybe they would prefer a more serious term—who are hungry for crime scene footage. Autopsy photos. The argument generally is that these photos can help solve a crime, that someone, somewhere, might see something and make a connection that ends up being important. Maybe that's true in some cases. But I've always had a feeling there are plenty who just want to see the blood in the bedroom, the head at the lakeside, every bit of a victim splayed out and dissected.

I turned my attention to the evidence box, resting safely on a table in the middle of the room, and thought about the woman we had no real name for. The urge to apologize, for all the invasion, caught somewhere before words.

Amy came out of the bathroom wrapped in a towel long enough to be a nightgown. But when someone's five foot two, towels tend to have that effect.

"You get a lot done?" She opened a tub of eye cream and started dabbing.

"About half. I'm taking a break. The photos are hard to look at. But I noticed something. Her hair is a lot longer than the artists' pictures. Shoulder length, at least."

Amy combed back her own wet, dark hair with her fingers. "I'll take a look. I think there's going to be a lot for us to reassess. But why don't you let me scan for a while? Take a shower. Rest. Then we'll watch something stupid on TV."

I did, and we did. I thought I might have that dream again, of the woods, the one that I'd had all spring, but I didn't. We turned off the lights in that humid little room, and I just slept.

———•———

After returning the files, we drove back to Missouri, to the lab of Dr. Jen Bengtson. She was an old friend of Amy's; they'd met in graduate school in the mid-'00s and bonded over veganism and a distaste for being patronized by men in their field.

Jen was originally from North Dakota and, like a lot of Amy's friends, had a collection of tattoos across her arms and chest. She had long, dark hair and an easy manner with her students, who were in the lab that week helping her on a project. Her true passion was archaeology, but she was a talented biological anthropologist, which was a good thing for Southeast Missouri State University (or SEMO). Her skills were needed. There were a lot of cases for her to handle and not much money to go around.

Kyana and Audrey were set to work with Amy and Jen on the examination of unidentified decedents from a variety of cases that Jen had in her lab: legacy, historic, and forensic. Within those cases were a number of historic remains that had certainly been in a museum at one point or another but had somehow ended up in the possession of a family living in a rural area of the state. It was going to be Jen's job to determine, if she could, where these human remains should lie: Should the decedents be repatriated? What else could be discovered?

When they finished reviewing Jen's cases, they planned to take a first, careful look at Ina Jane Doe in Jen's lab—not the formal analysis, but Amy wanted Jen's feedback. That's how she worked with her friends. The more eyes on any case, the better.

I was eager to learn as much as we could about Ina Jane Doe. The more detail we had, or thought we could guess at, the better we'd be at telling a story of who she might have been—a story that hopefully her family would recognize. But I had other things to take care of first.

While Amy and Jen and Kyana and Audrey set to work in the bone room, I walked the mile or so across the SEMO campus and into town, where I found a little drugstore. I bought every kind of poison-ivy treatment they had. Welts had risen up across my ankles and palms and, unbelievably, in a ring near my navel like some late-nineties piercing gone south. When I came back to the lab and began the slow work of ivy-scrubbing myself down in the faculty bathroom, I could hear faint echoes of bone talk up the hall.

" . . . it's fractured."

"This way, you see it?"

"Went clear through."

I turned on the sink, and their voices disappeared under the uneven stream of water. It would take a long time to clean up this mess.

CHAPTER SIX

THE METHOD: SKELETAL ANALYSIS

When I first started covering unidentified-persons cases, I thought that skeletal analysis was pretty simple: Age. Ancestry. Sex. Estimated height. Maybe a rough estimate of the PMI, or postmortem interval. I thought I could memorize some set of rules and then I'd understand how humans are identified via skeletal analysis.

But what I've learned in the years since I started doing this is that *every single part* of what is studied in forensic anthropology is always being examined, and reassessed, and debated.

Humans are as variable and complex in life and personality as they are in death and hard tissue. The accuracy of what is known, and what it is based on, and what can help or hurt an identification, is not cut-and-dried. Though the study of bones is one of the oldest forensic sciences, it is ever evolving: The more we learn about ancestry, sex, gender, and human development, the less we can rely on broad, sweeping standards. And there is an ongoing discussion of how much detail should be included in the biological profile—that's traditionally sex, age, ancestry (translated to "race" in many reports), and stature, and how that information could better be presented to law enforcement and other members of the medicolegal community to help resolve cases.

I'm certainly not here to teach you everything there is to know about forensic anthropology; I don't have enough degrees, and the ones I do have are in regrettably unhelpful subjects. But what I've begun to understand through my time spent following cases, and most especially working on the identification of Ina Jane Doe, has been enlightening, and fascinating, and helped me recognize how much identity plays a role in reidentification after death.

———•———

When it comes to the analysis of bones, much of the work of an anthropologist lies in comparing skeletal remains with different sources of knowledge: namely, what they understand about human anatomy and the skeletal system and can visually assess from the remains in front of them, and their knowledge of the data that has been gathered from museum collections and studies of other samplings of human remains.

There have been recorded measurement sets meant to help anthropologists separate decedents' remains by ancestry/"race" and sex since the 1920s.[1] If you have read a book or two about forensic anthropology, or maybe watched a few too many procedurals, you might have heard FORDISC mentioned; it's an acronym for Computerized Forensic Discriminant Functions. FORDISC is software that was first developed in the early 1990s and is one of the primary tools used by most forensic anthropologists today when determining a decedent's ancestry or sex. The program "uses discriminant functions to construct a classification matrix and assign group membership of the unknown cranium into one of the selected reference groups."[2] There are other measurement and grading systems developed by anthropologists, based on the study of collections of human remains, that are used during skeletal analysis—for instance, a list of features that help an anthropologist assess a pelvis based on morphoscopic features and use that information as one aspect of assessing the deceased's presumed sex.

A forensic anthropologist also examines remains for trauma and issues or disease in bone, and looks for recognizable features that can help identify a specific individual. In a skeletal case, forensic anthropologists can offer opinions on PMI; this can be estimated based on several factors, including the external appearance and internal state of the bones examined in the lab (for instance, looking at physical changes like the presence or absence of ligaments and fats), examining environmental effects and weathering, using context clues, and performing various chemical tests.[3] In some cases, those tests will need to be done with an outside lab, like the radiocarbon dating we talked about earlier.

When a forensic anthropologist analyzes human remains, they prepare a narrative lab report that summarizes the results of the entire exam. There is no single required format, but there are fundamental parameters that are observed; information on sex, ancestry/race, stature, and age is included, and the methods by which an analysis is made are noted.

We know that forensic anthropologists are tasked with studying bones and—basically—scoring them against known specimens and established norms to determine characteristics of a decedent, which can then be turned into a descriptive profile. But it's not as simple as matching up a skeletal feature to a perfect set of predetermined features and solving the puzzle. Even with a victim like Ina Jane Doe, who was found so soon after her murder, with so many "known" factors—skin color, hair color, indicators to gender identity—still present, there were many aspects of a full examination that couldn't be completed.

Ina Jane Doe's skeletal-analysis report, from 1993, is roughly two-and-a-half pages long. If Ina's killer hadn't worked so hard to obscure her identity, the report would almost certainly have been longer. But with only her skull and several vertebrae to examine, the anthropologist's observations were forcibly limited. There's a note at the beginning that "dental pathology and restoration"—something an anthropologist might discuss—"is not included" because a forensic odontologist was consulted and offered a separate report. Ultimately, Ina's report, written in narrative paragraph form, is broken down into six sections: *Sex*; *Race*; *Age*; *Stature*; *Pathologies and Individual Characteristics*; *Summaries and Conclusions*.

I've seen some older reports that include separate headings for *trauma*, *manner of death*, *time since death*, and other details; those are usually the purview of a medical examiner, who is trained to investigate cause of death. Perhaps those forensic anthropologists were asked to provide

additional information or were more involved in the original investigation than would be usual, or in an area where no medical examiner
operated. Each case is unique. In Ina's case, her remains were sent to the
forensic anthropologist for examination. But in other cases, an expert
might go out into the field with authorities.

For instance, in Georgia, the Georgia Bureau of Investigation (GBI)
called in a forensic anthropologist to help them with the recovery of a
skeletonized decedent in Twiggs County, Georgia. I got that file when we
covered the unidentified victim for *The Fall Line*. The presumed male
was discovered in 2003, in a culvert off a highway in Middle Georgia, when an armed forces fuel truck crashed. Apparently, a forensic
anthropologist arrived within hours to oversee the initial grid-search.
Although the case also went to the GBI's medical examiner, the anthropologist in question was able to provide a very thorough skeletal analysis,
including a long narrative introduction to the case. After all, he'd been
there from the start. He was able to offer the kind of detail that would
normally be contained in an incident report.[4]

Thankfully, nearly all the decedent's bones and clothing were recovered, too. Such a full examination would allow the anthropologist to
better estimate almost all the main characteristics, including age, and
stature, and possible trauma. But that doesn't mean that every answer was
simply at the expert's fingertips. For instance, between the medical examiner, the original forensic anthropologist, and a reexamination by another
anthropologist, the Twiggs County John Doe's ancestry estimation has
been updated several times.

What that means, on a practical level, is that he has been described
at various points as someone who might have appeared, in life, as His-
panic/Latino, biracial (Black and white), or white. That's not as unusual
as it may seem; improving, updating, or even eliminating estimations of
ancestry are ongoing conversations in the field.

And the remaining evidence? This may seem unrelated to anthropology, but it can actually be vital. The contextual details on items or clothing can help an anthropologist in a number of ways. The label and tags in
the Twiggs County John Doe's case were traced to a small chain of stores

only present in a few states; based on a conversation with the manufacturer, law enforcement narrowed down the possibilities to several shops in Florida. The closest was a Mr. Rags store in Pembroke, about six hundred miles from where the decedent's remains were recovered. The labels indicated everything he wore had been purchased in the United States, but in other cases I've worked on, clothing has helped place a victim's country of origin, or at least last residence, outside the United States.

It's something that forensic anthropologists Drs. Erin H. Kimmerle, Anthony Falsetti, and Ann H. Ross discuss as particularly vital in long-range unidentified-persons cases: contextual evidence that can place a victim who may have been a migrant, or unhoused, or otherwise distanced from their home of origin. Simply studying the deceased's bones only tells one so much—but with "contextual identification" methods, every aspect of an anthropologist's training comes into play.[5] When I spoke with Dr. Falsetti, he explained that even seeing the type of grave or burial site a decedent is found in can help an anthropologist better understand their context.

In some ways, Ina Jane Doe's analysis was straightforward, and in others, it was hampered by the circumstances of her murder and the scattering of her remains. Some aspects of the anthropological exam seemed straightforward to approach. But there was so much the experts were prevented from knowing, for sure.

When Ina Jane Doe was originally discovered, the coroner and law-enforcement officials estimated that she was "about thirty years old" at her time of death.[6] However, when the original forensic anthropologist on the case, Dr. Linda Klepinger, published a paper on Ina Jane Doe's skeletal analysis, she described her approximate age as follows: "The postmortem visual inspection of the face suggested an age span between the late twenties and late thirties." Facial features offer a suggestion, even after decomposition, but lifestyle and a number of other factors (skin slackening after dismemberment being one) can affect a visual estimate as well. Klepinger wrote in her report, "Because of the necessary reliance on cranial suture closure, osteological criteria for age assessment proved to be frustratingly imprecise, but suggested an approximate range of 30 to 50." So, Ina's age could not be narrowed down any more precisely based on her bones, and the range remained fairly wide.

That phrase "necessary reliance on cranial suture closure" is important because cranial sutures are not the best way to determine a middle adult's age. Amy explained to me that sutures can only give a general impression of age—young, old, or middle. Not that helpful when you're trying to narrow things down. We don't think much about cranial sutures after babyhood, when we know to be careful of a child's "soft spot"; the truth is, the bones of our craniums keep fusing for quite a while. There are bones that begin and finish fusing from early adulthood into middle age. It's not an exact timeline; for instance, one person's sagittal suture might begin fusing at eighteen and another's at twenty-one. But there are clear ranges that can help an anthropologist estimate a decedent's age at death.[7] In an older individual, sutures can look like faint, snaky etching across the surface bone while in younger adults, they look more like cracks in china. In general, an individual's sutures have closed by the time they reach between thirty and fifty years old. And the fainter, or "more obliterated," the suture lines, the older the individual. But that's not a universal truth. Some studies, for example, have shown clear sutures in individuals well into their eighties.[8]

For a forensic anthropologist, the ability to analyze a range of bones from a decedent, especially the ribs and pubic bones, combined with their ability to analyze bone matter on a microscopic level, will provide a better age estimation than cranial sutures alone. But with Ina Jane Doe, those chances were gone. In the skeletal analysis included in the sheriff's files, Dr. Klepinger's overall estimation—which she notes, again, is "notoriously imprecise"—is that Ina was over thirty years old when she died, and likely between thirty-five and forty-five based on suture closure and obliteration.

There's another detail in the report that seemed important to me. Though she left the full dental report to the forensic odontologist,

Dr. Klepinger took care to mention that the wear on Ina's teeth was "slight," suggesting a younger possible age than her skull sutures might otherwise indicate. That seems to correlate with what the pathologist, who performed Ina's autopsy, mentioned in his report; he said that, visually, she appeared to be "in her late 20s to early 30s."

Juvenile age estimation is more precise. For years, I followed the case of a child Doe in Dekalb County, Georgia—that's a metro Atlanta county—who was found in 1999. We covered his case on *The Fall Line* back in 2018, and we visited the Dekalb Medical Examiner's Office to go through his file or, rather, the *boxes* devoted to his case; the staff there had devoted hundreds of hours to the child they called "Dennis Doe." He'd been discovered in a local cemetery, laid out in the woods in a pair of new Timberland boots that were traced to a local Atlanta shoe store; they were double-knotted so they'd stay tied. He was seemingly well-cared-for, in neat, new clothing, and was well-nourished, and with no clear cause of death, though his autopsy did find evidence of cold medicine in his system.[9] He wore the same size shoes as my son. I was haunted by the thought of those little boots sitting in the cemetery for months.

Ultimately, "Dennis Doe" was estimated to be five to seven years old at the time of his death, which is a much narrower range than we'd see in adults. But a child's age is easier to estimate with accuracy; they grow at predictable rates, with teeth and other bones following known patterns of eruption and ossification. Sex and ancestry, on the other hand, can be much more difficult to assess.[10]

The Dekalb medical examiner announced in summer 2022 that they'd finally gotten a tip that led to the identity of Dennis Doe, twenty-three years after his body was discovered. His name was William DaShawn Hamilton, and he'd been six years old when he died. That put him directly in the age range set by the medical examiner and anthropologist who consulted on the case.

Though the cause of his death was never determined by authorities via their initial examination, his mother Teresa Ann Bailey Black's indictment "alleges that she caused her son's death by giving him 'a substance or substances containing Diphenhydramine and Acetaminophen' and by striking him in the head with an unknown object."[11] She was living in Arizona when authorities were contacted by a woman who'd known William and Teresa in the late 1990s and recognized the forensic art NCMEC released and circulated. This friend reported that Teresa and William had moved to metro Atlanta from Charlotte, North Carolina, in 1998, but Teresa had returned to North Carolina without him in 1999. No missing-persons report was ever filed.[12] While DNA testing confirmed the relationship, it was the forensic art that first led to William's identification. And though ancestry can be imprecise in children, NCMEC was able to capture his likeness and present him as the child that the family friend recognized: a six-year-old child who'd waited more than two decades to be named.

We all assess other adults' heights, and mostly based on our own. *Is this person shorter than me? Then they're short.* What is tall, or short, really? There are averages, of course, and we all know them, but accurately guessing a living person's height is harder than you might think. We tend to overestimate our own height, and probably always have . . . even before the advent of dating apps. Proportions make it even trickier; if you are particularly slender, you might look a little taller than you are. Maybe you have a short torso and long legs, or the opposite. And as for kids, well . . . are they three feet, four feet? Tall enough for the roller coaster at Six Flags?

I was asked for my son's height on a school form a few months ago, so we measured him when we got home, with my husband's big metal tape measure from his shop. My initial estimate, just from looking at him every day, was off by three-and-a-half inches. And even self-reported data can be inaccurate. When's the last time you got measured?

And we all have our own individual builds, too. My grandmother on my mother's side was a seamstress; in the 1990s, when so-called baby-doll dresses were a necessary fashion item and I was tall enough that the off-the-rack options were shirt length, she altered some longer dresses to fill the role. Not the most riot grrl thing ever, but thrift stores weren't kind to tall, chubby kids going for a goth-meets-Kathleen-Hanna look. One day she informed me, nonchalantly, with her mouth full of those extra-stabby little pins, that I had "low knees." It was something I had not yet been self-conscious of as I had no idea what that meant, but from about 1995 on, I was haunted by the concept of weirdly misplaced kneecaps ruining my whole leg aesthetic.

When I first started working with Amy, she told me that this actually translated to "unusually long femurs"—so basically, the majority of my height comes from the bones of my thighs, above the kneecaps. My calves are just chilling out, at an average length, probably wondering why the rest of my body has never been able to squat down properly without tipping over. If you're only looking at my femur, you're imagining someone who is six foot four.

Sure, bones can tell stories, but those stories are sometimes incomplete.

With complete or nearly complete skeletal remains, stature is fairly easy to estimate, within an inch or two; if experts are provided only a few bones, those estimates may become skewed or inexact. Forensic anthropologists can make the most accurate estimations from examination of the "long bones" of the legs, which generally make up around half our height. Barring those remains, the long bones of arms are also helpful in height estimation.[13] If there are no long bones of the arms or legs, stature is consequently more difficult to calculate. Human variation means that a single puzzle piece won't necessarily reflect the whole.

And what if there is only a skull, or cranium, like in the case of Ina Jane Doe, accompanied by several vertebrae? In Dr. Klepinger's 1993 skeletal analysis, she noted that "there are no satisfactory means of estimating stature from these remains." Besides the fact that Ina Jane Doe didn't have a large skull, which could correlate with a higher overall height—but wouldn't necessarily indicate that reality—there was nothing else for the forensic anthropologist to go on. Since then, there have been further studies using cranial measurements as an indicator for stature. Though combining ancestry information and age was able to create somewhat accurate range estimates,[14] experts hesitate to use those results in forensic cases. Some may offer a height estimate, but most, like Dr. Klepinger, are likely to offer the opinion that stature is not estimable.

It's also difficult to estimate weight during life based on skeletal remains. If clothing is found with a decedent, those sizes can give some insight, but even then we're operating on the assumption that the living person was wearing items that actually fit. There are a variety of reasons someone might have on apparel that is either over- or undersized. If there is no contextual evidence, forensic artists treat weight as they do age: They shoot for the middle range. That's what they did for Ina, in both cases.

———◦———

When Ina Doe was found, she was presumed to be a white female; her PMI was perhaps a few days to a week. There was never any real question as to her racial categorization by the investigators on the scene, the coroner, or the pathologist. When Dr. Klepinger performed the anthropological exam, she followed the standard procedures of a 1990s-era skeletal analysis for describing race or, more properly, ancestry/"population affinity"; she compared several features of Ina's skull and offered an educated opinion. Dr. Klepinger noted the features of Ina's teeth in regard to ancestry; she mentioned some "shoveling" of the incisors—roughly explained, that's a scoop shape, with the "scoop" facing the lingual side, or the tongue. This feature is less common in European and African population-affinity groups than in Native and Asian. Even so, that's a single characteristic; Dr. Klepinger notes other morphological traits that are consistent with European ancestry, and at least one that is consistent with African ancestry.

Depending on who is writing it and when it was written, a forensic anthropologist might reference a number of different measurements of the cranium and mandible, descriptions of a decedent's teeth, and of other features, and list their appearance or size as belonging to a range assigned to one of three or four major ancestry groups (depending on how old the report is): White/European, Asian, Native American, or Black/African.

The study of skeletally recognizable features—characterized by population affinity groups—became a focus of anthropology in the early

twentieth century when major studies of museum collections were under-
taken. Since then, further studies and data sets have been offered up, each
attempting to refine and improve the classification of human remains.
Forensic anthropologists talk about "discriminant function analysis
(DFA),"[15] which is "a statistical method of incorporating observations into
a mathematical formula to evaluate biological aspects of unknown individuals." There are manual systems of DFA, and, since 1993, the FORD-
ISC (Forensic Discriminant) computer program created at the University
of Tennessee.[16]

The idea is that by observing a number of skeletal features—i.e., counting them—and comparing how many of each category one has, one
arrives at their ancestry answer. It's not as simple as 1-2-3, but Dr. Jesse
Goliath of Mississippi State University described the classic method to
me this way: "The old way of doing it is you take the list of traits, and then
you put the group that are typically assigned to that trait. So, I have all
the skeletal traits. I see, let's say, narrow nasal aperture: European. Prominent jawline or cheeks and face: Asian. Black. And then you just keep
going down, and you literally are counting which group traits are most
represented."

When a forensic anthropologist inputs the data they've gathered into
FORDISC, like the measurements taken from a cranium, they should
receive sex and ancestry information that will help in their determination. That's an advantage, because some older methods depended on
having all the skeletal remains of a victim present to be able to make a
determination, and in many cold cases, that's not possible.

However, there are only so many people from any given ancestral and
ethnic group included in the FORDISC database; for instance, there are
a comparatively large number of European-ancestry decedents' data
included. Conversely, relatively few Asian and Pacific Islander decedents
have been entered, with those decedents not representing the expanse of
people who might be classified under such broad categories. How accurate and broadly applicable those results are continues to be discussed—
based on diversity of population, self-identification, multiple ancestries in
a single decedent, and more.

Some argue that FORDISC, though it is limited, is still the best standard; others insist that its limitations in regard to the actual variation and diversity of our actual population mean we should be looking for, or developing, a better alternative. It's been pointed out to me that FORDISC predominantly reflects just one method—metric—of doing ancestry estimation. The use of morphoscopic features in ancestry estimation is common as well; that involves studying traits "that are scored by their presence, development, or absence."[17]

After we discussed the Twiggs County John Doe on *The Fall Line*, and how his ancestry estimation had been updated numerous times, it stirred something in our listeners. They were especially interested to learn that the GBI had decided to release different versions of the forensic reconstruction in his case, to match the different estimations.

Before the Twiggs County John Doe case, I hadn't thought much about the inherent limitations of the process by which ancestry is estimated from skeletal remains. Mostly, I'd taken the police reports or NamUs listings at face value: Black female. White female. Sometimes a person might be listed several ways: White/Hispanic, or the "Other" that popped up in occasional reports. My understanding then was that each kind of listing depended a lot on who filled out a report, since forensic anthropologists weren't always involved. Sometimes the template itself was limited, and there weren't the categories available to express a decedent's possible ancestry. Occasionally, there would be a note: *Possibly biracial. Possibly Native American. White or Hispanic. Race Unknown.*

That's reflective of some of the conversations happening in forensic anthropology right now. Certainly, scientists are able to estimate ancestry from skeletal analysis, and they are good at analyzing bones; after all, they are experts. But some forensic anthropologists are now asking: Should ancestry be included in the biological profile at all? Amy explained the central issue to me this way in an email:

> Do our methods reflect the diversity of human variation? Do our databases reflect the diversity of modern human populations? Are our methods outdated and typological, doing nothing more than providing general

impressions of "race" that don't mirror the cultural complexity of human racial identity that is absolutely critical to how people perceive themselves and each other? There are underlying patterns in the skeletal midface and teeth that map onto ancestry groups, but can we ever truly account for the diversity of a person using skeletal methods? And if not—how can missing persons and unidentified decedents be connected? Are we losing an important factor in possible identification?

Since the mid-twentieth century, experts in various fields have discussed the idea that *race* is a social construct. Looking at the census and how the notion of race changes over, say, two hundred years can give us some idea of that; categories shift, change, are added, and taken away. Identity is an incredibly important concept, shaped by culture, family, society, place: how we are perceived and how we perceive ourselves. How one racially identified in life can also be tied into ethnicity, religion, history, and so many other factors beyond ancestry, and yet that nuance is not necessarily carried over into death. So, how does that affect our likelihood of being identified? With such a diverse population, are we so easy to sort into a few categories?

There are two broad arguments regarding ancestry in twenty-first-century forensic anthropology: those who believe that ancestry (population affinity) is not a vital aspect of the biological profile, and those who believe it is. The first camp may hold a variety of views for dropping ancestry from the biological profile, including inexact estimations, systemic racism in case handling, and/or widening the pool of potential matches for a given decedent. The second camp isn't necessarily in disagreement that there are issues with estimation practices, but they argue that ancestry can be—at least for most decedents—reasonably ascertained, and it remains a key factor to identification.

Then, of course, there are scientists who fall somewhere in the middle and hold the view that population affinity can be difficult to assess in an increasingly diverse society of individuals with multiple ancestries, and is not universally useful. But they point out that law enforcement and those working on cases need or expect ancestry/race information to work on cold cases, so they will continue to provide it. And as someone who writes about cases, I've always included that information when it's provided—which it always is.

I certainly don't have the authority to say whether or not ancestry should be omitted from skeletal analysis. But I can report that a growing number of forensic anthropologists are discussing how *useful* that information is—not only in terms of how cases are handled, but in regard to solve rates. And the best way to close the highest number of cold cases? If there's a conversation happening on that topic, I want to hear it.

Amy recommended I watch a webinar called "Blinded by the White: Forensic Anthropology and Ancestry Estimation," on YouTube, and I found the presentations fascinating. Some discussion topics that particularly interested me were touched on in the talks given by Drs. Phoebe R. Stubblefield (University of Florida), Jesse Goliath (Mississippi State University), and Meghan-Tomasita Cosgriff-Hernandez (Defense POW/MIA Accounting Agency). The first was a concern that structural racism will affect cases as ancestry estimates are made: if "missing white woman syndrome" and the centering of white cases is a phenomenon in life, then it makes sense it would carry over into death.

Another question forced me to reflect on my own research: Do we unnecessarily narrow a potential pool of matches by offering an ancestry estimation? How much do we assume about a decedent based on our preconceived notions, and how much, as researchers and scientists, do we learn about the areas where we work? Do we have a strong sense of who actually lives in any given place, and the nuances of how they may identify?

To learn more about this, I interviewed Dr. Jesse Goliath. He started where he begins with his students at Mississippi State: by explaining that it's difficult to turn any human population into a series of neat boxes based on distinct and separate features that can be set aside for ancestry groups. He told me,

In variation, there's a normal distribution. When you look at skin color, there's a normal distribution. When you look at height, a normal distribution. So, all those features, skin color, hair texture, eye color, all of those are not necessarily found in one group of people. It's a variation across landscapes, altitudes, or elevation. For example, I like to use the population in the Solomon Islands, where those individuals have dark skin, but they have blonde hair and sometimes blue eyes. You see Samoan peoples, Polynesian people who look African, who clearly are nowhere near the continent of Africa. [. . .] So, you can't say, all these features are European. All these features are African. All these features are Asian.

Another forensic anthropologist might respond to Dr. Goliath that, while variance certainly exists, experts have been able to estimate ancestry with a good degree of success for over a century. He pointed out to me, though, that the language we use to express and utilize that information across systems isn't consistent, which creates layers of confusion. Racial groups may be listed differently or even left out altogether. The term *Hispanic* is often used as an example in these conversations, because racially speaking . . . what does it mean? Ancestrally, a person classified as Hispanic might be of European, Native American, and/or African heritage, in combination or separately, and could identify in any number of ways. For instance, if three decedents are from the Dominican Republic, their skeletal remains might very well show the variety of that country's ancestral roots.

How would an anthropologist classify these victims? Would their friends and family recognize the descriptions if they were listed as White/Hispanic/Other, or Black/Biracial, or Native American? Dr. Goliath told me that the category "Hispanic" (or "Latino") doesn't exist in some systems at all; sometimes, he's left with "two or more races" as an option. How will someone reading that information translate it and use it? Will they look at their missing-persons report of a Mexican American male and think, *two or more races*?

Dr. Goliath also explained why, in his view, FORDISC is not the be-all, end-all of forensic casework. Because the tool is so useful, it's become the standard for DFA, but he worries that it doesn't have the capacity to correctly identify the variety of decedents a forensic anthropologist will encounter. As he points out, we are one country "on this global earth." And even more directly, he thinks it will be less effective in some states than in others: "If FORDISC is a nationwide system, we should have enough of each of those groups to then be used as a nationwide system."

So, in Dr. Goliath's view, in a city like Atlanta, or New York, or Los Angeles, the data set would be less helpful because the information contained in FORDISC wouldn't reflect the diversity of the population present in the area. Even so, he acknowledged that "we forensic anthropologists use it across the nation and across the globe. And so that's one of the problems that, when we talk about ancestry and the methods we use . . . they're historically racist and categorical. We're using white as the standard always."

Dr. Goliath proposed one solution: namely, that ancestry doesn't have to be omitted from a skeletal analysis—but it can be detailed in such a way that law enforcement considers more possible matches for a decedent. If a forensic anthropologist is required to or wants to include ancestry estimates, they can do so with more nuance. As he told me, "I have colleagues in other Southern states who list European, but then describe all of the known populations that would or might fit into that European category. So, they put North African, Eastern, Western Europe, the Indian subcontinent [. . .] and so it's a way to, one, give them the result they want, but also let them know as anthropologists, you can't say this person is a white American. All of these features that you're seeing are indicative of all these other populations across the globe."

I spoke to two other anthropologists who said they were offering similar information in their analyses. Rather than simply writing "white" or "Black," these experts are describing more possibilities, noting ethnic groups prevalent in the state or region, and generally adding more description to capture variation. Maybe that will become the new norm as forensic anthropologists continue to address questions and deep-rooted issues in their discipline. Law enforcement won't—for now, at least—stop asking for the information, and many forensic anthropologists believe that it should still be offered. But perhaps, as Dr. Goliath suggests, there are practical ways to reframe what it can and should mean, and to increase the chances of solving cases.

———•———

Sex has been treated as an equally important aspect of identification. Indeed, sex has remained an essential aspect of the biological profile since the development of the discipline of forensic anthropology. In general, anthropologists most heavily weigh cranial and pelvic aspects when estimating a decedent's sex, though they certainly prefer to examine as many skeletal features as possible. Though there are features that are traditionally judged as principally belonging to cisgender men or cisgender women, cases like Julie Doe's show us that basic human variation, the effects of gender-affirming treatments and surgeries, or perhaps chromosomal diversity might affect an estimation as well.

When Ina Jane Doe was found with recognizable features, her sex estimation was not a primary concern. Of course, as with ancestry, how a person appears to others—whether in life or death—doesn't necessarily indicate their sex or gender identity. But in 1993, with few context clues to indicate otherwise, Ina was presumed female. Dr. Klepinger was unable to examine all the features a forensic anthropologist typically studies before making a sex estimation; the skull is only one aspect that is studied in that particular assessment. In the note concerning sex in the skeletal analysis contained in the police file, Dr. Klepinger is brief: "Morphological traits of the skull indicate it is probably female. Metric discriminant function analysis of the cranium (Giles & Elliot 1962) also indicates the cranium to be female." That mention of Giles and Elliot is a reference to a DFA system—remember discriminant function analysis from ancestry analysis?—that was developed by the two anthropologists. Giles and Elliot's system is based on eight cranial measurements that include items like cranial length.[18]

In a case like Ina Jane Doe's, many of the features one would ordinarily examine—like a pelvis—were unavailable. If she'd been found in a skeletal state versus a few days after death, there would have been limited aspects to examine, and her sex estimation would have taken up more room in the report. That's often the case for experts. But some-times they would only have a femur, or fragments of a rib cage, or maybe a skull (cranium and mandible) to work with. In the case of a skull, the size of the mastoid processes, found on either side behind the ear, tends to be larger in males. So is the nuchal crest—it's the place where our neck muscles attach to the back of the cranium. The chin region, called the mental eminence, is generally flatter and less pronounced in females, and their glabella—the spot between the eyebrows—is also generally flatter than in males. Supraorbital ridges—the fancy way of saying the upper area of the eye sockets—are generally judged to be rounder and smoother in females. Overall, the cranium is smaller in females, and the mandible, or jaw, is larger and squarer in males. The list goes on. But as with ancestry, humans *are* variations. Ambiguity exists, and the less available evidence—the fewer remains—the harder one's sex may be to judge. This is why we see a pattern among younger decedents, even for post-pubescent adolescents: The younger the person, the harder sex is to determine—even after the onset of puberty.

A clear example of this can be found in the case of Kerry Graham. Kerry, fifteen, and Francine Trimble, fourteen, disappeared in December 1978 from their hometown of Forestville, California. They were suppos-edly headed to a local mall. According to the *San Francisco Chronicle*, the teenagers' bones were discovered seven months later, buried off a highway, but an exam identified the bodies as a pair of possibly related adolescents, one male and one female. Obviously, that didn't match up with missing-persons reports for Kerry and Francine. Both a forensic anthropologist and a pathologist worked on the case, examining both sets of remains. Those estimations remained in place when the victims' bodies were exhumed in 2000 in hopes that DNA might identify the pair.[19] Unfortunately, they would remain unidentified until 2016 when DNA tests confirmed the remains as being those of Kerry and Francine. It turned out that a local dentist, Dr. Jim Wood, had examined the teens' remains after the 2000 exhumation and had advised that both victims were female and likely not related, but for whatever reason, his opinions were not included in an updated report.

Bob Lowery Jr., vice president of the missing-children division for NCMEC, spoke with the *Ukiah Daily Journal* about the case, noting that "girls' bodies typically resemble those of boys until they begin to mature," which he said could have been a possible influence in their misidentification.[20]

Even adult sex estimations can be difficult in their own right. Though many forensic anthropologists' cases will generally fall into the category of "presumed male" or "presumed female," that's not always the case. I attended a presentation at a forensic science conference where a Michigan State PhD student, Alex Goots, demonstrated this via a case study completed in the MSU Forensic Anthropology Lab (MSU-FAL). She walked us through the skeletal analysis of an unidentified person, pointing out how each aspect of the decedent's skull was measured, compared, and graded. And depending on the aspect, the decedent's results scored differently. Some results made them more classifiable as natal female, and some more classifiable as natal male. But many fall in the middle range, making their sex indeterminate. The final estimation was undetermined, and DNA testing was eventually done in the case.

The point of Goots's symposium presentation was not to teach us all how to "sex" a skeleton—a verb I did not know existed until I read an anthropology textbook—but to point out that sex (and by extension, gender) is also overdue for reexamination in forensic anthropology. The presentation was part of a larger symposium on trans, intersex, and gender-expansive decedents, and the role forensic anthropologists can—and perhaps should—play in their identification and the treatment these victims are given, and in leading the change in the language regarding gender and sex in official forms and databases. The symposium, "Queered Science: Interdisciplinary Approaches to Gender-Inclusive Research," was arranged by Amy and her friends and colleagues Dr. Mari Isa (Texas Tech University), Dr. Samantha Blatt (Idaho State University), and University of Nevada Las Vegas doctoral student Taylor Flaherty, and featured a number of papers presented by academics across the United States. Graduate students studying forensic anthropology and an investigative genetic genealogist, Anthony Redgrave from the Trans Doe Task Force, covered

issues like misidentification of trans individuals in reports and dehu-
manizing and inaccurate language used in databases, as well as suggestions on how context clues and stronger knowledge of gender-affirming
surgery can be implemented to better identify and thus serve trans and
gender-expansive decedent cases.

The symposium also looked at how anthropologists could better assess
skeletal cases. Flaherty even talked about gender-affirming care, like hormone treatments' effect on bone. But their point went further than that,
since many trans and gender-expansive individuals do not seek medi-
calized gender-affirming care, and even if they do, the signs of that care
aren't necessarily present on the skeleton. Flaherty's suggestion, which
they elaborated on in an interview with me after the conference, is a more
holistically inclusive approach—a reframing.

> Right now, when a forensic anthropologist writes a report, what typically
> happens is they either say that the decedent is male, female, or we don't
> know so they are classified as ambiguous. And my fear is that a lot of peo-
> ple who are trans or intersex will be lumped into that ambiguous category.
> And then those become cold cases that may not get solved for years upon
> years [. . .] We try to pick a box for sex and a box for ancestry, and so
> on. Every single thing has to be put into a checkmark box. And we need
> to recognize that it's okay that we can't always do that [. . .] When we
> start to come to terms with that, people will start to recognize that we can
> expand our language, expand our reporting styles, and expand our meth-
> ods, because it's okay. Humans are complex, and not everything is per-
> fectly tidy.

Flaherty's solution is multifold: more informed education regarding sex variation, including intersex conditions and gender identity in
anthropology classrooms; engagement with communities outside academia who are affected by exclusion; conversations with the medicolegal community regarding contextualization of casework; and more detail
in reports. That's the simplified version, anyway. Flaherty says their biggest interest is in a "biocultural profile" (versus a biological one)—a term

anthropologists use to indicate the combination of biological and cultural factors, in context. It's a term I've seen used in papers regarding the identification of migrant and refugee decedents, and it can be applied to sex and gender, too.

In regard to skeletal analysis reports, Flaherty explained, "I analyze the skeleton before I look at pretty much anything else. The coroner's office sends us a cover sheet [detailing] where the body was found and what they want analyzed. And from there, I don't look at the autopsy photos, at the scene photos, et cetera. I do the skeleton first and then I look at other things, because I don't want anything else to bias or influence my reports."

"Then that's when you can start bringing in the cultural things," Flaherty continued. "You may say, 'I estimated this person as a male using X method, but now I see that they were dressed in all female clothing. Maybe I'm going to have someone come do a blind analysis of this pelvis and tell me how they sexed them. Maybe I'm going to talk to the investigators and see if there are any other indicators that the person might have been trans.' Right? So, integrating the cultural part, but not letting it influence you in a biased way too much is important."

Flaherty also noted that in UNLV lab reports, "we use 'assigned sex at birth' instead of just 'sex estimation' because it pulls in the cultural and biological aspects of it, making it more all-encompassing." The lab takes care to avoid checkboxes when possible, and instead collects what they describe as "bench notes": notes that will give law enforcement and other officials context that may not typically fit into a report template. In Flaherty's practice, forensic anthropologists haven't done away with analyzation of the major markers of sex, like cranial features and pelvic features. They're simply expanding to include more context.

Overall, the idea of biocultural profiles for decedents of any identity, ancestry, or country of origin seems like a net-positive concept; after all, context clues have served as crucial details in many identifications. More information, more chances, right?

It seems like we keep coming back to context—the more, the better. Forensic anthropologists carefully review human remains for a number of factors outside the basic profile; they want to learn as much about the individual as they can, and part of our individuality is our trauma. That finger you broke in volleyball in junior high? Poor nutrition? Radiation treatment for a serious illness? Hormone replacement therapy? That time you hit your head on the car door? Maybe it did leave a mark. It's easy to imagine that a broken bone or a medical implant would be spotted during a forensic exam, but all kinds of experiences leave unique marks on our bones and teeth. With some medical history of a missing person to compare against a decedent's remains, a forensic anthropologist can make a tentative identification to be confirmed by dental records or DNA.

In many initial Doe exams, though, the examining expert doesn't have any comparative material. So, they're searching for any individual characteristics—possible clues, you might say—that could lead to identification. But when you are working with just the bones, you don't always know for sure what the effects of an old injury, or an asymmetry, or a seemingly arthritic joint would have had in life. Would the living person's gait have been affected by a slightly shorter leg, or did they wear corrective footwear? Or perhaps, would it not have any measurable effect at all? We all have some asymmetry of our features; would that asymmetry look more or less pronounced when our craniums are viewed?

In Ina Jane Doe's case, Dr. Klepinger was probably working without the context she would have liked: namely, a better understanding of how Ina's vertebrae connected to the rest of her skeletal system. One of the most major findings of Klepinger's report was that Ina may have had what Klepinger described as "torticollis," a condition more commonly known as *wry neck*; this is a skeletal issue that can be congenital or can occur after trauma, like a car accident. According to Dr. Klepinger's published paper on the subject, asymmetries in Ina's remaining vertebrae, skull—particularly at its base—and in her mandible, which seemed to indicate more stress on one side than the other (as if she chewed on one side or favored one side of her mouth), were consistent with other documented cases of torticollis found in other, now-identified decedents.

The asymmetry Dr. Klepinger mentioned was something she considered marked, though she could not comment on how that asymmetry would necessarily have presented in life.

It's important to note that Dr. Klepinger *did not* diagnose Ina Jane Doe with any condition. She simply reported her findings, and then drew a line to possible conclusions. Her observations are never stated as fact, but as areas that might be explored by investigators when seeking a match.

Dr. Klepinger had also noted a few other important skeletal characteristics of Ina Jane Doe. Ina's overall cranial vault was described as "remarkably thick, particularly in the area of the frontal bone," which could be a sign of hyperostosis frontalis interna (HFI), a "usually asymptomatic condition." However, Dr. Klepinger observed that other features normally associated with HFI were not present, and that she didn't see signs of other syndromes or diseases that might cause a thickening of the frontal bone. As Dr. Klepinger explained, many cases are asymptomatic, and those with HFI may never know they have it at all. Still, "the disorder may be found associated with a variety of conditions such as seizures, headaches, obesity, diabetes insipidus, excessive hair growth and sex gland disturbances."[21]

How helpful could this be in identification? A forensic anthropologist can't see the future; they can only observe and record. For instance, the presence of possible HFI would indicate the likelihood, though not certainty, that Ina Jane Doe would fall into the upper reaches of her estimated age range: closer to fifty than thirty.

If Ina Jane Doe's postcrania had been available, there would have been so much to examine in detail: further healed antemortem injuries, perimortem injuries, more signs that could possibly help rule in or rule out torticollis—all things a family might recognize. Particularities of a person's skeletal structure are often immediately familiar to those who knew them—but only if the information lands in the right place. Sometimes, it's hard for those of us involved in the case on the receiving end to believe a decedent hasn't been identified, because each and every one of their cases seem unique.

CHAPTER SEVEN

THE CASE: NEW HAMPSHIRE

September 2021—Georgia and New Hampshire

By September, my family was used to my haphazard travel schedule. I, on the other hand, hadn't settled into it nearly so well. I was on planes often enough—flying to interview experts, to meet with Amy, to drive to visit law-enforcement offices hours or states away—that I missed things. I spent a whole afternoon getting TSA Pre-Check clearance, which for some reason involved sitting in a tiny indoor tent at a local Staples and being fingerprinted by a very bored college student, so I could spend less time in security lines at Atlanta Hartsfield-Jackson. But that only saved so much time. I still left early in the morning, in a Lyft or Uber that bounced along I-85 and dropped me at the terminal, and came back to Atlanta late at night, arriving when the whole house was dark and quiet. And then I'd find, in the morning, that my son had gotten a haircut or grown half an inch. It happened in his sleep, I was sure.

I missed him, and I missed being there for important moments. He got his yellow belt at karate, and I wasn't there to clap when he got home from class. I didn't even know because I was in the air, reading the police files I'd downloaded and making notes for podcast scripts. The pictures didn't load until my plane touched down. It was all right; my husband and son had gotten used to carrying on without me. That was supposed to make me feel better. "He goes right to sleep," my husband said. "The dogs pile in there with us. Don't worry."

And yet here I was again, saddled with mom guilt and, thanks to Delta, a growing credit card bill. Before I knew it, it was time to head back to New Hampshire. I needed to be on Amy's home turf for a few reasons: It was time for Ina's formal skeletal reanalysis, and I had the chance to go with her to visit a dentist who'd be examining teeth and loaning equipment for a few of her cases. There was also a private school nearby whose faculty had, literally, stumbled upon a mummy in the attic. Amy was helping them sort that case out, and there was no way I was turning that down. Oh, and she'd volunteered me for a panel at the university. And a lecture in her class. That's the thing with professors; they will get maximum mileage out of your visit to campus. Her friend Dr. Samantha Blatt—Sam, to me—who taught at Idaho State, would be in town, too. She was particularly interested in histology and teeth, and she planned to help us with the various analyses. I wasn't of much use when it came to microscopes and measurements, although they did appreciate my ability to find just about anything in the digital archives and consistently remember my own Newspapers.com password.

I promised my son I'd bring him something from New Hampshire that did not come from the airport. Boston had been a little shaky, what with the lobster T-shirt emblazoned with things like BOSTON COMMON and HARVARD SQUARE. I should have known better than to assume a seven-year-old would appreciate regional humor. I'd do better this time around.

I prebooked an Uber for the morning and bought the bus ticket I needed to get me from the New England airport to Portsmouth, New Hampshire. The university was actually located in a town called Durham, and Amy lived in yet another adjoining town, but it seemed the state was small enough that everything was fifteen minutes away from the next location. What a convenient arrangement; if it wasn't for the weather, I might consider relocating.

Before I left, Amy and I had a Zoom meeting with the DNA lab that would be working on Ina Jane Doe's case. I'd hoped that Astrea Forensics in Santa Cruz would be interested in helping us, because I found them interesting. I'd met the founding CEO, Dr. Kelly Harkins Kincaid, when she was a guest on *The Fall Line*. She'd come on as a DNA expert to discuss the SNP profiles necessary for genetic genealogical testing, and I'd immediately liked her. She'd managed to do an entire interview with feedback in her headphones—so essentially her own voice had been echoing back at her. I'd had that happen to me before; I couldn't get a sentence out.

Like Amy, Kelly had a background in biological anthropology, but she was also trained in paleo-archaeology and the study of ancient DNA. That meant her lab used techniques developed for highly degraded samples—sometimes thousands of years old—and applied them in forensic cases. But that wasn't the only way her lab was unusual.

Many other labs used prepackaged DNA extraction kits. That meant that the chemical agents came premeasured, and there would be a set process followed in each extraction. Astrea, however, had a "boutique approach": they created their own extraction kits for each sample that came into the lab, based on what the material was, its age, and what methods they thought might achieve the best sample. This allowed for greater flexibility and a higher chance at success in extraction and sequencing.

On the downside, it wasn't cheap. No testing is, but the costs were higher for this lab because of their custom approach. Amy and I might have had trouble scraping the funds together to cover both that testing and the genetic genealogy, although we would have managed it somehow. But there had been a fortuitous event in Ina's case that played in our favor. When Jefferson County went through all their evidence in Ina's case, they pulled Ina Jane Doe's hair—all of it, perfectly preserved—from the cold storage evidence locker. Officials sent the evidence to Amy so she could prepare a sample.

With the arrival of Ina's hair, Amy qualified for a grant that Kelly from Astrea was involved in via a company called Arc Bio. That grant covered cases that involved both bone (or teeth, in this case) and hair.

Astrea planned to test new methods alongside their proven techniques, and Ina was to be included. I'd been worried about whether the
level of antemortem decay in Ina's teeth might affect the quality of her
sample, but Astrea's definite involvement made me much less nervous.
I would go visit Astrea in November, but first I had to make it to New
Hampshire.

"Madam? Your ride."

Amy pulled the car over to pick me up outside the bus station at
Portsmouth. She'd cut her hair shorter since the last time I'd seen her;
it suited her high cheekbones. I threw my bag in the hatch and crawled
over a beauty subscription box and a few accordion file folders that were
scattered across the back seat. Like my own, Amy's car was something
of a traveling office and closet. Academics come in two flavors: neat and
armed with expensive pens they special ordered, and well-meaning
human whirlwinds who accidentally got hair dye or coffee on student
papers and had to note *not blood* in the margins. Amy and I were firmly
in the latter camp.

Joining us on our adventure was Sam, who sat in the passenger seat of
Amy's RAV4. Her thick, light brown hair was braided into a long rope,
and she wore glasses and an anthropology lab T-shirt. Sam was around
Amy's age—late thirties—and they'd met when Amy was leaving Idaho
State University and Sam came in as her replacement. They had similar
research and reality-TV interests, but most important, they both liked
teeth. A lot. Writing about them and looking at them under microscopes
and cutting them with tools precisely and discussing what might be
learned about decedents based on things like "Wilson bands" and other
mystifying scientific terms I had to look up on my smartphone while they
talked. Well, I guess friendships have been built on less.

It was a cool, sunny day in September, the perfect autumn afternoon,
and only a little past one p.m. Amy suggested we head into downtown
Portsmouth for some food and shopping before we drove to her house

and began our real work. That was fine by me. I had a guilt present to buy. Sam was willing to go if there was a used bookstore to poke around, which there was.

Portsmouth was a port town, to state the obvious. Everything about it screamed seaside but not in the way in which I was familiar; my father's side of the family came from Myrtle Beach, South Carolina, where the beachfront and the tourist traps spread wide, and I didn't see any airbrush T-shirt stands in Portsmouth, or snow cones, or rickety Ferris wheels trailing streams of sand. Everything looked narrow and old and compact, like the villages I'd seen in England when I studied abroad. No pastel condos in sight.

We went into a gift shop that sold everything you could possibly want from the ocean, and plenty of things you might not: sculptures made of oyster shells, commemorative sailor's knots, and fridge magnets fashioned out of driftwood. Amy and Sam helped me find a present worthy of bringing home: a hefty shell that felt like pebbled asphalt on one side and shined like mother-of-pearl in the interior. It was the perfect size for the trinkets a seven-year-old accumulated: acorns, string, interesting coins, rocks, and Legos that had recently been stepped on.

The store was in a tiny cluster of businesses surrounding a monument and memorial park that Amy wanted to show us. Before we got lunch, we walked through the paths and statues dedicated to the Portsmouth African Burying Ground. The park sits atop a cemetery that exists underneath downtown Portsmouth. The town was, literally, built on top of it. The burial ground, which dates back to the 1700s, had originally been on the outskirts of town. But Portsmouth had sprawled out and, consequently, over the consecrated ground. The park had been created where there had formerly been nothing—just road. Now there was a plaza, a marker, and bronze statues. A curving stretch of paving in cast concrete that the organizers called the petition line was printed with the words of a petition, delivered in the eighteenth century by enslaved people who demanded freedom. When I pulled up the official website on my phone, I learned that the burial ground, which had been in use until the early 1800s, had been unearthed in 2003. Experts had discovered at least thirteen people interred underneath the street, but they suspected there were many more; eight of the deceased were exhumed for examination, which confirmed their African ancestry. The ceremonial burial cover, decorated with a West African Adinkra symbol, marked a specific place: the spot where the eight exhumed decedents were reinterred after examination.[1]

The memorial space was laid out like an exhibit, with every element deliberately positioned. As I walked from one end to the other, it became clear that the committee that created the memorial park didn't want the public to forget what its original purpose had been. No matter how beautiful the space was, it was a cemetery. It should be treated as such.

We were quiet on our walk back to the car. After lunch, Amy drove us to a grocery-store chain I'd never seen in the South—Market Basket—so I could pick up enough keto-friendly food to survive in her vegan household for a week. Sam was happy to eat whatever chickpea stir-fries or fruit and almond-milk smoothies came her way, but I was tired of surviving on protein bars that lived at the bottom of my purse. I bought some salad and a rotisserie turkey breast that would ensure my status as Lucy the Pug's best friend, and then we headed over to Amy's neat little house, tucked into a corner in a residential neighborhood. It was surrounded by a big garden that Amy had already put to bed for the winter. She'd be using every available inch of space for her Halloween decorations. Those, she told us, took up most of the storage in the old carriage-house-turned-garage behind her home. It would all go up October 1st and stay in place as long as possible. When I saw the pictures, later, on Instagram, I wondered if any trick-or-treaters were brave enough to make it to her front porch. Really, a forensic anthropologist shouldn't be allowed unlimited access to Styrofoam zombie heads.

After we'd spent the proper amount of time greeting Lucy, we gathered around the kitchen counter, where Amy set out an alarming array of pumpkin-themed products she'd bought on her last Trader Joe's run: cookies, nuts, a popcorn thing, pumpkin samosas that actually looked good, and some sort of dip. People really took things too far in autumn. I held the dog for protection while Amy and Sam happily spiced themselves silly. Lucy snorted softly into my armpit and sun filtered through the kitchen windows as Amy ate her problematic hummus and told us about the experts she'd been consulting on Ina's case.

First, there was a local anatomist and medical illustrator, Dr. Steffen Poltak. He'd come to Amy's lab to examine Ina's remains, and he offered valuable observations that had set her off on another research tear. He was particularly interested in an area of Ina Jane Doe's cranium called the sella turcica. Amy explained—to me and, I guess, the dog, as Sam was already perfectly aware—that *sella turcica* was Latin for "Turkish saddle." It's a dip, or depression, in the sphenoid bone of the cranium; the sphenoid sits in the middle-front of the cranium, and is sometimes called the wasp bone, for its winglike shape. At its top is the sella turcica, the bony saddle that houses the pituitary gland. That, at least, was a term I was familiar with; I knew it had to do with growth. I said as much, and Sam and Amy gazed at me like proud parents whose child had finally learned a word.

"Very good. Yes, it does," Amy encouraged me. "But it also regulates a lot of functions, like hormone production. Sexual hormones, organ function, all kinds of glands and systems. In most people, the sella turcica will be kind of roomy, right? Plenty of space for the pituitary. But something I noticed right away was that in Ina Jane Doe's case, the bone is thick, and comparatively boxed in. That doesn't leave much room. And then the clinoid processes—that's just the bone that surrounds the sella turcica—also formed an abnormal fusion. Even less space for the pituitary gland."

That's what Dr. Poltak had been interested in; that this minor abnormality could point toward possible roads of investigation that might aid in Ina's identification while simultaneously contextualizing some of her other skeletal features. It was nothing definite, certainly, but Ina's pituitary arrangement may have affected hormone or glandular systems in her body in life, and if so, her family would likely know. In fact, it might be genetic. If the investigative genetic genealogists we planned to hire were able to track down an extended family—say, twenty to forty people, then information about possible hormonal issues could be key.

A lot of ifs, I knew.

Amy dipped an orange cookie into some suspicious maple-colored tub of goo. "Tell Sam about what you noticed in the file on your flight. What you texted about."

We had an exhaustive Google Drive folder built up by that point, full of research on everyone and everything mentioned in the police records. There were missing persons who'd been ruled out based on dental records, then possible matches who'd been explored, but a trail had run cold, or information was too vague for the sheriff's office to track them down. Sometimes, the person in question had been found alive.

"You remember that stuff about the POI they looked at?" I started. "There was a weird report tucked in there. Just a call someone made about a truck stop bathroom." The POI—person of interest—in question had been looked at for Ina's death because he'd bragged, while in jail in Texas, of murdering and dismembering a woman. But there was no evidence in his truck. The knife he'd told a cellmate about? There were only traces of deer blood. Authorities couldn't find any connection, forensically or logistically, to Illinois. But tucked in between lab reports and interviews was the lone report.

On March 6, 1993, an employee at the Big Wheeler Truck Stop in Mount Vernon called in a tip. He went into the men's restroom and saw something peculiar written on the wall, in black marker. He said it probably appeared within the past twenty-four hours. It was written in columns, with dashes that seem intentionally placed in the graffiti.

I passed my phone to them. They both looked as confused as I had when I first read it:

Serial Killer

3/93—-—-—- -

19 and counting

5 men 8 black

12 women 8 white

2 children. 3 hispanic

-----—-—don't worry, I'll get to the others!

"Did they get any more information?" Amy handed back my phone.

"No. I guess that's hard to follow up on. Anyone can write anything they want on a bathroom wall, right?"

The Happy Face Killer certainly had. He was a truck driver and a serial killer who actually had bragged about his crimes, in writing, in a similar fashion. But I'd seen sinister things written on bathroom walls dozens of times in my life—KEVIN NOW YOU DIE being a memorable entry from back home in Atlanta—and to my knowledge, none of them had ever been tied to a crime. There wasn't anything Jefferson County could do with a single piece of evidence like this, except look for others like it and hope something showed up.

"And who was the person of interest?" Sam asked. Sometimes I forgot that everyone around me hadn't been reading the file, over and over again, for the last three months.

"So, there was a guy in Texas, around this same time. March of '93. Kind of eerily close, right? Well, he got arrested in . . . I want to say it was Ward County. And his cellmate lets the guards know pretty quickly that he's telling these wild stories, right? He says he was traveling up and down the East Coast and through the Midwest, producing and selling bathtub speed with his friend, and that along the way they met up with a young woman who ended up joining them. They commit robberies, all kinds of stuff. The suspect says at some point he gets paranoid that the young woman is going to report on their activities, so he kills her in a really awful way, with a hunting knife, and dismembers her body. He leaves different portions of her body in different places over a few miles in what I believe was a rural area in . . . I think Illinois, and then traveled to Georgia or Florida, where he killed a deer and used that blood to cover up the victim's blood on his weapon and clothing."

"What???"

"That's not all. There was a major Satanic ritual at what he called a 'hillbilly festival' and he said they killed all the dogs in the area as some kind of sacrifice."

Sam just blinked. I couldn't blame her.

"What . . . uhm . . . did law enforcement do?"

"I mean, they looked into it. Got his vehicle, which he'd sold, and sampled everything. Foam rubber, hair, all that. Got his belongings he was arrested with. There was a knife with deer blood, and clothes. No trace of human blood. Nothing from the car that matched Ina Jane Doe. He was arrested for petty theft, and he had meth on him, but I think that after they interviewed the guy who'd been in the car with him, they thought everything else was fabricated."

"By the suspect, or the cellmate?" Sam had totally forgotten about the orange cookie she'd abandoned in the dip. It was probably better that way.

"I couldn't tell from the reports. But they checked up on the guy in the town he'd come from, where law enforcement knew him, where he said he'd picked up the girl. No one was missing as far as they could say. When the guy finally sat down with his lawyer, he said he'd been joking when he said all that stuff to his cellmate. Then he changed the story to he'd never actually said any of it. Then he took the fifth. But there was no evidence. Seemed like something he made up. They must have tested thirty or forty things."

"Creepy story, though."

"I don't think the cellmate made it up. But the other guy? Yeah. Whether he was high or thought it would be impressive, I don't know. But he sure scared the shit out of the dude who reported him."

Lucy whined from her little nest on the couch, snuffling around in the blankets, and I leaned down to scratch her head. I'd definitely be sharing my turkey with her that week.

———·———

Amy made a late-day pot of coffee and we planned out the rest of the week. We'd be in the lab on Monday morning for Ina's skeletal analysis, and then we'd drive out that afternoon to Orange, Massachusetts, to visit our colleagues at Redgrave Research. Then, on Tuesday, I was guest lecturing on true-crime podcasting in Amy's cold-case class. That afternoon there was a true-crime podcast panel at the university, arranged by Amy and another professor; I'd be there, along with my friend Josh Hallmark—if there's a more knowledgeable expert on the serial killer Israel Keyes, I haven't met them—and crime writer and podcast critic Rebecca Lavoie. Wednesday? Wednesday was going to be educational. We had plans to visit a nearby dentist, who was helping with full X-rays of Ina's teeth, and with a few other cases in Amy's lab. And then there was the matter of the private school and the mummified human body they'd stumbled upon in their attic.

That was how I'd described the situation to my editor, anyway, but a more proper and technical phrase would be *anatomical mummy*. After teaching for more than a decade and reading just about everything I could about the stranger and darker corners of academia, I thought I'd encountered just about everything. But then Amy told me about what had been discovered at the Tilton School, a private college-prep school upstate. The school had called the medical examiner for the state of New Hampshire, who eventually tapped Amy for help. She explained that there were quite a few mummies in the world that had not been preserved during death rituals as part of cultural religious rites. Rather, they'd been created by amateurs, and even professional anatomists, eager to practice their own mummification skills. These amateurs were often scientists, or professors, or perhaps "gentlemen scholars"—the kind of resource-rich leisure class who collected artifacts stolen from other cultures. And, apparently, people.

Where did they get the bodies? Nowhere good. The school had been able to check their archives, and they'd found references to the mummy *long* predating the Uniform Anatomical Gift Act of 1968. This law laid out clear rules for how bodies could be donated to science, and where and how bodies might be obtained for medical schools and other research endeavors. The school did as much research as they could. Really, they handled it beautifully, using the entire situation as a way to teach their students in a dozen different ways about complex issues and to spark conversations on ethics, death, forensic science, and much more. They even had their students visit Amy's anthropology lab and asked Amy and a colleague to give a lecture at the school about the mummy's possible history.

But they couldn't answer the essential questions: Who *was* the decedent? How had they died? Who had made the mummy, and why? A medical student, or an instructor, or rich dilettante who fancied himself a scientist? Had someone simply decided to play with the dead because they could?

The Tilton Mummy wasn't even the only unidentified and preserved set of human remains that Amy had charge of. We planned on taking another mummified human head to the dentist's office, along with Ina Jane Doe's remains, in hopes that he could do a panoramic X-ray of the individual's skull as well. This decedent's remains had been delivered to Amy's lab by another agency, accompanied only by the information that it had been donated to a private school sometime in the 1930s and was labeled "Amazon Savage." Besides the obvious issues with that designation—"Savage"?!—Amy didn't think the labeling was accurate, and neither did Sam. Mummification was not a popular method of human burial in humid climates. Amy thought that, unlike the Tilton Mummy, this decedent *had* been prepared for burial, not by a hobby anatomist—just not in the Amazon.

Amy's lab space was in an older building that housed all sorts of fascinating collections. In the hallway leading to her lab were tall, blond-wood cabinets that housed a massive entomology collection. There were trays of insects, each carefully labeled and stored in wooden boxes: roaches as big as my palm, butterflies and moths with tissue wings set against painstaking pins and labels, beetles shining like oil under glass. I'd never been afraid of bugs, but a few of those had me reconsidering.

Her workspace was full of large epoxy tables; there was plenty of storage space, and microscopes and other equipment lined the walls. Protocol for gloves and other proper care and respectful and careful handling of remains was strictly enforced. When we got in, Sam started messing around with some resin; she and Amy were already talking about teeth, and a paper they were writing, and most of it went over my head.

Amy offered to show me the "Amazonian" decedent's remains so I could see the difference between that decedent's preparation and the individual we'd see later at the Tilton School. Amy gingerly opened the protective material around the mummified head, and I peered inside. The style of mummification was quite different from anything I'd seen before, but I had seen very little; mostly, my experience was limited to educational programming on ancient Egypt. There was a thick, dark, tar-like substance that coated the desiccated skin of the decedent, and remnants of some kind of wrapping cloth or material as well as strands of hair.

To prepare for Ina's analysis, Amy had cleared a table and set up a photo box; she'd need lots of angles for her report. Kyana, who was lab manager that year, had lined it in a black velvet that made bone stand out against the light. I set up my field recording kit so I could capture everything she said, since I knew I'd have to look it up later. Amy would write her more formal report later, after she'd spent time going over each of Ina's features in detail, but these initial hours, captured before her students came in and turned the lab into a workspace, would make up the bulk of her report.

I fiddled with the volume knobs and set up microphones on either side of the long table. This might've seemed excessive at first glance, but Sam and Amy were both commenting, and a colleague, Dr. Leslie Fitzpatrick—she'd come on as a lecturer that year at UNH and specialized in isotopic testing—had joined as well. I wanted to make sure I had multiple tracks and could distinguish each voice.

Amy was interested in noting skeletal features, not in diagnosing Ina Jane Doe. She was already concerned that Ina had been over-pathologized by web sleuths convinced that she had particular neck conditions or paralysis, and that it had narrowed down the possible pool of missing persons who had been compared. It's not that Amy didn't think about possible issues—she just didn't want to limit our scope.

She'd actually told me I might have something interesting going on with my own neck. The night before while we watched TV and Lucy snored on my lap, I'd been rubbing the knobbiest point of my spine. I was getting the first twinge that signaled I'd need to take a shot of sumatriptan, my migraine medication. I experience what my neurologist calls "neck migraines," a fairly unusual form of the classic headache that actually originate in, surprise, my neck and knocks me flat for a day or two.

I'd mentioned to Amy and Sam that I'd need to give myself a shot of my medicine, and when I explained why, Amy narrowed her eyes in an assessing way.

"That's interesting . . . I'd love to see your bones."

"Thank you," I'd said. It seemed like the best answer.

At the lab, Amy put her gloves on and got her bench notation materials ready. Bench notes are the rough-draft notes a forensic anthropologist makes that are then translated into the formal report that enters a decedent's case file—the report that is sent to law enforcement. She might make note of something she plans to research, or a paper she knows she wants to cite, or a similar case she'd like to compare, or note a measurement. There's a lot of stopping and starting during an exam—taking notes, stopping for measurements, checking open books to consult various bookmarked reference pages. If Amy had Ina's entire skeletal system to examine, it would have taken much longer, of course; she took great care and time with her cranium and mandible. Because I was recording, she walked me through what she was writing down.

Amy told me that most people she knew only turned in their final reports to law enforcement, but she included all her calculations and bench notes, too. Her thinking was this: What if a bone was lost, sometime in the future, and more work had to be done? Then that expert, working on the case, would have her careful measurements and figures, and all that information wouldn't be lost. It was an interesting approach, and I liked it: not being too precious, thinking about a kind of future collaboration.

Amy tapped the paper with her pen to get my attention. I motioned to the microphone and then pointed to my headphones; I could hear her through them. She cleared her throat and leaned toward the mic, then away, then back toward it.

"Am I supposed to talk into this thing?"

"Just pretend it's not there. This is just for my transcripts. I mean, don't wander off, but you're not a morning DJ or anything. Do it however you normally would."

"When I prepare my formal report, there will be sections for all this information. But I make notes, now, of the preliminary information, so I remember to include it. Any important background goes first. So, I note from the pathologist report that the individual was supposed to be recovered approximately four to five days to two weeks after death, per original pathologist and remains were macerated at some point and they're completely clean. I note that when I receive—or in this case, transport and then examine—the remains, I was able to determine instantly of course, that the MNI, or minimum number of individuals, is one, because there are no repeating elements."

"Just one decedent?"

"Yeah."

Amy gently lifted Ina from the table, cradling her skull in a gloved hand. She pointed to the horizontal line cut during autopsy, which creates a cap so that the internal portion of the exam can be completed. There was another vertical set near the center jaw.

"Do you see this? I take notes on all of this, because in my final report, there's a space to note skeletal cleaning and preparation. I note that the skull was clean and free of debris upon my receipt of it, but that there were these hot glue chunks remaining on the bone, in many places. And that I did remove some of those when it was possible to do so without damaging the bones so that I could take better measurements. I will, of course, hypothesize that those hot glue remnants were for forensic facial reconstruction at some point in the past. But there's not much in the way of clay or anything over the glue, or in the bone, which . . . hmm. Okay, when you do see a clay overlay there, it's really hard to clean that off all the little bony crevices. So, I don't know if that glue was ever used for that purpose. We saw that clay reconstruction, but I don't know if it was actually molded on the skull."

I frowned. "You mean the artist might have looked at Ina as a model, and then built the clay sculpture free hand?"

Amy shrugged, still gazing down at Ina. "Right. Maybe. And the glue is so thick in parts that my guess is that maybe they thought that they were going to do a clay model on that, they glued the erasers or the tissue depth markers, whatever they happen to use and then they might have scrapped that plan. Because there are a decent amount of the little circular tissue marker kind of patterns on the skull, but there's not as many as you might expect. You can see the impressions of where they were. So, my guess is that they might have been like, 'you know what, let's not do this on the actual skull,' but again, that's just a complete hypothesis. I don't know for sure."

"And this would have been the forensic artist, with the glue, I mean, not the pathologist?"

Sam made a noise from her area near the sink, with all the resins and little rubber ice-cube trays, which I think signaled a *yes*.

"Yeah, so, look here. The mandible is sectioned. That happened during the autopsy, we can see that. The mandible sections were glued back together and the autopsy cut on the cranium, it has glue around parts of it as well. A pathologist wouldn't do that. That would be done for somebody after the skull is cleaned to try to do forensic art on it, whether they've successfully completed it or not."

Amy gently placed Ina back down, made notes, and started dictating to me again. I realized Kyana had entered the lab at some point—she'd gotten very good at sneaking around, excellent lab management skill—and she came up to the bench to watch as well. Amy pointed at the mics like she was being recorded by the CIA and kept dictating. "So, my third page of notes is adult skeletal inventory. I'm just noting everything that's present. You see this picture? This is what gets used in the report. I'd cross out the appendicular skeleton, because there's no post crania present. So, the only thing missing—that was presumably there in life—are the auditory ossicles to the bones of the ear. That just happens. Those can fall out during processing. They can also fall out postmortem, but this person was not outside for too long . . . as far as we know . . . But at any rate, I did not note auditory ossicles there, but everything else is present."

"What now? Ear bone? I thought they were cartilage?" This was one of the few scientific scraps of information I had managed to hold on to.

"You've got three little bones in each of your ears. We rarely find them in forensic cases, though."

"They tend to fall out." Sam's voice floated over from her workspace.

Amy looked at Kyana as she began on the next bit—she wanted her to pay attention. Kyana had already put gloves on. She'd even materialized a lab coat.

Amy tapped the papers again. "In most reports, you'd make notes so that you could include a traditional skeletal homunculus in your report. We probably won't include one, because there's no postcrania for the decedent. Is just kind of a holdover artifact from days of yore, but these appear in most case reports. I probably won't send something like this in, because it's not helpful in this case. We know what's present, right? But you would just shade what is present and note what's absent. Some people use this to draw trauma. But in this case, we have got good photos, so the homunculus is kind of superfluous."

"Anyway . . ." Amy bent over a form with a printed set of teeth on it, scribbling down notes in three different places. How she kept it straight, I had no idea. "So here we have the dental chart notes—I'm going to mark now all the teeth that are present, with notations on the teeth. All but third molars are present in the mandible, but the third molars are present in the maxilla. And on my inventory page and in my bench notes, we'll note which teeth are sampled for various things, including histology. That will be the Hubbard lab here, Astrea, and the tooth work Sam's going to do."

UNH'S Hubbard Center for Genome Studies was running a series of tests to discover if they might begin forensic work in addition to their current nonhuman DNA testing, and the COVID tests they ran for the whole university. Ina's sample was a trial; they planned to compare their results with Astrea's.

"I'm doing a basic inventory, but I'll need to come back and write in more detail. The dental inventory is complex. Calculus, fillings, caries, porcelain fused to metal crown, a root canal. Lots to describe and mark. The next page on the report would be for cranial osteometrics. These are just the measurements we take for FORDISC. So, they're all in millimeters. Some of them are bilateral. Here, Kyana, I'll measure and you make notes of numbers."

Although Ina was presumed to be both white and female—there wasn't enough context for much more nuance there—failing to do measurements for more information would have been poor practice. Amy and Kyana's measurements and results found Ina was, on average, consistent with FORDISC's data on females of European ancestry, but they still made detailed notes.

I waited until they were done to ask my question. "Now that you've had time for a visual inspection and you've done measurements . . . I'm thinking about how much has been made of Ina's possible asymmetry. All those people who wondered if she had a distinct or noticeable asymmetry in life. Can you see anything based on the measurements that makes you think that's more or less likely?"

Amy rested her gloved finger on what I thought of as Ina's brow bone, gently indicating the curve to me. "I mean, there's definitely some asymmetry. It's noticeable in death, in a skull. *But* you've heard my soap boxing on this. What does that mean for soft tissue? Sometimes a lot, sometimes not much at all. We can look at some of these numbers and try to get an idea. This cranial osteometry, just scanning numbers, you're not noticing much, right? But if you go to the bilateral measurements, look at those more closely. Go to numbers 15 and 16. These are orbital breadths and orbital heights; we're looking at eye sockets here. Those measurements do not match, with the right side being larger by one millimeter. Usually when I do this, I measure three times in a row just to make sure. So is one millimeter significant? I would not really say so. Then we drop down to number 24, mastoid length. I did note there's glue on both of those mastoids, but obviously my measurement doesn't take that into account. But that left side mastoid, so that's like the chunk of bone behind your ear. You feel that?"

I obediently reached behind my own ear and nodded.

"That's two millimeters bigger. Okay, now we're getting a little more significant, right? Maybe so, maybe not. So I just noted there's glue. In my notes, I'm careful to write that there's glue obscuring the left side, or maybe I'll just put 'obscured by glue.' That's my note to myself that I take this measurement with a grain of salt. If I say something like glue on both mastoids, that's my note to myself. That's present but it's not affecting the actual bony tissue that I'm measuring. You need to make small adjustments for the glue. Traditionally, the whole point of these measurements is to enter them into FORDISC and try to get into ancestry estimation. We're using them right now to help us discuss symmetry, but if we were trying to determine ancestry, I might be much more conservative, and just say, if there's glue, I'm not going to take that measurement. But in this case, I just noted when something might be obscured, by maybe the autopsy cut. Because of course with those cuts, you're losing bone because you're demolishing it. That affects a precise measurement. Even for symmetry discussion, there are some points where there is so much glue that the comparison is difficult. Numbers 32 and 33, and 30 and 31 on the left side, just too much glue, not possible to measure."

Amy used her finger to draw an imaginary line down to Ina's nasal cavity—that showed me her midline ran slightly off-center, so that the precise middle of her face would have been slightly to the left, through her right central incisor versus between her incisors.

"We can visually notice the nasal aperture is asymmetrical just by looking at it. Imagine a line bisecting the face down the middle . . . you can see the slight asymmetry in the midface. But would this have been subtle in life or very noticeable in the soft tissues? In the skeleton, sometimes we're looking so hard for something to note, to look different or 'nonstandard' that we may end up overstating something like the asymmetry we see here. In my opinion, I don't think this facial asymmetry would have been very noticeable in life."

Amy checked the numbers she and Kyana had recorded and run through the program. "So just as a reminder, with sex estimation from the skull, we are looking at a scale of 1 to 5 for various characteristics. Those characteristics that stick closer to 1 are considered more female; the closer to 5, the more male. Threes are 'indeterminate.' You can see here"—she showed me her notes—"I was equivocating between 3 and 4 on nuchal crest and mental eminence. That's the protrusion of your chin, right in front of your incisors. Everything else is 1s and 2s.

"When I write up the full report, I'll attach my FORDISC summary and what version I used, and include my sex estimation notes. I'd make a note in the sex estimate section that HFI may be present, which is generally an indication of middle-age or older female remains. My ancestry notes, too—I've got my notes on Hefner's macromorphoscopic traits that we can observe in the midface and make a qualitative score."

Amy paused and explained a few things to Kyana about using multiple methods, particularly for ancestry, and most especially when ancestry is ambiguous; gathering FORDISC quantitative data and Hefner's macromorphoscopic qualitative data, and using them together, was a more nuanced approach.

Amy flipped through her papers, pausing on a page and placing a sticky note. "Okay, so, antemortem trauma and pathological conditions. You could also use individual characteristics here; I know you've seen that. Some of this is going to be totally speculative and it will need to be framed that way. But as far as antemortem trauma? There's not much. She has a healed injury on the left parietal"—Amy pointed to one spot on Ina's cranium—"and it's about one and a half inches in length. It's a half inch from the sagittal suture, five inches posterior to the coronal suture. In layman's terms, the top of her head."

"So maybe an old injury?"

"I'd say so. Something we could ask family when we find them. If. When."

"Could be childhood, maybe? Or maybe she didn't even tell anyone she hit her head. I've done that. Banged my head on the car trunk and forgot about it six hours later."

"Exactly. And the extent to which that would be a soft tissue injury, it definitely would, you can't have a skeletal injury and no soft tissue component, that'd be very hard to do. But did it require stitches or staples? No idea, right? It could have just been something like you said, she suffered and just didn't even think to say anything. There's really no other ante-mortem trauma. We can't unfortunately speak to postmortem because we don't have her vertebrae, though according to Klepinger, there appeared to be cut marks. But I'll include this injury in this section. I'll include the thickening of her frontal bone as a sign of possible HFI. I'll note that her clinoid processes of the sella turcica are fused. Though, that in and of itself . . . people have different feelings about what that translates to in life, if anything. And I'll mention the caries in her teeth."

I'd eventually learned that *caries* was science speak for cavities. What threw me off was that they always used it in the plural. I tried describing a single cavity as a *cary*, and they all looked at me like I was failing the course.

"Her asymmetry is so mild that it may not be linked to a particular condition or diagnosis in life. Because . . . what does it mean? Human variation? We don't know. Do some of her skeletal features differ from the absolute norm? Yes. But did that affect any aspect of her health, her appearance, or any other aspect of her life? It would be a mistake to assume that. While the features are different, they are absolutely in the range of normal variation."

"So you don't see anything that could have fueled the online speculation about her?" That was what I'd been waiting to hear about. Since day one, I'd had the feeling Ina wouldn't be identified based on her art, because everyone was looking in the wrong direction.

Amy sniffed. "There's certainly nothing that would warrant any of that extreme speculation. The original anthropologist's potential diagnosis was misread as unassailable fact once it hit the internet. Her paper was used out of context—not something she could have imagined would happen. And then there were leaps made by online researchers who wanted to connect possible physical trauma and mental disability."

Well, then.

Amy and Kyana worked their way through possible antemortem trauma notes, which was limited; without the presence of Ina's vertebrae, there was little they could note. She did write up the lack of taphonomic changes in the bone—so no weathering or animal activity—and what she'd noticed about Ina's hair, which had arrived just that morning at the lab. There were still leaves and debris caught up in her hair—an enormous envelope of it had been sent to her, perfectly intact in two sealed envelopes. They noted Ina's broken tooth; Amy postulated she'd had a filling or a weakened enamel area but wanted to speak to the dentist for a second opinion.

Amy looked back up at me. "We'd also provide more detail here on the possible HFI. Not that she had it or didn't. We can't and shouldn't diagnose. But we'll note that she has a remarkably thick frontal bone and occipital bone. The parietals are on the thick side. I have the measurements here. The gist is that hyperostosis frontalis interna is an overgrowth of the frontal bone. And then interna, well, there are some internal features that she should present with if she has HFI. When you go back to Dr. Klepinger's report—and I agree with her finding—she points out those internal features are not as striking. Ina doesn't have the ropy appearance in the internal bone that most people with HFI have. But this thickening in the right spots in the cranium, that's textbook. Her skull is unusually heavy, too. These are features we normally see in a postmenopausal woman. Not in all postmenopausal women, of course. That's just the group where it's most likely to occur. But HFI can occur in younger women. It can be congenital. What we're doing here, when we record all this information, is we're working backwards from what we see in a skeletal presentation and trying to make a few educated guesses as to what could have been happening in her life."

"What can you do with that?"

"Write my report very carefully, and very thoroughly. You don't want to phrase things in such a way that investigators think they're looking for a single, narrow type of person, with some specific condition, or appearance. If Ina had HFI, she may not have even known it. Asymmetrical skeletal features? We might notice them if we ever see a picture. But that's because we know how to look."

"Sort of like . . . my right eye is smaller than my left. If I point it out to you, then you see it."

"Exactly. And I'll remember that, thank you." Amy smirked and went back to her fiddly numbers. I turned off my Zoom and began the process of dissembling the mic stands. Amy and Kyana had more to cover; there were observations to record about possible cause of death, and perimortem trauma. But I had made an agreement with law enforcement not to record or report on those details. If Ina could be identified, then Jefferson County would need information held back.

Amy wouldn't be finalizing her report anytime soon. This was just the start; as we continued to work on the case, she'd revisit it again and again, adding to her notes. Her report would differ from that of the original forensic anthropologist in some ways; that was natural as they were different scientists, studying thirty years apart. So far, Amy's major takeaways were that she couldn't comment on the torticollis that had interested so many online sleuths. The asymmetry that had been so prominent in the forensic art—Amy was confident that Ina's features would have been mildly asymmetrical if at all. She was also interested in the thickness of Ina's skull, which might signal a medical condition she'd be aware of, one that could identify her. Her extensive dental issues—Amy suspected thin enamel because Ina had dental work done in her life. Fillings, and on her front teeth—that would be rarer. All these observations would go into Amy's final, full report. But they'd also go to the forensic artist who'd agreed to work with us. And if we hadn't been able to afford DNA and genetic genealogy? This reanalysis, and the art, would have been the best bet of identifying Ina. Maybe radiocarbon dating or isotopic testing if Amy could scrounge up the lab funds.

As Amy and Kyana worked out descriptions and muttered to each other, and Sam cut something with a very small, very loud blade near the sink, I looked at Ina Jane Doe sitting on the layers of protective paper that kept her remains safe in the box Jefferson County had entrusted to us. The pages piled up around her. Of what remained of her. All the scientific language and observation . . . it wasn't a far stretch to imagine someone I loved in her place. Or me. Amy. Any of us. Taken down to our pieces and studied, hour by hour, by strangers who were trying to make us whole.

Most of the rest of the week was a blur. Guesting in classes where students asked some questions I could answer, but some I couldn't. Like: *Why were there so many movies being made about Ted Bundy all at once?* "No idea, kid." *Do you like (fill in the blank podcast)?* "Yes." If I didn't, my blanket answer was always that I'd never listened.

We visited the Redgraves at their office in Massachusetts—that's a story in and of itself, better told when we really dig into DNA. The podcast panel went off without any major disasters. We all went to Josh Hallmark's podcast meetup afterward at a local bar; his intensive, obsessively thorough investigation into possible further murders committed by Israel Keyes had attracted a loyal listenership, and they showed up with good questions. It was an interesting conversation; Josh had a lot of fascinating information up his cardigan sleeve, and I never got tired of talking to him about his work. The rest of the evening was relaxed: Amy found vegan corn dogs on the menu, and no one asked her about bones.

We had most of the next day reserved for two main tasks: our visit to the Tilton School to examine the anatomical mummy they'd discovered in their attic, and our after-hours trip to a local dentist to make use of his panoramic X-ray machine. For the trip to Tilton School, which was about an hour northwest of UNH, we all piled into Dr. Les Fitzpatrick's minivan. She'd brought a tool bag with her, including a small Dremel tool; Amy had warned us that the anatomically prepared decedent had been coated in a strange material—a resin, maybe—that would likely make any future analyses difficult.

It was a cool, drizzly day; Atlanta wouldn't see this kind of weather until November, at least. When we pulled up to the school, it was more like a college campus than somewhere children might attend classes. I'd never been to a private university in the Northeast, but I'd seen plenty of them in movies, or at least campuses pretending to be them. Lots of grass and trees and windy roads, and buildings named after alumni who'd endowed this or that. All that made sense, considering it was close to two hundred years old and had been everything from a junior college to a seminary; now a co-ed prep school, it looked like the perfect setting for a YA novel with just a little magic involved. Maybe a school for alchemy? Some of the older buildings had that feel, with the high-peaked roofs and all the brick. The light sprinkle of rain and mist probably helped with that, too.

Amy Despins, executive assistant to the head of school, met us at the top of a curved driveway. She had bright, reddish hair and was smiling through the mist of rain as if she patiently waited for people in inclement weather on a regular basis. The school's administration had been nice enough to allow me to record the whole trip—there was no way I'd take decent notes in an attic—but she did want to introduce us to the Dean of Teaching and Learning, Katherine McCandless, first. Moving through the buildings was an interesting experience; some portions felt straight out of a British boarding school, with a *Narnia to the left* kind of feel, but the administrator's offices were modern, enclosed by glass walls. After meeting with everyone in the main office, Amy Despins took us on a winding trip up a steep old staircase toward the attic.

On the way up, she explained the shock when they'd made their discovery. They'd come upon the anatomical mummy—the decedent—stored inside a large wicker case, standing upright in a corner, and were at a loss. Should they call the medical examiner? A coroner? The police? Get a death certificate? As a fellow educator, I could relate; there was nothing in any handbook I'd ever seen that covered this kind of situation. After they called local authorities, it became clear that everyone would need more information in order to proceed. That's where my Amy came in.

To Amy Despins's credit, she did her part, too; she dug up every bit of archival material that she could find that might mention this "mummy," in hopes of discovering when, and how, it came to the school. She hadn't been able to pinpoint either. Students had involved themselves in the research as well, and in long conversations about history and ethics; the school had used the discovery as a major educational moment, whereas some institutions would have chosen to quietly hush things up. They hoped to discover everything they could about the origins of the individual whose remains had been stored at their school. If enough information could be established, the deceased could be returned to their place of origin, or their people. But answers remained elusive.

Based on mentions in school annuals and newspapers, the decedent's remains would be considered historic versus a forensic case, though that wouldn't preclude the necessary return of remains. Amy Despins found mentions dating back to at least the 1930s, long before the Anatomical Gift Act. There had even been mention of the decedent's remains being used as part of a haunted house at one point. Tiny strands of synthetic black hair—from a wig, no doubt—had been discovered alongside the remains. But beyond that, school officials had very little information to go on. Amy, Sam, and Les hoped to get samples that could be tested—if not for DNA, at least for radiocarbon dating and isotopic testing, to learn more about where the deceased might have originated, and when they had died. Their visual inspection would be just as important, too.

When Amy Despins opened the attic door, she warned us: "There's not a lot of light. And . . . there are bats." Based on the droppings I saw scattered all over the floor, I believed her. We edged in, gingerly, and I was taken aback by the sheer size of space. I'd read *Flowers in the Attic* as a preteen, which was a book passed around my fifth-grade class like it was *Lady Chatterley's Lover*, and when I imagined the eponymous attic in the book, it looked something like this in my head: an enormous space, stretching back so far that the edges disappeared into darkness, with corners and boxes and trunks and bureaus you could spend months exploring. Just imagine all the things that a school founded in 1845 might accrue in its attic.

Instead, I plugged up my shotgun mic, put on my headphones, and stuck the Zoom recorder in my purse. My podcast's producer would silently weep if she'd seen this arrangement, but it would be good enough to get a transcript for my own notes. Amy Despins told us to watch our step as she led us over to the large, weather-worn wicker container that they'd found. It was propped vertically against a load-bearing wooden post. The basket seemed small for what it was: a makeshift tomb. Just a little to the right, Amy Despins gestured to a table that had been put together out of an old door and two sawhorses. The mummified human remains had been placed there, away from the clutter of the rest of the attic.

"We thought this would be easier," she said.

Our Amy nodded. "We would have needed to move the decedent for sure. This will work well. We can get around on both sides. We'll just need a little more light." I took out my phone and turned on the flashlight function. I ended up moving slowly around as the anthropologists gazed down, mic in one hand, flashlight in the other. The air was thick with dust, and though we didn't need to, everyone was speaking quietly. It felt right, considering.

The body laid out before us . . . I'd been in the presence of a number of deceased persons over the last five years. Some in the early stages of decomposition—even only hours dead—and many more mostly or fully skeletonized. Sometimes, I'd feel sick, or sad, or both. Standing over the makeshift table in the attic, shivering a little in my thin sweatshirt, I realized what was wrong. The decedent at Tilton had been preserved in such a way that they didn't seem real. Not at first. Whatever the amateur scientist or hobbyist—and even I could tell this was the work of someone without real training—had done to this individual, it had been done badly. The result was a skeleton that looked like an artificially aged movie prop.

So, *this* was what Amy called "anatomically prepared," though it was not even remotely what I'd expected. I'd seen pictures of traveling museum shows like *Bodies: The Exhibition* and anatomical skeletons in classrooms. But this person's remains had been almost plastered over. What I saw was something like a skeleton with skin, stretched tight over its bones, that had been cut bilaterally, to allow for a view "inside"—a kind of macabre viewing box into the human body.

It was as if a person had been desiccated down to skin and bone, and then lacquered back up until they resembled a plastic-cast model from a kitsch '80s horror movie; I thought immediately of *Return of the Living*

Dead, where the zombies could talk and weren't supposed to look quite real in the first place. The decedent's face, throat, the area where their lips should have been—all were ridged with spiderwebs of interconnected red resin-ish veins. I'd seen venous and arterial systems displayed before, but not like this. It was haphazard. And, Amy said, the colors were irregular. They should have been done in red and blue.

At the chest, there was a dramatic change in presentation: an open rib cage and a torso that was as hollow as a carved-out log, coated with that same thick resin—clear-ish this time. Sam shined her phone's flashlight down into the decedent's chest cavity as she slowly moved to the far side of the table. Amy followed behind her, then Les. I was looking everywhere at once, not sure what they'd spotted that I hadn't. Amy Despins, the Tilton staff member, stood some feet away, letting the anthropologists work. After all, she'd already spent a lot of time with this mummy.

Suddenly, they were all putting on gloves. Anthropologists always seem to somehow have pairs everywhere, like magicians pulling those colorful ropes of scarves out of every pocket. Amy reached in and delicately pointed out two little lumps low in the carved-out torso of the mummy, so I could follow along. "You see those? They're organs."

"Been dried out," Sam explained.

"And just . . . tossed back in?"

Les was bent over, looking very closely at one organ in particular. "Nah. They're filled with air, and then put back inside. This would have been something used as a model, right? So they'd want the organs on display. Most are missing, though. I see the bladder. And is that . . . that's the uterus, right?"

Amy and Sam agreed.

"And I see there's still remnants of a vulva." When Amy was really working, she started muttering, so I was following her around with the mic as closely as I could without getting in her way. She stopped short, sending up a tiny cloud of dust with her shoes. "Laurah, shine your phone right here." She pointed at the decedent's pelvic area.

Sam or Les, I couldn't tell who, saw what Amy was talking about and let out air through their teeth. "Pubic hair."

That was troubling for reasons I couldn't logically explain. Making a mummy out of a person's corpse without, I had to assume, their permission, was horrifying. Haphazardly cutting them to pieces, with some skin preserved, and some bone jaggedly exposed, that was bad, too. But this? Not to mention, she didn't have any hair left on her head at all—probably because the man who'd prepared her, and it was almost certainly a man, based on the time period, had wanted to show the vascular system across her cranium.

"Is this . . . an adult?" I asked. I'd been so taken aback by the sight of the mummy, I hadn't really noticed her size. She seemed very small, but maybe the table, or the mummification process, had deceived me.

"Probably," Amy said grimly. "But we haven't measured yet. Not that height is necessarily the indicator." Amy looked at Les, who went to her tool bag and got a measuring tape. The mummy was approximately sixty-two inches—or five foot two. Just about exactly Amy's size, actually. She seemed much smaller.

"Could be an adult or a subadult," Sam told me.

"What counts as a subadult?" Amy Despins spoke up for the first time in a while, startling me. I'd totally forgotten she was in the corner.

As our Amy explained, "Ranges vary, but essentially anyone under twenty-five . . . ish would be a subadult." She pulled on my sleeve, and I refocused the flashlight more closely down on the decedent's rib cage so she could point something out. "What we want to see, and we can't because of this preparation on the bone, is what essentially looks like jagged lines in the bone. They're called epiphyses." Amy laced her gloved fingers together with a faint squeaking noise. "That's when your bones are still fusing together to make one solid bone."

Les was over at her tool bag, digging out her Dremel and an extension cord. I could see bits of dust floating around her gray sweater and blond ponytail in the uneven light. She was looking for something—electricity, I assumed. There were already a few cords strung across the attic floor and running in different directions, so there had to be a plug by the door.

"But we can't see that with all that resin stuff," Amy finished. "I'm not sure exactly what it's made of. But it's thick."

"And did you see this?" Sam asked. She was still near the decedent's feet. There was less of the resin on the toes, so they planned to take a bone sample there, in hopes that the bone was less degraded. But Sam had trained her phone's light back on the pelvis again. "A wire's been driven straight through."

I couldn't see Sam's expression in the dimness, but I could hear the distaste in her voice. When we all put our phones together, we saw it. There was indeed a thick, rusty length of metal pushed up through the skeleton, based in her pubic region.

"That would have been to hang her up for display," our Amy explained to the room. "For . . . *education*."

That attic was full of teachers, all of us trying to show our students better things, and to learn better things ourselves. I tried to imagine the instructor who would bisect this tiny person and practice their homespun mummification skills for the sake of their students. I wish I could say it was difficult. But I knew enough about American history to picture it with perfect clarity.

When Amy moved on to examine the head of the Tilton Mummy, I backed up to give her a little more room and brushed my hand in the wrong direction along the side of the makeshift table. A thin wooden sliver slid neatly down into my thigh, right through my jeans. The denim took most of the impact, but it was still sticking out of my leg like a tiny stake. I hissed under my breath, stuck my phone in my back pocket, and pulled it out—not really the time to ask for a Band-Aid, what with a mummy situation at hand. I'd find a little purple welt, like a single vampire fang mark, when I took a shower at Amy's house that night.

Amy was calling me. "Light!" she said over her shoulder. When I limped into place, I understood why. She'd found that the cranium hid another surprise: Another organ had been tucked inside. Not the brain. After a few moments, the anthropologists agreed it must be the decedent's heart. Probably it had fallen off the model at some point, and there had been some thought of reaffixing it, and—well, that never happened.

This was my first real close-up look of the deceased's face. The "scientist" had fixed in false eyes, made of some kind of ceramic or glass. They were absolutely eerie—not because of the mummy herself, but because of the incongruity. These were life-size doll's eyes, blank and cold, gazing up into the rafters, into nothing.

Amy and Sam were murmuring about teeth, so low that the microphone wasn't picking up what they were saying. I had to turn up the volume and scoot up closer, pressing my sore leg against the wood. They were gathered on either side of her head.

"Laurah, shine your phone down on her mouth, please." Sam leaned so far over that her braid was dangling in front of her face. She pushed it back over her shoulder in irritation. She and Amy both had streaks of dust on their shirts and pants, but their gloves were still holding up.

"Teeth aren't worn," Amy muttered. Not being worn, I guessed, had to do with possible age at death. Most of what they'd be using to estimate age was obscured by all that coating. If the skeletal system had held any remnants of trauma or cause of death, that, too, was obscured by the trials the decedent's body underwent.

Amy glanced at Sam. "You see this, right? The placement . . . it's strange. They may not be hers. And if they aren't, obviously, we can't test them."

Sam nodded slowly. "Yeah. Maybe misalignment of the jaw and teeth, right? Do you think it's another mandible and teeth, or just teeth? Or maybe we're just seeing how badly the teeth were put back in."

So, the mummifier could have used teeth from another skeleton—just how many human bodies or parts of human bodies did he have access to?—and constructed a piecemeal model out of multiple people's remains. I'd actually seen that once before, in a FOIA fulfillment I'd gotten from Florida. I was sent a picture of a cranium and mandible that didn't look quite right; when I zoomed in, I noticed the metal hinge. There was even a forensic drawing, of a presumed Asian male, included in the file. The art was skewed, but how could it not be—the artist was working with not one person's remains but two. When I showed it to Amy, she verified that: There was no other way. All the other anthropologists I talked to agreed. I'd sent an email to the department with that email to let them know I'd seen a notation in the file about sending off a tooth for DNA testing. If they pursued that, they'd want to do upper *and* lower molars. But I'd never heard back.

After a few minutes of consulting, Amy and Sam decided that the teeth were likely original to the deceased. The odd placement—protruding from her mouth as if they didn't quite fit—probably had more to do with the mummifier's lack of skill. After examining the resin and coating in different areas of the remains, our crew decided to take a number of samples from her: a tendon, a tooth, a fingernail, part of a toe, and a portion of the fourth rib bone—if they could be cut through. It was the least invasive way to try to discover what, if anything, hadn't been degraded or damaged by the treatment. At least not damaged so thoroughly that testing was impossible.

The rib bone could help with an estimation of age at death. Radiocarbon testing could be done and isotopic testing as well. Les explained that analyzing multiple types of tissue could create fuller pictures, or isotopic landscapes called "isoscapes"; essentially, we could learn about a decedent's diet, possible regions of birth, and adult long- and short-term stay. It was easier to rule places out than to rule them in—to say "The deceased was definitely not from the Southeastern US," for instance—but it was certainly a start. It would depend on what funding the school had for testing, and whether, upon lab examination, the anthropologists thought the samples were viable. It would also be easier to really study everything with good lighting and a microscope.

The scientists had to work carefully, pulling items one by one from Les's bag; I discovered her kit was a patchwork mix of actual home tools, the sort I kept under my kitchen sink, and what I imagined an archaeologist might carry. They used a tiny chisel to chip away a single tooth from the cement that held it in place. The rib cut was the most difficult; Les dulled a blade on the resin, and tiny fragments of it flew everywhere. I was pretty sure that whatever it was, there'd be a nice dust of lead and something like arsenic, all very nineteenth century. Finally, Les started using the blade like a tiny manual saw, slicing back and forth with applied, precise pressure while Amy braced the sides of the decedent's rib cage, gently, so nothing would be disturbed or damaged. At last, a tiny chunk of bone was freed. It had a thin layer of the resin around it that reminded me, despite myself, of the jawbreakers I wasn't supposed to bite through as a child but always did: powdery and pale, with a bleached-away candy coating.

Amy made a few more notes directly into my microphone—measurements she'd want to look up later—and said we'd done what we could. So, I switched off the Zoom and started fiddling with the cord of the shotgun mic. But as Les picked up the tools, including her Dremel—which was totally shot at this point—I noticed Amy was still standing by the table, quietly reflecting on the small figure laid out there.

"Should I turn this back on?"

She hadn't taken off her gloves yet.

"No. Nothing official. But . . ." Amy gestured at the wire thrust through the decedent's pelvis. "I'm not going to leave her like this. With this stuck through her." She glanced at Amy Despins, who nodded. She didn't need to get a vote from the rest of the women in the room. We were all in accord. As Amy carefully slid the wire out from between the deceased's lacquered skin and bone, we remained silent. Amy left it sitting on the makeshift table, beside the small body, a twisty little hook that curled at its end, like a snake.

CHAPTER EIGHT

THE METHOD: DENTAL COMPARISONS AND ODONTOLOGY

The board certified forensic odontologist who first examined Ina Jane Doe, Dr. Rodney Brown, was struck by the unusual nature of her dental work—so much so that he personally wrote to the *ADA News* and asked that they publish a notice on her root canal "in hopes that some dentist might help" with her identification. He enclosed a drawing of tooth 19 alongside the following description:

A decapitated head was found in Jefferson County, IL, near the city of Mt. Vernon IL, in January 1993. This was a white female, aged 30 to 60 years. Tooth #19 (universal numbering system) is *UNIQUE*.

    1. Three rooted lower left molar.

        Mesial facial root.

        Mesial lingual root.

        Distal Root.

    2. Endodontic treatment on all three (3) roots.

    3. Distal root has a post inserted.

    4. Tooth has an all-porcelain crown.

Due to gross rampant caries in remaining dentition, it might be assumed tooth #19 was treated years prior to death.

If you think this might be your patient, contact. . . .

So, what does this mean? A dentist would read this information and, unlike me and probably you, actually understand it. Based on several dental textbooks, it seems that it's normal for tooth 19—also known as the first molar on the lower left quadrant—to have two large roots. Ina's had three. That's not totally remarkable; some people do have three roots instead of two, but it's just unusual enough that, combined with other factors, a dentist might remember her. She also had a root canal that treated all three roots, with a metal post and a porcelain crown with a filling that a dentist described to us as a "silver point," which was a method that would have fallen mostly out of favor by the late 1980s or early 1990s.

It was a specific enough treatment on an unusual enough tooth that Dr. Brown thought the practitioner who had done the procedure, or treated her afterward, would recall it. A notice in the American Dental Association's publication was a good idea; it was a smart way to reach many practitioners in a time when the internet was largely limited to AOL chat rooms and clunky message boards. Amy told me that this was a fairly common practice among forensic odontologists, at least when they came upon a unique enough tooth or dental aspect in a case.

The dental decay Ina Jane Doe experienced was extensive, too, but it would be difficult to say when it had occurred. A combination of significant dental work, like she had—numerous fillings, and a crown, plus removal of the wisdom teeth—and extensive decay, which was present in her molars . . . that could mean a significant change in life circumstances. That was the prevailing theory on Reddit, and I could see the logic in it. Trouble was, of course, that there are always multiple logical answers to any question.

For example, I was born with thin enamel—what my maternal grandmother would have called "soft teeth." I've had cavities and crowns and root canals despite scrupulous dental hygiene and religious attendance to the dentist's office. I've managed to crack a few crowns, too. But my son inherited his father's teeth: They're strong. He hasn't had a single cavity. When the pediatric dentist compliments us for an excellent routine, I smile at her with a mouth full of disintegrating fillings and think, *Genetics*. My teeth also got worse during my pregnancy—with him.

What if the same had been true for Ina? We had no idea if she had a child, or several; if she'd already had issues with her teeth, then pregnancy, or an illness, could have brought on serious issues. Or she could have experienced the same problem many Americans do: She might have had dental insurance for a time, or access to dental care, and then lost it or the ability to pay for it. Amy and I must have talked this through a dozen times. We tracked the theories that people offered online, which were mostly well-meaning. They wanted her case solved. But we kept coming back to the same conclusion. All we could really say about Ina Jane Doe was what Dr. Brown had written in that notice for the American Dental Association: *Tooth #19 is UNIQUE.* Someone should recognize this work *if they see it.*

——————

For close to thirty years, the best chance of identifying Ina Jane Doe lay in her teeth. It's strange, but our dental records, which are so vital in rule-ins and rule-outs in missing persons and Doe cases, are not kept in any organized, standardized way. It's a topic I've discussed with Todd Matthews of the Doe Network at length; though not a dentist himself, he's passionate about the valuable role dental records play in the potential identification of victims, and how trauma to families can be reduced if only law enforcement are proactive in seeking those records. Because, of course, dentists' offices are not federally regulated agencies—or even state regulated—in terms of the way records are kept. A dentist has to have a license to practice, naturally, and standards of care must be met, including certain HIPAA expectations, but there are not laws pertaining to how long a patient's files should be stored or any mandated reporting. In other words, if a missing person is in the system, there's not a function that would find their dental records at a practice in their state.[1]

We've already talked previously about parents in the 1980s and '90s who kept copies of their children's fingerprints; it was an initiative pushed in many states. But how many of those families have dental X-rays or charts stored away? Amy pointed out to me that it would have been prohibitively expensive back in the days when hospitals and dentists had to develop their own film.

I've also spoken with dozens of families of long-term missing persons for my podcast, and many have had trouble remembering which dentist their loved one saw, or the last time they even went. When I've gone to look for those records, the offices are often closed, and the practitioner retired or even passed away. The chance to find a chart or radiographs from decades ago is gone.

Todd Matthews has been talking about this issue for years. Though a civilian, he knows a *lot* about dental comparison; his work at Doe Network and NamUs taught him. I think it bothers him so much because dental comparisons are an incredibly practical, reliable, and low-cost method of identification, and yet we have not organized a system for utilizing the information that we—as a society—already have. Obviously, not everyone has access to dental care in the United States, and there will not be records for all individuals, or there will be outdated records; it's symptomatic of systemic inequality that affects us even in death. But the records we *do* have could, Todd argues, be put to greater use. He worked tirelessly in his home state of Tennessee to have the Help Find The Missing Act passed and enacted in 2017.[2] This law requires that "law enforcement agencies request the missing person's next of kin to supply dental records. Then, if the person is not located within 30 days, that information must be passed along [to] the NamUs." In unidentified-persons cases, "law requires the regional forensic center supply both the TBI and NamUs with fingerprint cards, dental records, DNA records and other identifying information."

This may seem like a no-brainer, but in many cases, even when that information is gathered, it's not uploaded to NamUs. But Todd wants the law to have more teeth, in more ways than one—and there isn't any clear consequence built in for failing to meet the standards it outlines. As he explained to me, "Now, in Tennessee we're not really following the state law, even with the proclamation, so I'm having to go back now and look, what's the teeth going to be? What's the punishment if we don't use it? Is it an audit finding? Because in my factory days, I worked [in] audit and quality control, that type of thing, and I know what punishment phase is. If you don't carry out certain procedures, it's an audit finding, and it could affect your fund, so maybe that's what we have to look at. Did you enter the dental records in NamUs? No. Did it impact the identification when remains were found? Yes."

He brought up an example that had recently come up with a case that the Doe Network was covering in Tennessee, one that he was following in NamUs:

> I put the records and NamUs on a boy that was recently found here. [Law enforcement] didn't go back and use NamUs. They made the family wait. They recollected the dental records from the dentist and made the family wait an additional two days while they went and redid something that was on their desktop had they been using it for state law. Yeah. I'm a little disheartened about that because they made them wait, so maybe that should be a finding. Why didn't you just use the records that were there? I don't know what their answer would be. The dentist even told them, "They've already come and got the dental records." The family did. That's one of the first things they asked the family to do to spare them some time. Law enforcement redid it when a body was found. We did it before the body was found, months. Why didn't they just use what was already there? There's no answer for that. I didn't know about it. Well, why didn't you? It's state law, and there [were] trainings across Tennessee, so who failed to make sure you went to your training? I mean, two days of suffering is a long time for a family that has a missing person. That's a *long* time.

And it's not just about X-rays. You know, the kind where you put on a lead vest and grip a plastic bit while a technician clicks away from the safety of an alcove, getting all those angles of your teeth, ferreting out cavities invisible to the human eye—or even the newer, glossier panoramic ones. Most insurance pays for those at least once a year, but your dentist has other records, too. There is valuable information stored on a simple dental chart, printed on paper or digitally maintained, and filled with notes about your teeth: They're keeping a watch on tooth number 18, for example. You have a ceramic filling on number 32, and an amalgam filling on 30 that will need replacing one day. A crown is noted on number 16—there was a root canal, too. A chipped central incisor—number 8. That's one of your front teeth. Your mouth is like a fingerprint, in its own way, if the records of its upkeep are available. Wisdom teeth removed? A bridge? Dentures engraved with serial numbers, or even a name? There's a mountain of evidence there. If I ask Amy, she'll rhapsodize about the general identifying architecture of the roots, their positioning in the alveolar bone, and the shape or positioning of teeth. Trust me, once she gets going, it's endless. Respectfully.

Before I began to work alongside and learn from forensic scientists, I assumed that forensic odontology was a field practiced separately from dentistry; that while of course the training was the common ground, I incorrectly thought a practicing dentist wouldn't also participate in forensic work. In reality, however, many forensic odontologists consult on criminal cases alongside their everyday practices. One forensic odontologist told me that he'd come home from his family practice in the evenings to receive overnight shipments of human remains and dental charts from law-enforcement offices that needed his expertise.

Officially, forensic odontology, like forensic anthropology, requires specific certification and many hours of training post-DDS; in areas where there is not a forensic odontologist available, I've seen files where a local dentist has been brought in to examine a decedent's teeth. Similarly, forensic anthropologists can offer opinions as well—but if there is a forensic odontologist on hand, their insight is invaluable. Like forensic anthropologists, forensic odontologists are called to crime, recovery, and especially disaster scenes. They are particularly vital because they can make positive IDs on the ground, based on available dental records. Forensic odontologists were on the scene at the different crash sites on 9/11, at wildfires in California, in the Southeast in the aftermath of Hurricane Katrina, the devastation at Waco after the Branch Davidians' compound burned—so many different tragedies. Sometimes, they are even working with human remains that have endured extreme conditions. Burned bodies whose jaws no longer open. Partial remains. Bodies driven into the ground by the force of a plane crash. A single tooth found, yards from an accident scene, that has to be matched to a decedent.

Last time I spoke to Todd Matthews of the Doe Network, he was running errands in his small Tennessee town. He'd had to call me back a few different times because customers kept coming into his family business, Sweet Pea Fashions Boutique. Like most of us, Todd has a variety of professions.

We had to finish our conversation while he picked up some prescriptions at the drive-through pharmacy window. He told me that I should really speak to a friend of his, Dr. Richard Scanlon. They'd known each other a long time because, like Todd, Richard had worked on cases at NamUs. If I wanted to know more about teeth, Dr. Scanlon was the man to interview.

"Rich, now . . . he actually made a dental cold hit. He saw a missing person's dental records, and he said, 'Wait a minute, I've seen this dental pattern before.' He remembered a John Doe case that he coded. In his living memory, he does what I'd love to see a computer do, a dental match database." Todd paused momentarily while he spoke with the pharmacy tech, who knew him. Everyone in town did. To me, he added, "It had been years, but Rich recognized that pattern. Sure enough, it was a match."

When Todd tells me to interview someone, I do my best. Amy's interest in teeth meant I was somewhat ahead in the game in decoding Ina Jane Doe's forensic odontology report, but she'd encouraged me to seek out a specialist to tell me more about odontology, and Dr. Scanlon certainly fit the bill.

When I attended a forensic-science conference in 2022, I listened to several talks on teeth, and one of the most interesting concerned how forensic odontologists assisted in identifying the victims of Canadian serial killer Bruce McArthur: "Dental Identification in a Case of Purposeful Commingling of Remains by a Toronto Serial Killer Operating in the Gay Community of Toronto, 2010–2017: The Bruce McArthur Case."[3] *Purposeful commingling of remains* was explained in the presenters' slide show: McArthur, who murdered members of Toronto's gay and primarily immigrant community, used his job as a landscaper to dispose of and scatter victims' remains without arising suspicion. Skeletal remains from multiple decedents were combined and hidden in large flowerpots and planters used in residential clients' yards. Upon his arrest, Canadian law enforcement searched at least thirty properties for human remains.[4] Because of McArthur's obfuscation, a variety of experts were needed to link his victims to missing-persons reports but also to sort the decedents' skeletonized and decomposing remains. Dental records were a vital component in the process; antemortem records were obtained for seven of the eight victims discovered at the recovery sites. It took the combined efforts of lab testing, fingerprinting, skeletal exams, and dental comparison to help fully separate and identify all eight victims.

Before the advent of DNA technology, fingerprint comparison and dental comparisons were the standard for positive identification, and they are still used in many cases today; a dental ID is low cost, reliable, and can be done in the field. But Dr. Scanlon told me that, in his opinion, the need for field ID via dental records will decline. With the advent of rapid-process DNA technology and machines that can be transported on location, Scanlon wonders how much work there will be for odontologists.

It's hard for me to imagine that the field would fade away; I'm not even a novice, but I saw so many conference presentations on new dental advancements and interesting approaches to dental technology that I left convinced that science was still invested in teeth. And from a practical standpoint, while many of the cases that make the headlines are DNA solves, there are dozens more that come into labs or ME offices and are solved quickly via positive identification through dental charts. Still, Dr. Scanlon has watched the field grow and change for decades. He was on the ground during 9/11, working at one of the crash sites. He has personally identified many people and studied a *lot* of teeth.

Dr. Scanlon patiently answered all my questions, even the strange ones about dubious experimental techniques (this can happen when you start reading too many research papers very late at night, and everything starts sounding like a good idea). One of the first things he explained to me, though, was that when he began in the field, few medical examiners or other such officials had the kind of equipment needed to take radiographs

(X-ray films) that he'd need to properly examine a decedent's teeth. Sometimes, offices might've had MRI or CT scans but not the equipment to show him what he needed to see in order to do a true exam. That's why a few decades ago, a forensic odontologist might find themselves in the position of needing to either travel to an office or receive remains by mail or courier. After all, they often were, and still are, the ones who own the necessary equipment, in their own practices. Now, with digital records and improved technology available to all professionals, things are marginally easier.

Throughout the years, Dr. Scanlon has received all kinds of records from law enforcement, including some more helpful than others. Sometimes, he told me, it's that no one has explained precisely what a forensic odontologist might need. So, say that even though there *are* dental X-rays available for a particular missing person, perhaps an officer who hasn't been briefed goes in and just picks up a dental chart instead. A chart lists teeth and conditions but doesn't provide the necessary photographic visual. Or dentists believe that they can't release the records, and it needs to be explained that, in the instance of a crime, the dental forms are cleared to share. My guess is that the obvious is true: Law enforcement have less familiarity with which dental records are needed because dental records' use in identification is not their primary use. Unlike fingerprinting, these kinds of X-rays weren't developed for forensic purposes.

One of the first things Amy checks for when we're reviewing new cases is the presence of dental charts or radiographs on NamUs. After all, she can do a rule-out based on that information. If they're absent, they may still exist somewhere, but they can't help her in the moment. That's what Todd Matthews wants to change: To have those records uploaded for missing people would mean that so much could be accomplished with a simple database search.

Dr. Scanlon told me that records exchanges are much simpler now with the advent of digital radiography; dentists no longer have to agree to send their original radiographs or else inferior photocopies. They can upload direct digital versions of the high-quality files and email them to forensic specialists like Dr. Scanlon, or send them to the law enforcement, who can input them into NamUs.

Of course, when Dr. Scanlon started, there was no NamUs; he, like Todd, was working in the field long before the database existed. Perhaps that's why he wasn't as impressed as Todd and I were with the story of the case he'd matched from memory when he'd seen a missing person's dental pattern and remembered a Doe case he'd seen in the past. Naturally he remembered it, he said. It was an unusual pattern. That was Dr. Scanlon's general attitude about the work he'd done over decades—*matter of fact, no big deal*—but the stories he told me were eye-opening. Of all the forensic experts I interact with, I've had the least contact with experts in dentistry, so hearing about how they work, and under what conditions, was fascinating.

We talked a good bit about field work, including mass casualty situations, whether they be accidents, terrorist attacks, or the like. In casualty situations where identification is needed, Dr. Scanlon explained the difference between an *open population* and a *closed population* scenario. In a *closed population event*, you know who is there—like on a plane manifest at the site of a wreck. You then have to identify and separate the remains of the deceased. The terrorist attacks at the World Trade Center would actually be considered an *open population event*, because while there would be records of who worked in the Twin Towers, forensic investigators couldn't know who else might have been in or around the buildings: delivery persons, people walking on the sidewalk, someone who saw the first plane hit and ran toward the building to help . . . all those possibilities widened the field. There were also missing persons who were not verified to be in the World Trade Center at the time of the attacks, whose families still think that they may have died during the collapse. One such case is that of Dr. Sneha Philip, a physician who lived nearby and who was reported missing after the attacks. Although there's no concrete proof that she was at Ground Zero, there have long been theories that Dr. Philip saw the first plane hit and ran toward the Twin Towers to render aid. After a series of court battles and eventually an appeal that overturned a judge's ruling that Dr. Philip most likely died on 9/10, not 9/11, she was officially declared the 2,751st victim of the World Trade Center attacks.[5]

If Dr. Philip did die during the attacks, she would certainly not be the only victim whose remains were not recovered; as late as September 2022, experts were still working at the New York Office of the Chief Medical Examiner (NYC OCME) to identify human remains from the attacks. Surprisingly, there are more than a thousand victims known to be at the World Trade Center who have not been positively identified—roughly 40 percent of the total number killed.[6] The 9/11 memorial in New York honors them, and their loved ones, and the open-ended grief the families face.

Per ABC News, "For these families, who have yet to receive any remains of their loved ones, the closest they can get is a special section of the National September 11 Memorial & Museum located at what was once the foundation of the north tower of the World Trade Center. There, behind a blue wall with the message 'No day shall erase you from the memory of time,' lies the remains of unidentified victims, along with a room that only victims' families can access to pay their respects. It includes a window that looks on the rows of cabinets that contain the remains." The NYC OCME is still testing the remains contained within that memorial, and it's difficult; the assistant director of the office explained to ABC News that "heat, fire, jet fuel, water, sunlight, mold and bacteria present following the attacks has left many of the remains extremely fragile for analysis so his team has had to grind up tiny pieces of bone to extract DNA." To make it more challenging, there's often a single chance at testing.

Dr. Scanlon's work concerning the 9/11 attacks was more immediate. He was one of the experts who worked at the Pennsylvania crash site, where forty-four people died.

"It wasn't a very well-populated flight," he told me. "I was there after the plane hit the ground and it was literally a smoking hole. The hole was about 25 to 30 feet deep. And then 40 feet beyond that, in the ground, they found the black box. The plane hit the ground approximately 600 miles an hour, upside down."

Dr. Scanlon and the other experts had to comb through wreckage and human tissue to find single teeth—not sets of teeth, but a singular tooth. That's the kind of work they did to slowly begin comparisons to dental records. "Even after they suspended operations, official operations, and the FBI left, there was an anthropologist that worked there, and he brought his students down, and they did a fingertip search. And they found one tooth. And so he said, 'Rich . . . we found a tooth . . . I'm going to send it down to an AFIP (Air Forces Institute of Pathology) for DNA, but it's got a filling in it. Do you think you can do anything with it?' And I said, 'Well, okay. Send it down. And who are you sending it to?' And he told me. And so I talked to him and he said, 'Sure. We can do X-rays like that. What do you want?' I said, 'Since it's just a tooth by itself, X-ray it around. Every 45 degrees.'"

Dr. Scanlon received the scans and began his work. "And I looked at it and I said, 'Well, because of the dental anatomy, it's most likely a second bicuspid, lower right second bicuspid.' So we have a search program. I went down to the lower right second bicuspid, which is tooth 29. I said, 'Who has a restoration on 29?' And two people popped up. And I looked at both of the X-rays, and one was . . . the metal restoration was a perfect match for this one woman. And so I called them back and I sent both of the X-rays down so he could look at them visually and compare them. And I said, 'Her dental records show that she had this tooth restored. So this radiograph of the ante-mortem and postmortem tells me that it's her.' He said, 'Well, Doc, we can get DNA. They could do it down there in three days. I'm going to still run the DNA before we do anything.' I said, 'That's fine.' Came back. He called me. He said, 'That's her.'"

It turned out that nothing else of the victim would be recovered. Her single tooth was all that remained, matched by an odontologist and verified by DNA.

Dr. Scanlon would go on to lecture about the experience; it's an excellent example of how powerful a tool dental identification can be. "Again, that's a closed population, which allows you to do that. In lectures, I explained that. I said, 'I just didn't look at all the people that had tooth 29. Maybe I made an error. Maybe it's the left second bicuspid. Or it could even be an oddly shaped first bicuspid.' So I went through every other tooth on all of the passengers that had a tooth like that. All the other bicuspids, upper and lower bicuspids. I looked at all the bicuspids. And that was the only tooth that had that restoration." He pointed to an issue that I hadn't even thought of: There were unknown variables on the plane, since, obviously, there were no available antemortem dental records for the terrorists who died on the flight. But the victim had such good dental records that all the experts agreed the single tooth's restoration exactly matched hers. Dr. Scanlon added, "If there would've been no DNA available at that time, we could have made that identification, if the coroner thought it was solid, just by that one tooth."

Dr. Scanlon also told me about another mass fatality scene where he assisted in identifying victims. In 1994, USAir Flight 427 out of Chicago crashed in Hopewell Township, Pennsylvania. Authorities eventually determined that the plane experienced a rudder malfunction so serious that it changed the design of future planes—but it took years for that information to come to light.[7] At the time Dr. Scanlon and his team went out to the crash site, there were no answers; all that was known was that all 132 individuals on the flight had died. The coroner was concerned that identification might be difficult—it had been a horrible, plummeting impact—but Dr. Scanlon saw something almost immediately that helped him form a suggestion. He discovered a gold crown, still attached to the mandible, that could be matched with certainty to dental records, once they had them all assembled. Dr. Scanlon recalled, "I said, 'You need a dentist on every search team.' He looked at me. Then he said, 'Bring them up.' Long story short, at the end of 13 days, we made 78 identifications based on dental."

He also explained the importance that dental identification can play when there's been a fire—whether accidentally or purposely set—and remains are fragile. In the days of early DNA testing, conditions had to be close to optimal to get a good sample, and a dental ID might be the only shot. Dr. Scanlon worked on a number of multiple-person fire fatalities and was able to successfully identify the victims via dental comparison. But he's also done plenty of individual casework, too, on unidentified decedents for different medicolegal entities across the United States. At NamUs, Dr. Scanlon noted a distinct and early focus on DNA confirmation versus dental confirmation; though he did casework for NamUs while it was based out of UNT, that work was comparatively minor when you consider how many possible dental comparisons might have been made.

But DNA science has been both a boon and, some might say, treated as the answer when it might not always be—or, at least, when it is only *one* of the answers. I'm certainly not suggesting that agencies avoid testing, but if there's limited funding for these kinds of cases, then the lower cost of dental identification, spread across more cases that would not have otherwise received DNA review? Seems like a win-win. A dental match, like a DNA result, is considered a confirmed ID. The bottom line is: It can resolve a case. We can still build and use and celebrate rapid DNA sequencers because they truly are a marvel; we shouldn't forget to utilize the simple and effective method of recognizing a filling in a molar when the option arises.

That's what they'd hoped for in the case of Ina Jane Doe. And maybe if the internet had been just a little further along back in 1993? They might have gotten their wish.

CHAPTER NINE

THE CASE: A TRIP TO THE DENTIST

September 2021—New Hampshire

That week in September when I flew out to meet with Amy, Sam, and their colleagues, we talked a *lot* about teeth. After all, Ina Jane Doe's teeth could have identified her if the right person with the correct knowledge had come across the description of her "unique" tooth 19. We knew that she had significant decay present, but we weren't willing to make a guess yet as to her life circumstances before her death; there were still too many variables. And guessing? Well, that was a short trip to tunnel vision.

Teeth could have been our best shot with the mummified woman found at the Tilton School, too. Amy had the samples, and the school was more than willing to pay for testing; Amy was worried about what the labs would say about the resin coating on the decedent's bones. It was even on her teeth. There was a strong possibility that even radiocarbon or isotopic testing would be impossible. The students of the Tilton School had hoped to discover the individual's identity so she could be properly buried or returned to her people if she had them. They didn't like calling her "the mummy"; they knew she'd had a name and hesitated to assign her anything else in the interim. But it felt too cold to keep calling her what amounted to "a body." So they'd done research and found a list of the most common names for women in the nineteenth century. That was the era, they thought, when it was most likely that she had died. Of that list, they chose Mary as a placeholder. It might not be culturally accurate, depending on who she'd been, but without any more information, that was their best guess. Maybe the labs would tell Amy something promising, and "Mary" would be replaced by her true name.

On the way home from Tilton, we stopped at a Mexican restaurant for a quick meal. I missed most of the conversation that happened between placing our orders and the arrival of the plates; I had a bad habit of zoning out when I was working on a single case, and now I had two to think about. When my fajitas landed in a steaming skillet on the table, I blinked. The basket of chips to my right was half empty, the guacamole was gone, and my friends were immersed in the tail end of a discussion of a particularly graphic story that included the phrase "extreme blood loss." Strangely, no one was digging into their newly arrived plates of food.

I cleared my throat, eager to bring focus back to Ina. "So, I know you extracted and prepared two teeth today for Ina's case. One is going to Astrea, with Ina's hair. But Sam, explain again what you're working on?"

Sam was doing something complex with salsa and a tortilla, but she paused, spoon in hand. "It will be sectioned for dental histology. You know what that is, right?"

"Sure. You're going to slice off a very small piece and look at it under a very strong microscope." I'd googled that enough times that I had the stock image that popped up memorized.

"We're going to be looking specifically for stressors at key points in life. Amy's told you about Wilson's bands, I think?"

"Stress marks that show in layers, right? Like when the enamel's forming? So they can line up with things that happen in life?"

"Pretty much. Short-term stressors that are microscopically apparent. Imagine rings inside a tree, kind of, but they mark events, not age. They might line up with illness, shifts in nutrition, things like that."

The waitress brought me another Coke Zero, and I paused to take a sip. "But you can't use these for identification, right?"

"Nah." Sam leaned against the back of our booth, framed in a weird halo cast by the flashing beer sign that had stuttered on and off at odd intervals. "The extra information could help to narrow the field, though. And once a decedent has been identified, the events can add context to their life story. Medical records can be examined and compared for instance. Maybe we'd have better insight as to when a possible medical issue developed in a person."

Amy had slowly begun turning my rice and tortillas into very sad little tacos. She added, "I'm interested to hear what Dr. Albee—that's the dentist—has to say about Ina. Especially those hypoplasias."

In the lab, the anthropologists had studied Ina's top teeth and noticed what looked—to me, at least—like pockmarks: as if hail had hit the surface of metal and left little, round indentations. They were in some disagreement as to what could have caused them. Maybe they were the result of braces? Caries, or cavities, could form under braces. These marks weren't accompanied by any kind of decay that I could see, but they were clearly a kind of damage. Whether that was congenital or situational, we didn't know.

After dinner, we drove back to the lab so that Amy could securely package the individual decedents' remains that needed radiographs done. Les backed her SUV straight up to the door of the building so that we could carry the secured boxes from the lab and to the vehicle without the danger of trips up and down stairs, through heavy swinging doors, or anything else that could cause an accident. I saw Amy stuffing a few handfuls of gloves into her jacket pocket, which honestly made me feel better; I'd begun to think she was manifesting them from thin air. This was the first restock I'd actually witnessed.

———— •—•—— ————

By the time we made it to Suncook Dental in Pembroke, New Hampshire, it was after business hours. That was a good thing. I have to imagine that Dr. Andrew Albee, accommodating as he turned out to be, would have preferred to keep his patients' teeth cleanings separate from forensic tooth examinations.

Suncook Dental's office was bright and beautiful. The lobby's sweeping front counter and tasteful gray aesthetic reminded me more of a salon than somewhere I'd go to get my teeth cleaned. This was, in my book, a definite plus.

"Hello!" Dr. Albee practically bounded into the lobby to greet us; he'd met with Amy before and was very pleased to consult again on a case. He was tall and slim, with spiky dark hair, and was probably in his late thirties, but I'd never been good at guessing ages. Dr. Albee liked talking shop, and Amy'd brought him two new experts to do it with. And then there was me.

Dr. Albee led us down to the basement area where the radiographs were performed. Basement isn't really a good description of the area; it looked as clean and lovely as the upstairs, but there was the addition of a staff kitchen, and a large flat-screen TV on the wall. I'd soon learn that it was used for projecting digital images for study.

Our main goal for the trip was to have Dr. Albee and one of the dental hygienists, Amelia, who had volunteered to stay late, to operate the panoramic X-ray for Ina Jane Doe. Dr. Albee had examined Ina's teeth once before, but he went over his findings again in more detail. This was partially for my benefit; understanding what he saw would help me search the archives and missing-persons reports. But also, Sam and Les were interested, too; Les dealt with teeth often enough in her isotope work— so there was a lot of dental talk to be had. Amy had also arranged for Dr. Albee to examine the mummified head that had been delivered to her lab as the "Amazon Savage," plus a partial cranium of a presumed female discovered on a nearby mountain that Amy wanted to x-ray to check for lead wipe, and the remains of a John Doe decedent whose "extreme alveolar resorption" Amy wanted an opinion on. I had no idea what the latter meant but hoped they'd tell me. "Lead wipe" I was more familiar with: a bullet—a projectile—that has passed through bone can leave behind residue or fragments that may not be visible to the eye but will be evident on a radiograph, or X-ray. While we were getting Ina Jane Doe's panoramic X-rays done, we'd check to see if the decedent recovered on the mountain showed evidence of projectile trauma.

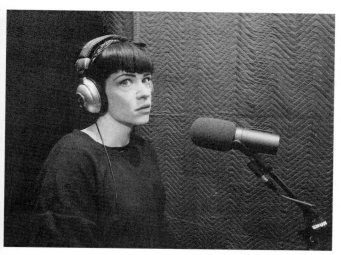

Author, Laurah Norton, waiting for Dr. Amy Michael to get on for a recorded phone call

Medical illustration of Ina Jane Doe
Dr. Steffen Poltak

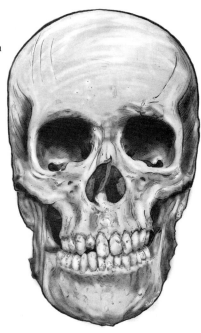

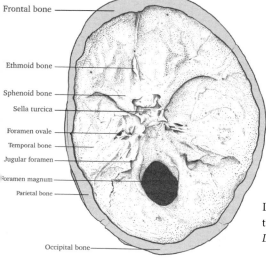

Frontal bone
Ethmoid bone
Sphenoid bone
Sella turcica
Foramen ovale
Temporal bone
Jugular foramen
Foramen magnum
Parietal bone
Occipital bone

Labeled internal skull illustration of Ina Jane Doe
Dr. Steffen Poltak

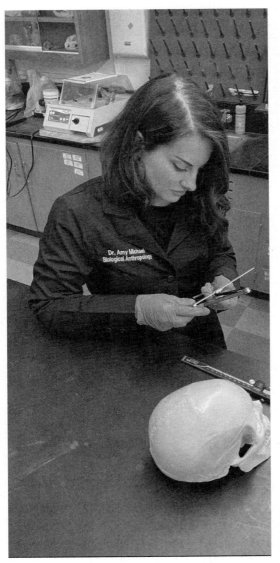

Dr. Amy Michael in a class
demonstration using artificial
human skulls

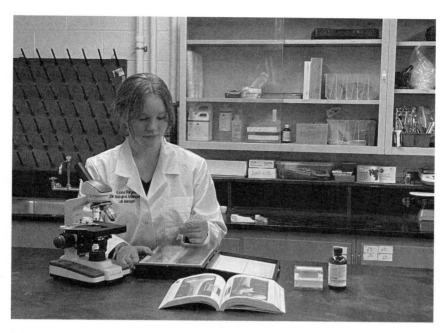

Lab manager Kyana Burgess practicing measurements on artificial skull

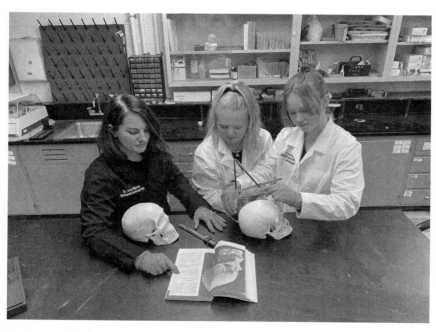

Dr. Amy Michael using artificial (plastic) human skulls to teach students about cranial measurements

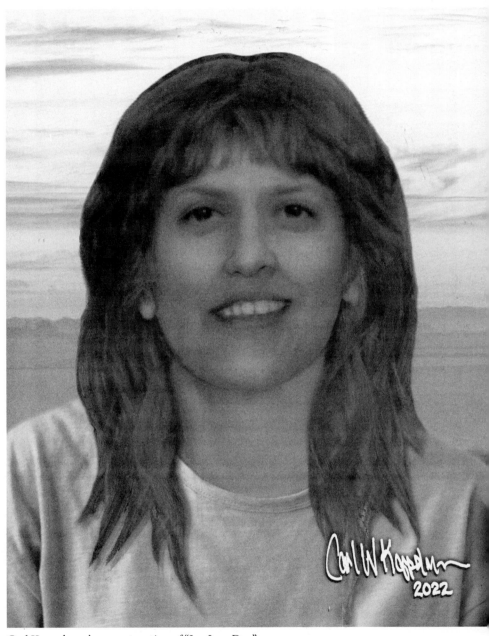

Carl Koppelman's reconstruction of "Ina Jane Doe"
Carl Koppelman

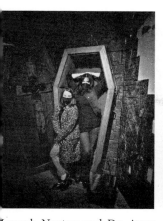

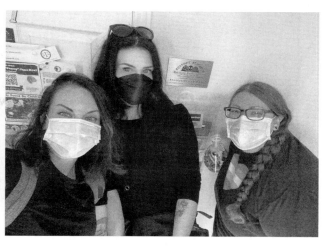

Laurah Norton and Dr. Amy Michael visit the Museum of Pop Culture in Seattle, February 2022 (during the American Academy of Forensic Sciences conference)

Laurah Norton, Dr. Amy Michael, and Dr. Samantha Blatt outside Redgrave Research, September 2021

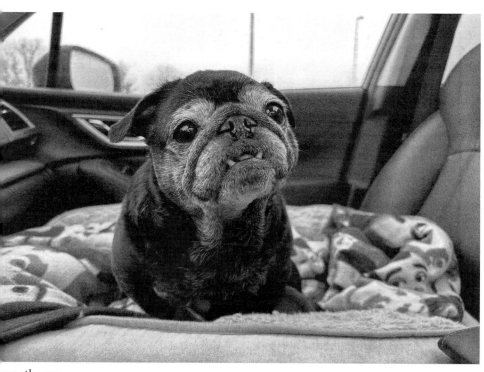

Lucy the pug

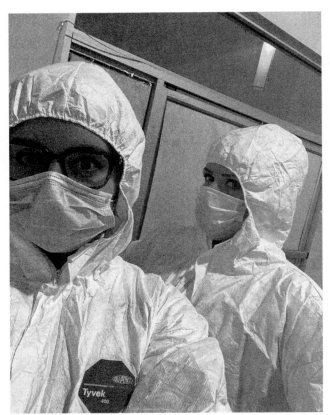

The Fall Line producer Maura Currie and Laurah Norton at Astrea Forensics Lab, November 2021

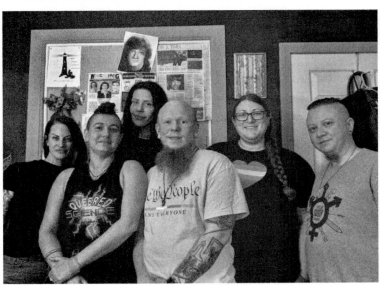

At Redgrave Research, September 2021. From left: Dr. Amy Michael, Viktor Veltstra, Laurah Norton, Anthony Redgrave, Dr. Samantha Blatt, Lee Redgrave

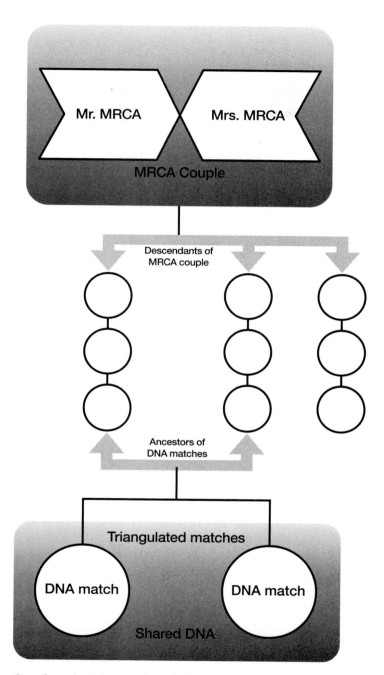

Genealogy chart showing the path from the Most Recent Common
Ancestor to the Doe
Anthony Redgrave

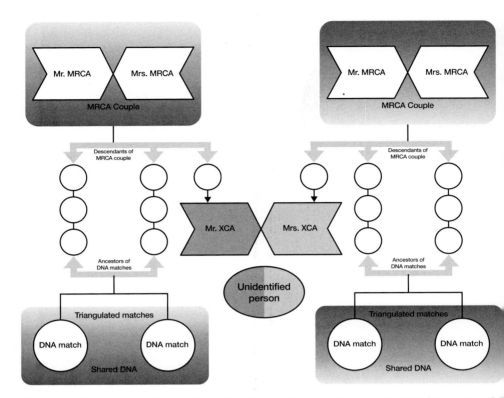

Genealogy chart showing the path from Most Recent Common Ancestors to XCA (Union Couple) to the Doe
Anthony Redgrave

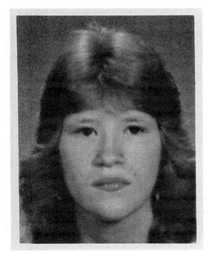

Senior photo of Susan "Sue" Hope Minard, from the Highland High School yearbook

Dr. Albee was practically vibrating with energy as he led us to a little table laid with sterile tools and, yes, more gloves. If we had to perform emergency field surgery on a dozen or so people, we'd be well-equipped in the clean hand department.

He nodded at Amy. "Want to pull some chairs up?"

Amy and Dr. Albee posted up at the table, and the rest of us formed a row opposite out of the overstuffed lobby chairs, like an audience. The dental hygienist who'd offered to stay late, Amelia, was young and friendly; she told us she'd never done anything like this in school. She disappeared into the back to turn on the machines. That's when I caught sight of something else, in the corner: A giant stuffed frog propped up in a chair. Unfortunately, it had its own set of very human teeth. I decided not to mention it. But I kept eyeing that frog. If it was meant to encourage children into brushing their teeth, well . . . I could see why it had ended up in the basement.

I needed notes on everything they had to say, and there was no way I'd be able to spell everything correctly, much less keep up with the speed of their observations. With everyone's permission to record, I dug around in my bag and pieced together a super-basic recording rig. I didn't want to put mics on the little table, especially when delicate human remains would be examined, so I'd just have to hold a shotgun mic and balance the Zoom interface on my lap. It was the kind of sound that would give my podcast's producer, Maura, a migraine, but this was just for my personal use. It always felt funny to be sitting in a room full of people going about their business while I wore headphones and pointed a microphone at them, though. Very *Only Murders in the Building* of me.

While Amy carefully unpacked each skull from their respective boxes, I leaned over to Sam, who sat on my left. She was looking at pictures of her dogs that her fiancé texted in a steady stream while she was out of town.

"What was that reabsorption thing Amy mentioned?"

She rested her phone on her jean-clad knee and leaned toward me.

"It's 'alveolar resorption' you're thinking of. So, that's a by-product of tooth extraction. Imagine when a tooth is removed, and nothing is put in its place? Empty socket, right? So, imagine that over time up to half of the bone from the empty socket is reabsorbed into the upper and lower alveolar ridges. Those are the bony borders covered in skin that hold the roots of teeth in place." She tapped her upper lip. "If you feel with your tongue, you can easily feel the upper portion—it's that bumpy bit above the front teeth."

The difference between scientists and scientists who teach, I'd realized, is that the latter immediately know that people need clear examples. I felt my ridge with my tongue, then nodded.

"Too much reabsorption can make restorative work—like dental implants, that kind of thing—difficult."

"Got it." I kind of got it.

Amy was ready to go. I asked her to dictate what they were doing so I'd have good notes. Dr. Albee spelled his name for me while Amy snapped on her gloves. She cleared her throat and began dictating like a champ.

"We're at Suncook Dental, with Dr. Andrew Albee. It's September 22nd, 2021. We're here to discuss the dentition in several cases, starting with the decedent we're describing as a mummified head discovered at a private school. The deceased was recovered sometime in the early eighties. The decedent's remains have been in the possession of the New Hampshire state archaeologist. The office is currently seeking to determine whether the remains should be repatriated, if we . . . can determine that information. But currently we know nothing."

Dr. Albee looked around at us. "This is great. A real pleasure to help."

I decided to like his frog with the human teeth.

Amy continued, "This person was accessioned by a school, in 1933. One of their alumni donated it. And the donation records list 'severed head of an Amazon Savage.'"

Dr. Albee winced. "That's, uh . . ."

Amy nodded. "It is. So now the State of New Hampshire will pay for testing, if testing is possible, to try and determine more about this individual. Because their view is that it's unethical to have this individual's remains in storage if they can be returned, and if they are Native American and need to be repatriated, that's law. So, they want to pay for

AMS dating and Strontium Isotopes analysis to determine how old the mummy is and where they originated from."

Dr. Albee asked, "And would the next step be to contact authorities, like the embassy representing the country . . . ?"

Amy nodded. "Exactly. If the individual originated from outside the United States, they'd work with representatives to begin repatriation."

Dr. Albee whistled. "This is fascinating."

Amy gingerly handed him the decedent's head so he could begin his examination. "I'm glad you think so. Otherwise, this was going to be embarrassing."

Dr. Albee selected a small mirror. It was a delicate business, to examine the teeth he could see: the deceased's mouth was firmly closed in such a position that forcing it open could destroy the remains. Their skin still clung to their head in a dehydrated kind of sheaf, but it was gummier than the Tilton Mummy's resin coating; I could see the remnants of some kind of bandage wrapping and the marks of the hair Amy had shown me earlier, even in the light of the dentist's basement. Dr. Albee was unwilling to risk damaging the individual's mouth by inserting the little mirror farther than a few centimeters—but he was able to make some observations. Amy held a small flashlight for him to maximize visibility.

Dr. Albee glanced at the three of us who were still sitting in our lounge chairs. I pointed the shotgun mic expectantly.

"So, you guys are hoping for some good information from me, huh?" he said after a moment.

Amy snorted. "Yeah, no pressure, but I did bring guests."

He laughed. "Okay, so, when we number teeth, we start in the upper right. I think you guys do the same thing. One, two, three, four, all the way to thirty-two."

They all nodded. I decided to nod, too.

"Looks like they're missing a second molar on the upper right, tooth 2. And either missing or an impacted wisdom tooth in the upper left. Two molars on the lower left. A lot of front teeth are broken off, but that damage looks like—you'd call it postmortem, right? I'll say that. As if they fractured after death. So, this person had all their teeth. Really heavy grinder, which could be parafunction. Or more likely, diet. Eating stuff that's tough on the teeth."

He pointed out that the wear on the decedent's teeth was mechanical, but there was no sign of decay. He and the anthropologists discussed possible diets that might have created that wear—*preindustrial preparations* of grain, which Sam translated for me as "stone ground."

As he used a probe to gently touch one tooth, Sam said from her seat next to me, "I actually clean a lot of teeth, too. Well, to collect dental calculus in cases."

Dr. Albee was having an excellent night. "Oh really? What does that tell you?"

"Diet. The evolutionary change of oral flora and sometimes migration. It can be a lot."

I had an uncomfortable moment imagining what could be discovered about me after my six-month cleaning. Probably a lot relating to coffee intake.

Dr. Albee delicately set the decedent's head back on the table. "All I can say now is that it looks like maybe they broke one tooth off from an injury and had a few impacted wisdom teeth. That's in life. The wear, though—largely, that just looks like someone who's eating a really fibrous diet."

"Any guesses about age at death?" I realized I was pointing the mic directly into Sam's ear and shifted position.

Dr. Albee frowned, thinking. He was up again, walking around in a tight little circle near the large monitor. "It's considerable wear, so I would put that person well at or above their thirties. Even with the diet."

Amy asked if they could try a panoramic exam; Dr. Albee was game, but he needed Amelia's help. They figured out a system to create a test patient file to store the radiograph, and Dr. Albee held the decedent's head while Amelia ran the machine. There wasn't enough room for us to crowd back there while they accomplished it, but they talked us through what was happening. Since they were already doing the X-rays, Amy began the process of carrying each decedent's remains to the back, one by one, so they could complete the radiograph process; then, we could view all of them in one go on the big screen. Ina Jane Doe was the last. Once all were finished, we crowded back in to review.

Dr. Albee finished the mummified decedent's exam first. When he pulled up the radiograph, he was able to confirm the impacted wisdom teeth he'd suspected, but we weren't able to glean much more information.

For the second and third cases Amy had brought, things went quickly: She got the radiograph she needed to test for lead wipe—there was none—and then Dr. Albee did a brief examination on the John Doe decedent's skull with what Amy had described as the alveolar resorption. He examined a few different points in the decedent's mandible; Amy told him the individual was a presumed white male.

"This is extreme bone loss. I'd say you're looking at someone who was probably a longtime denture wearer," he said. "That can certainly contribute to the loss."

Amy made notes for the three cases and repacked each decedent's remains into their respective protective containers; she'd add this information to her case file on each. She stuck her pen back in her bun for easy access later on.

Finally, Dr. Albee turned his attention to Ina Jane Doe. I'd been waiting to hear his opinion; when Amy first spoke to him, she'd called me, excited, on the drive home, but I'd had trouble parsing all the tooth talk as her signal cut in and out on the New Hampshire highway.

Still, every time I saw Ina Jane Doe's skull sitting out on a table, it bothered me. It's not that the experts weren't doing what they could to help identify her—that's exactly what was needed. It's why I'd been flying up and down the East Coast and driving across the Midwest with Amy. But seeing her, with the autopsy cuts across the cranium, and the glue, and thinking about all the eyes that had already been on her . . . she needed to be at rest. The other cases felt easier because I knew less about them. But it was all the same.

Ina's radiograph was on the widescreen, showing us the details we'd examined again and again—but now, we were looking at them from an entirely new angle. Amy began speaking for my tape, going over what we knew and letting Dr. Albee add in his thoughts as she went. We knew that Ina's dentition was rather unique. She'd definitely had dental care, but it had dropped off sometime in the last few years of her life. When she died, she'd had significant decay in a number of teeth, especially her back molars, which were so damaged that Dr. Albee said they likely would no longer have been painful; it was past that point.

Dr. Albee estimated that she'd gone at least five years without significant dental care; her tartar buildup suggested that, and then there was the significant decay. But perhaps she had thin enamel to begin with, like me.

We were particularly interested in a series of notches along Ina Jane Doe's anterior, or top, teeth across the upper right quadrant: Those were the possible hypoplasias the anthropologists had discussed. Amy was more in the "possible braces" camp, but Les thought they weren't caused by dental gear.

Dr. Albee took a look. "These notches indicate to me, at least, that she probably had braces. The straightness of her teeth indicates that she had braces and then maybe didn't wear a retainer."

Les asked, "Do you think they could be pitting enamel hypoplasia?" She explained for my notes, "Depressions, basically. They could range from microscopic to visible pits in the tooth. So, pitting hypoplasia are developmental defects of the enamel that become apparent during childhood, right? They can be scattered or form patterns." They'd all risen from their chairs to stand in front of the table by this point, so they could look from Ina's teeth to the radiograph display.

Dr. Albee considered. "Absolutely, I think it could be that. But the teeth, developing at different times—they're not necessarily going to line up like this. Tooth number five came in when she was twelve, but braces aren't a foregone conclusion."

We wouldn't know for sure until we positively identified her. But I'd begin looking for cases where the missing person was described as wearing braces, or having had them, and flag those if they fit in our other parameters.

Dr. Albee turned his attention to Ina's root canal—"silver point filling," he called it—and showed us what it looked like on the big screen. I'd seen one of my own crowns and root canals in a radiograph before, and he and the original forensic odontologist were right; this was distinctive. It almost looked like a straight, sharp pin shot through the root.

"And she was found when?" Dr. Albee asked.

"1993," Amy said.

"Okay, so, that would make sense, especially with the estimation that she's at thirty-five to fifty. She could have older work. You also see these more in the military. She could have been a military kid or military personnel herself."

I perked up. "Why do you say military?" The major theory online had been institutional, public hospital work. Amy told me that wasn't the route she thought we should pursue, but I was interested to hear alternative theories.

Dr. Albee shrugged. "Maybe that's just modern dentistry, but a lot of the silver points that I see now are from the military. It was probably cheaper."

Sam had been quiet for a while; I only realized it when she suddenly spoke. She was squinting up at the radiograph. "Are those teeth in wrong?"

"Which?" She was looking back and forth, and now Amy and Les and Dr. Albee were, too.

She squatted down next to the table so she was eye level with Ina. "Right here, see? . . . because the right and left don't look like they're correctly situated . . . the mesial side should be the flat side. And the distal side should . . . is that winging or something? No, they're just in the wrong spot."

"Holy shit," Amy said. "You're right. That's not a crooked tooth." She pointed to show me the central right incisor. "See this? It's been switched with another tooth, glued in the wrong spot."

I could only think of one reason for that. "Maybe . . . her tooth or teeth were removed for testing?"

"Maybe, or for other reasons. Or teeth fell out and had to be glued back in."

Amy looked at me. I knew we were both thinking of the forensic art of Ina that had been circulating for decades. There was the asymmetry we didn't think was present—not to the degree it was portrayed, anyway. We weren't convinced of the wry neck syndrome that was so prominently featured. And now, the distinctive presentation of a crooked, jagged smile? It was based on two misplaced teeth and another that had broken postmortem. That wasn't the fault of the artists; the only image available to share was becoming even further removed from what she had actually looked like.

"It's not going to come out," Amy decided, after gently testing the tooth. We don't want to risk it with all the glue. "Good catch, Sam."

Sam smiled. She *was* very good with teeth.

"Anything else we should note based on the panoramic?" I wanted to know.

"The important facts are confirmed, I'd say." Amy glanced over to Dr. Albee for confirmation. He nodded. She pulled the pen from her bun and started pointing at points on the screen; I did the same thing in class with my dry-erase markers. "We have pitting across the upper right quadrant, possibly from braces, or pitting enamel hypoplasia. There was a composite restoration that had replaced most of her lateral incisor. Good dental upkeep, and then significant decay. Wisdom teeth removed. An old-fashioned crown, with the silverpoint."

"So, I have a few new avenues for research. That's great. I'm going to turn this off so everyone can chat without feeling like they're being, uhm, recorded."

As the flat-screen went dark, I considered Dr. Albee's points about braces and the military. *Had* something happened to cut off her access to care? Or was I falling into the same rabbit holes I'd been trying to avoid online?

We each carried a box to Les's vehicle and then walked back to the entrance of Suncook to say goodbye to Dr. Albee and Amelia, who were locking up the office. I'd been thinking about saying something for the past few minutes and had decided he was so welcoming that I could chance it.

"So . . . ," I started. "That frog downstairs?"

He laughed. "Yeah, the kids love that thing. It's been manhandled by a thousand of them."

Les had apparently missed the frog. "What was with the frog?"

"It had, uhm, human teeth."

"Oh no."

Dr. Albee wasn't at all offended. "You wouldn't believe the stuff we've collected that has teeth."

"I think it's cute," Amy offered.

She *would*.

"Of course you do, because you have *puppets*. It's exactly the kind of thing Amy would have at her house," I told Dr. Albee. That was the truth. I'd been sleeping in her office on a very nice inflatable mattress—Sam was sleeping in the only spare bedroom, down in Amy's basement. But staying in her office also meant I was spending a lot of time with her *unique* collections.

Amy cut her eyes at me. "Don't mischaracterize me. They're *ventriloquist dummies*."

"That's worse," I told her.

Sam and Les nodded vigorously. Dr. Albee gazed at us with polite confusion, like that young, fun uncle who was willing to play along with whatever game the kids came up with. Really, he was a very nice man.

CHAPTER TEN

THE METHOD: FORENSIC ART

Every artist has reconstructed the human face. Every *person* has—once you pick up a crayon, a pencil, a piece of charcoal, and attempt to capture reality on paper, you've joined the ranks of those who want to transmit and transfigure. Create, sure, but isn't it really re-creation—of a real person, or even the picture you see in your head—to try to move that image from your mind to the paper in an uninterrupted flow?

I minored in art in college, mostly because I liked it. Drawing people had always been my favorite thing to do—though I wasn't overly fond of "naked model" sketching sessions—but I could never *quite* get it right: the way skin dimpled in over the elbow, or the crinkle at the corner of an eye. It was a good thing, my instructor said, that I was not a major. I could produce a competent portrait, but you'd never look at that sheet of paper and feel a shock of recognition: *There they are. I know them.*

But forensic artists, the best of them? They are specialists who can do that on a whole other level. They aren't using models, not in the traditional sense. And their imaginations must work backward rather than forward. They are not just creators; they repair and reconstruct what once was there, often without any blueprint beyond the suggestions left in the clefts and the angles of a human skull.

Whether they work in pencil and paper, or clay, or 3-D digital modeling, the process is much the same: Correctly estimate how the math of the human bone structure would have added up into a face and re-create that face so that it looks and feels like a person. Then, it might be recognized by those who knew the human it represents. Few artists take their work lightly. But those working in death reconstruction—it's difficult to imagine higher stakes. Creative success means case closure. Get something too far off the mark, and there's the danger an unidentified person will never be recognized.

The story behind Ina Jane Doe's forensic art isn't covered in her police file. There are actually three separate reconstructions in existence. There was an early sketch, done by someone in Illinois, and then a more detailed forensic drawing circulated to the public. Later, a clay bust was released. We were unable to access the name of the sculptor during our work with Jefferson County. The artist who drew Ina Jane Doe's original, circulated sketch is well-known; Charles Holt, a former law-enforcement officer, has trained many other officers and even departments in art. He's one of the artists who worked with my friend Todd Matthews of the Doe Network on an initiative that Todd launched years back called Project EDAN: Everyone Deserves a Name. He got forensic artists from around the country to donate their time and create art for cases that had no professional renderings—and Holt was able to assist between receiving training at Quantico and teaching his own classes.[1]

All this to say—Charles Holt is certainly no amateur. That's important to point out, because Ina's sketch has appeared on a number of "most shocking forensic art" posts and listicles. Some of the art that is included is there because it's considered—by those who gathered it, at least—to be bad. That's not the case with Holt's sketch of Ina Jane Doe; his drawing skill is evident. Rather, the art is considered memorable, and probably shocking, based on the features that both he and the clay reconstructionist were tasked with interpreting. *Interpreting* is the key word here: There are so many choices a forensic artist must make. And in Ina Jane Doe's case, they had, in some ways, less information—no postcrania—and also a lot of skeletal detail to interpret.

Ina's teeth, which Sam noticed had been glued in backward, and the tooth that had been broken off postmortem? Those were features the

artists had to take at face value; they had no notations regarding dentition, as far as we know. They also had to make calls based on Dr. Klepinger's report: How much asymmetry should they show in the decedent's
features? Should they display the possible torticollis she noted? How old
should they make the decedent? In those cases, both artists chose to show
asymmetry, and torticollis, and hedge closer to the outer reaches of the
age range; that was the expert opinion at the time. There's always an element of chance involved, even if they'd had access to postmortem photos
as well as Ina Jane Doe's skull for reference. A face in death is not a face in
life, and she'd experienced postmortem violence.

I'm a bigger fan of forensic art than some of my friends; it might be
all that time spent in creative writing workshops. Suggestion, I think, is
a powerful thing. Amy has come to appreciate art more than she once
did, but she and many others—even some artists—prefer the term
"approximation" to "reconstruction." Amy put it to me this way: "Forensic reconstruction makes it sound like the image produced should precisely replicate the person during life. We cannot possibly know exactly
how they looked, since the skull tells us nothing about hair color or style,
eye color, or how they wore makeup. 'Approximation' better describes the
intent which is to, as close as possible, approximate the reality of what the
person *could* have looked like."

And for Amy that makes perfect sense. She works with skeletonized
decedents. She knows, of course, that there are cases where the artist does
have some of that information—when, say, a decedent is found hours or
days after death—but their photo can't be used in the media. But even
then, there will be unknowns. Decomposition, the effects of the manner
of death, and even the slackening of muscles can change the visual presentation of the face. And, as Amy importantly pointed out, how we look
in death is often not how we look in life.

That's another guessing game forensic artists must play: how best to
present this creation, to catch the eye of the right person, to spark a memory. Should you use color? What about including clothing? There are
arguments made on both sides as to whether specific choices can neg-
atively affect identification. A colorful and arresting image may catch

someone's eye; but they may focus on some small detail that is incorrect, and not see the forest for the trees. If a drawing or composite is in black-and-white, perhaps they won't discount an approximation because the shade of hair or skin tone isn't quite right. But, then again, it's much less likely to be shared on social media and run repeatedly by the media—and that's where people will have the best chance of seeing it. Then there's the choice of medium: a sketch versus a digital image, which can be so lifelike that the viewer can mistake them for photos—which, again, can be good or bad. A composite of available features. A forensic clay bust, most often shaped upon the skull.

Many of the techniques forensics artists use now—the manual, hands-on work, at least—have existed for a century or considerably more. For instance, measuring tissue depths to re-create the proper angles of a human face is a craft that took decades upon decades to perfect. That doesn't mean techniques have failed to evolve to meet the needs of forensics; 2-D re-creations, or manual drawings, have necessarily shifted to meet the unique needs of an artist working from bone, or burned flesh, or partial remains. Innovation has been necessary, and in that regard, artists have pulled forensic science forward. They've melded classic techniques with digital developments to provide the most accurate reconstructions possible.

Karen Taylor is perhaps *the* most influential forensic artist in the United States. Maybe in the world. I spot her book, *Forensic Art and Illustration*, in the office of every forensic artist I meet. Some anatomical artists, too. Taylor's book covers technique, but it also delves into the history of the discipline. She describes, for instance, the 1932 case of Isabella Kerr, who was the longtime romantic partner of an English doctor, Buck Ruxton, and mother to his three children. The couple were known for their fiery arguments. After one such fight, Isabella and her maid, Mary Jane Rogerson, disappeared.

There were no leads for weeks—that is, until "grisly remains were found near the Scottish border." Apparently, the remains recovered were difficult to distinguish: human bodies—likely two, because two skulls were recovered—had been dismembered, and then packaged into more than fifty parcels.[2]

To ascertain that the bodies belonged to the missing women, a new technique was employed. Photographic superimposition of Isabella's face and a picture of each of the skulls was arranged. Then, some of the best doctors and anatomists in England were invited to examine the results. They were able to line up the features exactly.

In the 1980s, Karen Taylor developed a similar method to use on unidentified decedent cases in her own work; she devised a use of the pictures that were helpful even when there was no possible comparison to be made. She sketched the faces of the deceased directly over photographs of their skulls.[3] Her method, which gained widespread popularity, is not so different from the 3-D computer programs in use today: Using measurements, artists are able to take CT scans of skulls and fill in missing pieces. They can then build—virtually—the faces, bit by bit, until a distinct and unique human emerges.

The technology might be new, but the practice isn't. Contemporary forensic artists may work toward different goals, but there's ample evidence that a number of early civilizations created art upon human skulls, building up representations of human faces—sometimes realistic, sometimes with modified or exaggerated features—all over the globe.[4] And think of the funerary masks of ancient Egypt, or the death masks of the Western world, which were popular through the dawn of the twentieth century and the availability of the camera.

Many famous faces were captured in death: Dante Alighieri, Mary Queen of Scots, Ludwig van Beethoven, John Keats, William Blake, Napoleon Bonaparte, and even Charles Dickens were all cast in wax or plaster. Some of these masks were used as the basis of statues, like the bust in the Dickens Museum;[5] others, cast of the infamous or obscure, might be forgotten on dusty shelves in mortuary storage or university labs.

Death masks served practical purposes, too; they were also produced as a medical record. The Somerton Man's plaster cast indirectly identified him as Charles "Carl" Webb. And when you think about how scientists preserved examples of anomalies, growths, and other conditions before photography was widespread, molds were, along with illustrations, practical.[6] Those are the models likely to turn up in forgotten corners of university labs. They tend to shock the students. And some police morgues discovered in the nineteenth century that the practice could come in handy in preserving the image of the dead—until, of course, cameras were plentiful. But conditions needed to be ideal. Otherwise, what one needed, truly, was a reconstruction. A death mask, or a picture, wouldn't help in identification if a person no longer looked like their living self.

The first true forensic reconstructions of unidentified skeletonized people were also attempted in the late nineteenth century, when archaeologists and anatomists began to examine data sets based on historic skulls, and also the various tissue depths found in the facial features of the recently dead. By gathering significant data on both subjects, scientists were eventually able to come up with average tissue depths for various facial features, which they grouped by age, sex, and race. Though these numbers have been further honed and expanded, the use of tissue-depth measurements as a guide to creating something more lifelike—a true reconstruction—is a long-standing practice.[7]

Modern facial reconstruction builds on such concepts. Whether produced in 2-D sketch, 3-D clay upon a skull, a digital image, or even via 3-D printing, an artist must use their knowledge of anatomy and how hard and soft tissue connects—how to measure and estimate the depth of that tissue, how it might lie across the bone. Skill plays an important role, as in any art form, but the stakes here are even higher: The choices a forensic artist makes can be the difference that resolves a cold case.

Nowadays, there are more tools available—even DNA phenotyping, like the process used at Parabon NanoLabs here in the United States, which allows us to predict to reasonable certainties what a person might have looked like in life based only on their DNA. Their analysis can give an artist information that practitioners thirty years ago only *dreamed* of. When I spoke to Dr. Ellen Greytak of Parabon NanoLabs, she explained to me how the company's Snapshot Advanced DNA Analysis Service— which, among other things, provides DNA phenotyping—aids in the art they provide in both perpetrator and unidentified cases. As Dr. Greytak clarified, "For unidentified remains, the phenotypes predicting the person's appearance can be very useful. I mean, of course, if you don't have a skull, then getting a reconstruction is very, very difficult. [. . .] And what we've seen a lot, especially, is that the ancestry is often different from what was predicted from the anthropology."

With the addition of DNA phenotyping, a reconstruction can be more precise in regard to the victim's ancestry groups, including (but not limited to) traits like eye color, hair color, and skin tone. Whether they're presenting an unidentified decedent's reconstruction, or a perpetrator's possible features, the artwork is framed in an interesting way: You can't forget that it is not a final product, but rather, a possibility based on averages and interpretation. Along with the digital image of a perpetrator or unidentified decedent's face, we're presented with ancestry origin results, sex, and in the case of decedents, age estimation and body mass (if known). Parabon offers a scale of graduation of shade and a confidence in prediction. This is very helpful when you're looking at the reconstruction, because you're forced to remember the nature of approximation.

I first became aware of Parabon's use of phenotyping in forensic art when I saw their reconstruction of a young woman formerly known as the Anne Arundel County Jane Doe.[8] The Anne Arundel Jane Doe's remains were discovered on June 14, 2017, in Glen Burnie, Maryland. Law enforcement found the partially skeletonized remains of a presumed young-adult female "covered up by a tarp," and noted, consequently, "foul play was suspected in her death."[9] The Anne Arundel County Police worked with Parabon on a forensic reconstruction of the victim that combined both skeletal analysis and "DNA predictions in order to generate an image of how the victim may have looked when she was alive." The Snapshot predicted the decedent was primarily of African ancestry (West and South), with a small percentage of Northeastern European ancestry. Her age was pictured at approximately twenty-five, and the Snapshot predicted her skin color as brown or dark brown with 99.4 percent confidence, her eye color as brown or hazel with 87.5 percent confidence, her hair color as black with 100 percent confidence, and her likelihood of having zero freckles at 90.6 percent confidence. The resulting forensic art was circulated to local law enforcement in surrounding areas, and the Baltimore City Police Department responded; they had a missing-persons report for a woman named Shaquana Caldwell, twenty-six, who matched the description. She was last seen a month before the Anne Arundel Jane Doe's remains were discovered. This tentative identification was verified via dental records, and later on, Shaquana's boyfriend was arrested for her murder.[10]

Even though Shaquana's case was solved very quickly, Dr. Greytak cautioned me: Like any other forensic art, a Snapshot should not be treated as a photograph. It's a *prediction*. There are variables outside our DNA and skeletal features that can affect appearance that an artist or scientist simply can't account for: weight, hairstyle, health, previous injuries. Nothing is a sure thing. But science and art, together, can get us a little closer.

I'm lucky enough to be friends with a forensic artist, and one who I consider to be one of the best in the country. Am I objective? No. Am I right? Definitely.

Kelly Lawson, the renowned second-generation forensic artist, first caught my attention when I saw what she did for the mother of a long-missing child, whose case we were covering on the show. Kelly created something that in two years of true-crime research I'd never seen before: an age progression of a baby of whom no photograph existed.

At the time, my podcast *The Fall Line* was covering a long-running series of infant abductions associated with Grady Memorial Hospital in Atlanta from 1978 to 1996. Kelly had recently completed a sketch of one of the two infants—who would now be adults—who were still missing. Because Raymond Green was just five days old when he was kidnapped, his mother, Donna, had no pictures of him. Kelly needed to use alternative methods to imagine Raymond, whom she drew as a toddler, and then as an adult man. She did this by studying the Green family, both in person and in photos, and tracing their growth.

She then compared those images with Donna's memories and began her work. The resulting portraits were startling and beautiful, drawn in Kelly's signature color palette: muted pastels, soft earth tones, plenty of light in eyes, across the cheeks. She had re-created Raymond, or as close to him as she could—he looked like a member of the Green family. Donna could recognize him. The adult picture was for forensic purposes. But the toddler? That was for Donna. To give her something to hold on to. Now that she has seen these versions of Raymond, she wonders less about the faces she sees on the street: *Is that my son? Is that him?* It hasn't stopped. But it's better.

Over the past four years, Kelly and I have stayed in contact. She's one of the experts I trust the most. She can tell the work of other artists without seeing a signature, and she's always able to explain technique to me, or why a certain approach was taken. I've been in to watch her build a clay reconstruction for a decedent; after a quick trip to the art supply store for more hot glue and such, she let me practice cutting tissue-depth markers from the long, skinny, pink automatic-eraser refills I hadn't seen since middle school. She had a special tool to measure them precisely, and handed me a razor blade to use as I worked from a tissue-depth table—not so different from the kind of information that is kept in FORDISC. It gave average depths and widths based on ancestral groups, and though I followed the chart as exactly as I could, my efforts were . . . well, let's just say, she didn't use my tissue-depth markers. I maintain her measurement tool is designed for right-handed people and that I was at a marked disadvantage.

I've been to Kelly's office a handful of times now, and we've done formal interviews at the GBI headquarters, on the phone, and even at her mother Marla's house, which is a pretty big deal. Absolutely *everyone* in Georgia knows about Marla. She started as a typist in the Atlanta Police Department, and eventually she began doing sketches for the department because they didn't have anyone else—anyone else probably being "a man" in that context. But Marla was good. *Very* good. And soon, she was driving all over the state to do sketches and clay reconstructions. Eventually, she would become the GBI's full-time forensic artist.

When Marla started, there was no program, no blueprint. She had to design everything herself—she was the first. Not the first professional forensic artist, of course; she was aware of the other big names in the field, like Karen Taylor and Betty Pat Gatliff, whose classes her daughter Kelly would later attend. But as far as the GBI was concerned, Marla was the first person to create perpetrator sketches, reconstructions, and age progressions full-time. And she worked that job for decades.

Around the time Marla was looking to retire, Kelly was at a turning point in her own life. She had an art degree from Brigham Young University, in Utah. She'd grown up learning from her mother and watching her work. Marla was having trouble finding a replacement; no one she considered was up to her standards—until Kelly became her mother's next job applicant.

Kelly once told me, "[Marla's] very old school. She says exactly what she thinks. If she feels like you're wasting her time, she tells you. So, she approached me one day, and she said, 'Kelly, can you draw a face?' She threw me a mugshot. And I drew it on the paper as best I could. She said, 'It ain't great, but it's better than what other people were doing.'"

Kelly got the job. She began training under her mother and eventually took over as her mother retired. In the years since, she's come to love the work. It's such a part of who she is that she can't imagine doing anything else. She is at home in that lab, where bones sit in marked evidence bags on shelves, waiting for her to sculpt life into them, or to imagine their features onto paper, exact enough so that someone, out there, might recognize the person they'd been. It feels like magic, what she is able to do for these people.

Kelly's office at the GBI is more like a lab than a studio, with cabinets and counters lining the walls, and a storage closet to one side. However, it's been adapted to the needs of an artist: a drawing table at the center of the room. Supplies stacked—charcoal, pencils, pastels. The space is low ceilinged but bright, with lots of windows to give her the light her art needs, even if the view was less scenic and more parking than she might wish. Every time I visit her, our conversations are punctuated with the slamming sound of the parking-level back door and the echoes of the stairwell just above her space.

Kelly's portraits decorate walls, clipped up on bulletin boards and pasted to white-painted cement, some in black-and-white, others in color.

There's a permanent gallery, and then the cases she's working on: suspects, drawn from witness descriptions. John and Jane Does she'd built up from skeletal remains. Sprinkled throughout her collection are celebrities, like Biggie Smalls and Tupac—projects to keep her fresh between cases. Not that she's ever had an abundance of free time.

As the only forensic artist working for the GBI, Kelly might be called to travel anywhere in the state. She might assist local law enforcement or a regional bureau office. With little notice, she would need to be packed and ready to go. But sometimes, her subjects come to her: skeletal remains, delivered by agents or couriers. These she stores in that closet area, where she works on facial reconstructions, meticulously measuring clay to match estimated depth of tissue. After more than a decade in the field, she can picture the decedents' faces—how they should look—in her mind. Work had slowed down some, for a time, during the early days of the pandemic; perpetrator cases were made more difficult to sketch because of masks. But Kelly did many more unidentified-persons sketches from 2020 to 2022, more than she'd done in the previous eight years put together. I'd wondered about why that was, suspecting that maybe departments finally had time to go back through their files.

It's always easy to spot Kelly's work. Marla's, too. Her portraits don't look like mugshots. In her imagination, unidentified people are as they might have been in life—smiling, looking over one shoulder, their hair moving, their eyes crinkling at the corners. It's a style reminiscent of, yet distinct from, her mother's; both can get life into paper, into clay, where others can't quite manage it. Kelly prefers pastels, and Marla did a lot of pencil work, in grayscale; they're both versatile. Even so, anyone who knows forensic art can spot a Lawson piece, even if they can't see the signature.

It's even more impressive when one realizes what they're working with. You might imagine that Marla and Kelly Lawson received well-preserved skulls, in one piece and ready for reconstruction. But that was only sometimes the case. More often than not, forensic artists are given mere pieces: a jaw (mandible), a few teeth, fragile sections of cranium that must be unpacked with care and laid out on soft cushioning to protect the bones.

We'd been lucky with Ina Jane Doe that she was well-preserved and whole.

Kelly sometimes worked even more indirectly. There had been times when all that was left were photos of remains, or a living person, and she'd have to make do with those. Not too long ago, Kelly told me a story about one of those situations. In this case, she was looking at a victim who'd been discovered in Brooks, a rural county in South Georgia. After a traveling fair packed up and departed from the tiny town of Dixie, GA, a young woman had been found, both stabbed and strangled. A fair employee, George Newsome, was eventually convicted of her murder, but her identity remained a mystery.[11] When law enforcement reviewed the case, they came to Kelly for updated art.

The photos that Kelly was given to work with were likely the ones taken at the funeral parlor, where Jane Doe's body was displayed for as long as possible. Then, a local philanthropist funded a proper burial for the decedent—including a cement vault, and a headstone marked with the words: "Known Only to God."[12] That vault would prove to be a valuable choice, later, when DNA testing needed to be done.

After close to thirty years without an identification, the agent in charge of Jane Doe's case asked Kelly if she could update the victim's portrait. "I got these Polaroids there in black and white and I redrew her. Now, there's a lot to be desired from the photos and it's difficult to get a completely accurate view of what she would've looked like. But really, I just kind of followed my intuition and produced for them what I deem to be a very beautiful, full color, almost three-quarter profile drawing of what this girl looked like. And I gave it to him, told him they could do with it as they will. I filled out my little report and I moved on."

But that wasn't the end of it. A year later, the same agent called Kelly again. "He said, 'Kelly, I'm just letting you know, you're going to be on the front page of the paper down here.' And I thought, 'Well, that's interesting. No one's come up here to take my picture.' He said, 'Oh, no. We got some stock photos we're going to use, but you're going to be on the front page.' I said, 'Well, why am I going to be on the front page?' He said, 'You remember that drawing you did for me last year? . . . Well, we aired that drawing. And a woman who went to school with her, who lives in a totally different part of the country, saw that story online, called down here, and said, 'I'm pretty sure I went to school with her.'"

It turned out that the woman *had* been a classmate of the decedent, who had been considered a missing person for decades. Shirlene "Cheryl" Hammack had left her family behind in Thomaston, GA, in 1981 so she could take a job with a traveling fair, but she'd stayed in regular contact, as her mother and sister told reporters. They'd heard from her several times a week. When those communications ceased, they knew something was wrong, so they filed a missing-persons report. Unfortunately, there were no real leads in Cheryl's case—not until her classmate saw Kelly's drawing, all those years later, and called the GBI. Cheryl's body was exhumed, and in January 2020 her positive identification was announced.[13]

That solve came down to simple recognition: Kelly's ability to capture likeness with pastel and charcoal. She's interested in all the advancements in forensic art, but she remains a classic portrait artist. It's in her training, and probably her blood. When Marla Lawson started, decades ago, there were no computer programs, or 3-D printers, or labs like Parabon, or digital initiatives like the Forensic Anthropology and Computer Enhancement Services (FACES) in Louisiana, which creates phenomenal digital art. There were bones, and the supplies she could dig up at a hardware store. There was no one to teach her. Sure, there were anatomy books, and her texts on forensic art, and data sets of tissue and bone—but she would have to figure out how to transform a skull into a face on her own.

I first met Marla in person in 2018 to talk to her about a case she'd worked on: the reconstruction of a toddler, "Christmas Doe," who'd been found in the woods down in South Georgia. Brooke and I drove out to meet Marla at her house. She and Kelly and the rest of the family had just been to church and came home for a meal. I think we might have been expecting a nice, neat suburban Southern house—something with an emerald square of lawn. Maybe a fancy mailbox in a tasteful shade of beige brick that didn't interfere with HOA requirements.

Instead, we pulled up to the archetypal artist's home: tall, and full of windows and light. The yard is absolutely bursting with plants—crepe myrtles grown to the size of trees, great broad green leaves that brush your face as you walk under them, flowers jutting up wherever they please.

I'd recorded my conversations with Marla to use on the podcast, of course, but so much of what I captured then wasn't included. It was several hours' worth of introduction to forensic art, and what it was like to work on cases in the 1980s and 1990s. I could have listened to several more hours of Marla's memories, to be honest. Marla told us that whenever she got a new case, the bones would arrive in a paper sack—like the kind you might pack a child's lunch in. Moisture was the enemy of her work, and any material other than a brown paper bag could cause the remains to further degrade.

The job was never easy, and the harshest critic a forensic artist often has is themselves. According to Marla, a major part of the job was questioning oneself—and questioning the doctor or anthropologist's determinations, too. You had to know that being wrong could mean a miss at identification—a case never closed. You needed to judge every choice you made, about the shape of the face, the set of the jaw, and in bigger things: race, age. You had to try your best to get it right, even though you know that, sometimes, you'd miss.

She also told us how she got started on a new clay reconstruction. "What I did was go to Home Depot and assemble some little stands with plumbers' pipes on them, so I could just sit the skull in front of me." She gestured, spreading out her fingers as if they were spanning the distance of a human face. "There are a series of markers, which are erasers that are cut in different tissue depths."

She wasn't talking about the pink erasers at the ends of pencils that children use in school, but rather the same ones I'd bought with Kelly: long strips of cylindrical eraser that are sold in office supply stores and used to fill mechanical pen-like contraptions. Those strips were a mainstay in Marla's reconstruction. They could easily be carved into pegs of varying length, to match the tissue depth of faces. Those numbers had been established through cadaver studies, by doctors using rods to measure and establish norms. Forensic artists still use these erasers—or sometimes wooden pegs, measured to those same depths—to help them mold clay to a skull.

"Now, they have all sorts of wonderful things like CAT scans and all sorts of machines that'll get up under there and give you the tissue depth thickness. But then? You got your little erasers and you glued them on the different landmarks of the face." Marla said that she'd experimented with this for six months, never quite happy with her work. Then came a revelation: the material was the problem. The clay she'd been using was too fragile. As she shaped one part of the face, another would be dented or damaged in the process.

She decided to go to the craft store, where she found a kind of air-dry product, Creative Paperclay, that held up better—it didn't show fingerprints, or crumble under her touch. She could actually paint it, and get closer to victims' skin tone and eye color. It was a vast improvement. To this day, as far as Kelly knows, she and her mother are the only artists that prefer that particular kind of clay. Marla was able to sand it, too, and smooth out most imperfections—and what she couldn't manage to grind down, she could mask with the right lighting. She managed that by learning her way around a camera—she had to take her own photos, too—and positioning the reconstructions just so.

Marla made a circle with her thumb and forefinger, in front of her own eye. "After we get the markers filled up in the little flesh on the face, what I like to do next is put the eyes in the holes. You have to allow enough room around the ball for muscles if you're a human. Because as you get older, the muscles get weaker and your eyes sink back in your head."

That started a new intrusive thought cycle for me that continues to this day: With each birthday, I now wonder how much farther my eyes have sunk back into my head.

And then I thought about the different reconstructions I'd seen of Marla's, a John Doe in Twiggs County, another in Barrow. Both had been anywhere between twenty-five and fifty. How would an artist know just where to position those orbs? If they were too far back, how much would

it "age" the reconstruction—perhaps too much—so much that an identification might not be made? The pressure to get it all right was staggering.

Marla has had many solves in her career, and Kelly has, too—but there
are the cases they still think about. Perhaps the most frustrating ones
are the most solvable: a victim, found soon after death, whose likeness is
captured exactly, but who remains unidentified. That's what happened in
2019, when a John Doe the GBI called "ACE" or "The Riverdale John Doe"
was struck by a car in Riverdale, Georgia, near the intersection of Valley
Hill Road and Mockingbird Trail. The nickname came from the word
ACE tattooed on the victim's forearm. He was a Black male under twenty
years old, most likely between fourteen and nineteen. The person who hit
him was charged with vehicular homicide, but investigators still had no
knowledge of his identity.[14]

Kelly was the one who drew his portrait; when the story ran in the
Atlanta Journal-Constitution, I recognized her work immediately. And
I couldn't stop looking at the beautiful face of the teenager she'd drawn.
Close-cropped hair, dark brown eyes, long eyelashes. In the portrait,
he's smiling, a little, and gazing off to his left. Someone somewhere must
love him. You can see it in the time she took in the shading, in the life
she brought to his face. NCMEC, the National Center for Missing and
Exploited Children, did a digital portrait of this unknown child, too—
pictured a little younger, perhaps, than his age at death. Both were circulated, along with a photo of the tattoo that spelled out *ACE*.

And finally, in February 2022, it was enough. NCMEC reported that
a tip was called in; someone had recognized the boy. Dywimas Autman
was only fifteen years old at the time he was hit. He'd only been living
in Georgia for a little while; he'd come from Mississippi to live with
his father in Riverdale, a city in the metro Atlanta area. Based on local
reporting, Autman's father told officials that his son had run away in
2019, and that he'd both reported him missing and looked for Autman
on his own;[15] it's unclear why the connection wasn't made between a local
hit-and-run victim and Autman, considering his disappearance was close
to the time of the vehicular homicide, but some on social media have
claimed that the missing-persons report was actually filed in Autman's

home state, Mississippi, not in Georgia.[16] Autman's mother and relatives back home didn't recognize the tattoo; he hadn't had it when he left.

It was the tattoo that ultimately identified Dywimas Autman, but without Kelly's art and the art from NCMEC, the "ACE" tattoo wouldn't have been circulated widely—and, I suspect, he would still be unidentified today. Cases without art attract less attention, from media and citizens, whether we're scrolling social or pausing on an article. Volunteer genetic genealogists at the nonprofit DNA Doe Project have told me time and again that cases without artwork raise fewer funds; that's why they work with forensic artist Carl Koppelman to reconstruct as many of their case files as possible. When people can connect a face to a case, they're more likely to click Share, to donate a dollar, to forward the image on to someone else who might have the answer—or know someone who does.

That's what we hoped might happen for Ina Jane Doe. Though we were pursuing investigative genetic genealogy and other testing for her, there was always the chance that circulating new art could be enough to bring in the right lead for Jefferson County—before Astrea had even finished its analysis.

CHAPTER ELEVEN

THE CASE: THE RECONSTRUCTION

Once Amy's skeletal analysis was complete, and the samples of Ina Jane Doe's hair and her tooth had been sent to Astrea, we needed a forensic artist to complete an updated approximation for Ina Jane Doe. This would serve a few purposes, the primary one being that the Jefferson County Sheriff's Office could circulate it widely, along with a press release that new avenues of investigation were being pursued in the case. They'd get calls, and social media conversation would start up, too; I'd be able to track most of that. The local pages—news outlets, the sheriff's official Facebook page, TV stations—that's what I was most interested in digging through. I knew locals would have something to say about the art, and they'd share their memories of January 1993 when Ina's remains were found in the park. While theories were as likely to spring up on these threads as they were on large, international message boards, and unhelpful suggestions ("Run fingerprints!") would undoubtedly pop up here and there, people who'd lived in the Ina and Mount Vernon areas for decades would have memories. And hopefully, they'd be shaken loose by just the right reminder.

But first, we needed new art. Most artists, like Kelly, worked for departments or state or federal agencies and needed to be formally requested by another agency to lend assistance. If there was an artist operating in the region where the case was located, I knew Kelly would follow their lead; she didn't like to step on anyone's toes.

When I emailed Carl Koppelman to ask if he'd be interested in completing updated forensic art for Ina Jane Doe, I hoped I'd hear back from him in a week or two. I included all my contact information, reminded him that we'd had some contact in the past through a colleague when discussing another case, and hoped for the best. But he was busy—I knew that.

You can imagine my surprise when, ten minutes later, my phone rang. I didn't recognize the number, but I had a rough idea of where Carl lived, so I answered.

"Hello? This is Carl."

As luck would have it, he was interested.

Carl Koppelman was the second forensic artist I'd ever spoken to at length. My friend Kelly had formal training twice over, both from her years in art school and from her mom's training, since Marla held the job before her. But Carl's life had taken a decidedly different path. Carl graduated in 1993 and was working in LA as a CPA by 1994. It was an interesting place to be in the mid-1990s, and one of the most formative events of those years were the murders of Nicole Brown Simpson and Ron Goldman, and O. J. Simpson's subsequent arrest and trial. If you weren't alive in the mid-1990s, it's difficult to describe how focused everyone was on this case.

Like many LA residents, Carl occasionally found himself at the edges of the storm. At one time prior to the trial, Carl drove by Nicole's house on Bundy—the crime scene—and stopped when he saw a crowd. Reporters were discussing hoax evidence that had been planted a little earlier, a "bloody knife" meant to look like the murder weapon. One of them saw Carl, and asked, *Hey, if you were going to get rid of a knife, where would you stash it?*

"Oh, I'd drop it in somebody's gas tank," Carl remembered saying. "That was back when the gas filler caps weren't as small then as they are now. You could take off a gas cap and you have a fairly decent-sized hole in there. You can just drop a knife right down in the hole and it'd go into somebody's gas tank, and nobody'd ever find it. So I said that to the reporter, and I ended up getting quoted in the *LA Times*."

Watching the case progress interested Carl, but then, he'd always had a general interest in true crime—particularly unsolved cases. With the advent of the internet, it made keeping up with developments in cases like these easier. His introduction to forensic art, though, wouldn't come until he discovered the Websleuths discussion forum. Websleuths, a message board for unsolved true-crime enthusiasts, was founded in 1999, which is practically ancient in internet terms. Carl stumbled upon it when he was searching for more information on the Jaycee Dugard case, in the mid-'00s. Like so many others who were concerned for the kidnapped girl (and this was before she was rescued in 2009), he occasionally checked for updates, particularly when he was at home caring for his ill mother without much else to do.

Carl didn't find any updates on Jaycee's case. But he did find a thread about her on Websleuths, which led him to other threads. That's when he stumbled on an entire subforum devoted to John and Jane Does. "It never occurred to me that that was a thing, that there were a lot of people on Websleuths who were collaborating to try to solve these unidentified remains cases," Carl later told me. "And that became fascinating, because there were a couple of cases that the sleuthing community had just solved at that time. There were a couple of long-term Doe cases that were solved by people matching up missing-persons reports to unidentified remains cases. And I thought, *Wow, this is something I can do while I'm sitting here taking care of my mother*."

As Carl dug into the cases, he noticed that many of them had art that was either missing or poorly rendered. Few departments were lucky enough to have access to artists like Kelly Lawson, Karen Taylor, or Betty Pat Gatliff. Many had to rely on composite kits or whoever had enough talent to create a sketch—but even then, drawing and forensic art were two very different skills. Carl had always enjoyed art, though he had never formally studied its forensic branch. But he began to think seriously about how he might contribute to this art issue.

The truth is that many unidentified-persons cases, particularly those before 2000, don't have DNA on file, or have it on file in a limited capacity. Only with those SNP profiles can investigative genetic genealogists do the new work to solve cases, in public DNA databases. That means new testing, and more funding. New art is far less expensive . . . but someone has to actually *do* it. So, Carl Koppelman decided to teach himself how.

Using Corel Photopaint and Corel Draw software, he began to experiment. He used a combination of drawing and photo layering, using details of a case file—like a description of a victim's Philadelphia Eagles football jersey—to find pictures online. Then he incorporated edits to photos that had been released in a case, like shifting eyes from closed to open, or adding a lifelike expression. His first attempt made it onto the Doe Network's website, and soon, he was experimenting with more difficult tasks, like skeletal reconstruction, which required him to work with proportion and measurement based on skeletal features. For human features, Carl used photos of people, from celebrities to friends to stock photos, to set basic shapes and structures that matched what he'd deduced from the cranium and mandible. Then he built upon them until the base—the foundation—was no longer discernible.

The first forensic reference photos that Carl worked with he found online, either released by the departments or NCMEC, or posted through less official means. Maybe some anonymous person got them through FOIA and decided to scan them—though few departments offer pictures when they send out files. Perhaps they were printed in papers. After a little practice, Carl began posting his artwork for the public, mostly on Websleuths and other groups devoted to Doe cases.

Carl's art got noticed. Posters asked him to do more art, for more cases. And then law enforcement contacted him. Not to reprimand him, but to make their own requests, for art in cases that needed it. Soon, the forensic photos arrived straight to him, by email.

Though he sought out formal training via workshops with artists like Karen Taylor, Carl continued to do art for free. He would accept payment if offered, but he never required it. Soon, he'd done over 250 portraits, after which point, he stopped counting. His work was featured in *AARP Magazine*, and he was inundated by requests, both from private citizens and law enforcement. Now, he primarily works with departments and nonprofits like the DNA Doe Project, where he's created art for a number of high-profile cases: the Sumter County John and Jane Doe, James Paul Freund and Pamela Mae Buckley; the John Doe who used the pseudonym "Lyle Stevik," whose family preferred his name not be released; and "The Lime Lady"—eventually identified as Tamara Lee Tigard—just to name a few.

When the cases were solved by the DNA Doe Project, Carl was able to compare the likeness and judge his approximation. He'd see things he'd gotten right, or nearly so, and aspects that were off. Weight could be a problem; with skeletonized remains, it was often a guessing game, unless clothing was present to provide size. And even then, a decedent might have worn clothing of various sizes during their life.

He'd find that his accuracy varied. Often, it came down to what he was working with—the angle of a cranium photo that only allowed him a limited view. Missing bone that left much up to his best guess. Or simply human variation: approximation *is* approximation. Look at any group of siblings and see how many ways similar features and bone structure combine and shift in ways that are both similar and subtly but strikingly different. Take a look at acting families like the Baldwins or Wayans. Really study their photos, and you can see how much variation exists in similarity.

In the years since Carl started making his reconstructions, a number of cases have been closed (either in part or in whole) due to his creations, including a 2016 case in Spokane, Washington. A presumed white male was found in the river, his body badly bloated, but with a few discernible features: a gray beard, a balding head, and a thin frame. Carl completed his reconstruction, and the staff of the local homeless shelter recognized the decedent as Donald Nyden, who was a regular visitor at their organization. When they identified Donald, Carl was able to see his photos—and realized he'd been much more emaciated than his postmortem photos had implied. The bloating had hidden that. Still, the likeness had been clear to those who knew him, and Carl's art solved the case.

I was hopeful that Carl would help us in drawing renewed attention to Ina Jane Doe, too, especially since her forensic art had made the rounds for years. He was as keen as Amy and I were to see the old art replaced. Jefferson County approved Carl's participation, and soon we were on a Zoom call. He had access to skeletal photos taken in Amy's lab, autopsy photos from the original file, and consulted with Amy and the anatomist and medical illustrator Dr. Steffen Poltak, who'd also examined Ina Jane Doe in person. They encouraged Carl to be cautious in interpretation of asymmetry in Ina's features. If the last round hadn't sparked a tip, maybe a new approach would.

One particular advantage we had in Ina Jane Doe's case was access to her hair. Jefferson County discovered that they had retained all of it, and not just a small sample, so precise measurements were gathered of the varying lengths of each lock. Based on that, Karl was able to better approximate that Jane Doe's hair hadn't been cut in a chin-length bob, as the previous art had presented her. She'd had a long shag-style cut, shoulder length or so, and auburn red. We weren't sure on eye color, but brown or hazel was the tentative original guess, and Carl went in that direction.

During our conversation, I asked him how he picked which inspiration photos to use for his base drawings. He explained, "It doesn't have to look exactly like the person you're dealing with. It's mostly just for the purpose of adding color, lifelike color, to a lifeless face. Because a lifeless face doesn't have good color to it. So, you need a good living photo of somebody to return the lifelike color to the face and muscle tone as well, maybe smile lines and that sort of thing."

"So you could have used me? Or is my face shape too different?"

"Oh, yeah. I could have used a photo of you if there was a good frontal photo of you. I just need a photo of a woman, about 30 to 50 years old. In this case, Caucasian. I overlay it over the skull and now we have all the eyes, nose, and mouth in the position where they're supposed to be."

In Ina's case, Carl started with a photo of actress Shelley Duvall. I was expecting to *see* Shelley Duvall when he first told us that, but he'd layered and painted and shifted and stretched her face in his programs so that the photograph had somehow become someone else entirely—the forensic representation of skeletal features I'd seen and heard described dozens of times. He built out her features over several days, refining, shaping eyes and nose and lips, stretching skin over bone. He made a slight adjustment for a very mild asymmetry around the mouth. Then he aged her into the midrange of the estimation of thirty to fifty and portrayed her as of medium build.

Kyana, Amy's lab manager, had spent a good deal of time measuring and studying Ina's hair before samples were sent to the lab; she was able to give us a better sense of length and color than previous artists had access to, and with that information and postmortem photos as a guide, Carl tried to approximate her haircut and length as closely as possible. Kyana and I spent a few hours one late November day pulling example photos of what Kyana thought of as a "wolf cut" and what I remembered as an extremely popular haircut in the 1980s and '90s: lots of layers, with shaggy bangs, that some women hair-sprayed into gravity-defying forms that could withstand an entire Bon Jovi concert. We had no idea how Ina had actually styled her hair, but the varying lengths of her hair samples indicated she was a redhead—probably natural, since there was absolutely no regrowth at the root—and that she had layers and bangs that she wore much shorter than the rest. That would have been shoulder length. Carl may have spent the most time on her hair; we only had a few photos and the samples to match by, but he wanted to get the color as close as possible.

There was no clothing to incorporate, but Carl picked something that was appropriate to the early 1990s. Finally, he chose a background for his art—a setting that subtly evoked Wayne Fitzgerrell State Park. Then, all that was left was to share it with our working group and fine-tune the details. He prepared a version of Ina with and without makeup. When Jefferson County eventually made their announcement, they would decide to release both.

Later, I asked Carl about his choice to put landscapes in his forensic reconstructions. I'd never seen another artist do it.

"I've had other people, who are in the industry who are paid forensic artists, say, 'Oh, you shouldn't be putting backgrounds in there, and making them all colorful.' And I said, 'Well, the whole point is to try to get people to look.' You can make something very technically accurate and make all the fine details perfect. But if people aren't going to look at it, then there's no point in putting it out there. The idea is to make something so visually appealing that people will stop and look at it and then say, 'Oh, that's an interesting image. What's the story?' And then they read it and share it."

Considering that I had discovered Carl in precisely that way, when I'd clicked on a picture of Julie Doe . . . he had a point. Whether or not other forensic artists liked his style, the reconstructions never looked like death masks, or mug shots, or wanted posters. You weren't quite sure what they were: illustrations of a person, partly photograph, partly digital image, smiling at you from a dreamy location, sometimes frozen ten years, or thirty, or forty back from the present day. And you wanted to know more about them. And you clicked. And then you read.

———— • ————

Carl was finished with Ina Jane's reconstruction by late December 2021. By then, Ina Jane Doe's samples had been assessed at Astrea Forensics, and the investigative genetic genealogists at Redgrave Research were in communication with the lab, ready for the results. They'd be able to upload Astrea's data as a "kit" to GEDmatch and, if necessary, Family Tree DNA, and they were ready to begin their work. Things looked good: We hoped, even felt confident, that Carl would see a photo of the real woman behind Ina Jane Doe's case file so that he could compare his drawing to her reality.

In the meantime, Jefferson County released their press statement featuring Carl's artistic renderings. And as I hoped, the news caused a stir in the Mount Vernon area—and the whole true-crime community online as well. Internet sleuths who'd followed the case were ready to post the reconstruction and updated information. There was buzz: News that a skeletal reanalysis had been performed and a lab and genealogists were involved meant answers were on the horizon. That's what everyone wants to hear about a cold case.

But that's not where I spent my time. We wanted to know what the locals were talking about. Facebook can be handy, as much as it's been abandoned by anyone under thirty. The day after Jefferson County's press release was posted, and it had begun to make the rounds at local stations and newspapers, I posted up on my couch with my laptop and a big cup of coffee. My son was just back at school after the holiday break, but he'd left reminders of his vacation inhabitation all over the living room: Christmas presents that hadn't quite made it upstairs, half-filled-in Mad Libs pages, and lots of single socks tucked into furniture crevices. It took me several minutes to get situated and ready to read because a tiny mechanical voice kept screaming from somewhere under a pile of pillows. *FEAR THE CLAW! THIS IS A RESCUE MISSION!* I finally found a velociraptor-rescue-helicopter combo toy stuck halfway through its transformation. Honestly, it looked painful. I stuck it very deep into the toy bin, stacking some books on top of it.

On the JCSO's posts and on local news sites' social media that featured the announcement, I picked through the comments, looking for anything that might be worthwhile. Mostly, it was people who remembered the case from 1993. Some offered up possible matches pulled from websites. Some, I saved. Others I knew were rule-outs; we'd seen the dental charts on NamUs, or a quick records check told me the dates didn't match up. There was a comment from a friend of the girls who'd discovered Ina; she said she'd gone to school with them and could still remember what it was like after they'd come upon her remains at the park.

I was relieved that she didn't mention their names.

And then, a hundred or so threaded comments in, I saw something interesting: a link to a news story. An old one, actually; I was surprised it still loaded. It was posted by a reporter who said she'd written about another dismembered female body part—but one found in Indiana. After a few calculations, I realized it was only ninety minutes away.

When I read the story, I texted Amy. She was used to receiving paragraph-long iMessages from my laptop.

> LE found a white female's arm in 1993 or 1994 in Indiana. Vanderburgh County Coroner. They aren't sure; the records are lost, so no one knows who brought it into the coroner's office. They serve a lot of different departments. Even Illinois. And they make mention of thinking it might be related to a decapitated head, but that case being solved. Except there were two dismemberment cases in Illinois that year, close together. Remember the other woman found in the park? Maybe they thought that Ina's case was solved and not Lynn's. Worth checking out.

It took her a few moments to reply.

> Long shot, but we should email. I'll contact them tomorrow.

It *was*, admittedly, a long shot. But the arm of a presumed white female, found that close to the discovery point of a murder victim's head, in the same timeframe of her discovery? There might be something there. Moreover, Amy was familiar with the area, and when she looked at the map, she realized: The Vanderburgh County Coroner's Office was big, and close to the state line. In addition to Indiana cases, they'd likely be handling some work for Illinois counties that didn't have the facilities. And that was their difficulty—it wasn't just Indiana law enforcement that could have brought the remains in to be examined. In the article I'd found, the then-coroner explained that the victim's fingertips seemed to have been removed, which further complicated any attempts at identification. Amy said that could have been animal predation, and that she'd ask the current coroner to take a look.

Amy's email got a quick response. When she reached out, she discovered that they were more than willing to provide a sample. Officials had been wondering for years about the hand and forearm that had been floating in formalin (formaldehyde in water), sitting in their office, with no paperwork to identify it. They were up for doing an examination and sending her a sample for testing. The formalin, though, was going to be a problem. It had soaked into the flesh and bone, destroying most of what could be tested under normal circumstances.

Fortunately, the University of New Hampshire had its own lab, the Hubbard Center for Genome Studies, that was interested in beginning work on some forensic cases. In fact, they were testing their first whole-genome sequence in a forensic case with a sample from Ina Jane Doe; they would compare it with Astrea's, and if all was well, they'd be able to help with some of the cold-case work Amy performed for the state. After a meeting with the center's director, Amy thought it would be possible to try to make a comparison, as long as some DNA was extractable.

A local Indiana anthropologist met with the Vanderburgh County coroner, and they began the careful work of dissection, selecting a bone that was most protected within the hand—as much as anything could be, with the formalin solution. As they studied the victim's arm, it became clear that her fingertips hadn't actually been manually removed; there were indeed signs of carnivore activity. However, there were marks on the bone that showed evidence that it had been severed by a sharp instrument. This process—from finding the article, to contacting the coroner, to arranging for the samples and testing at the Hubbard Center—took months. It's funny how quickly weeks can be summarized when you're remembering them—but it was March 2022 by the time the bone arrived at Hubbard and graduate students in the lab began the arduous process of attempting extraction on formalin-damaged tissue.

Ina's testing was much faster. Not *fast*—it takes time—but things moved along quickly.

I should know; I was there when it began.

CHAPTER TWELVE

THE METHOD: DNA ANALYSIS AND INVESTIGATIVE GENETIC GENEALOGY

The Golden State Killer. Babes in the Woods. The murder of Carla Walker. The case solves that come via the combination of DNA profiles and genetic genealogy roll across our news feeds and can seem effortless: magic solutions to cases that were previously unsolvable. Unseen wizards behind curtains, twisting this knob or that, and with a swab or a sample and a few clicks of the keyboard, maybe a trip onto Ancestry.com or 23andMe? Boom. A case is solved.

But none of it is quite that simple. Though it feels as if we've had this technology forever, the truth is that the first solves using forensic or investigative genetic genealogy—both perpetrator and unidentified-persons cases—were announced in 2018. Genealogists like CeCe Moore, Dr. Barbara Rae-Venter, Dr. Margaret Press, and Dr. Colleen Fitzpatrick had all recognized the value of home DNA tests when they hit the market. DNA gets complex—*surprise!*—but to really simplify things, the basics of what they recognized was this: Single nucleotide polymorphism (SNP)–based genetic testing can allow for connection to farther-flung relatives than the classic short tandem repeat (STR) tests like the ones used in CODIS. STR DNA testing can be used to locate familial information, too, but it's less stable over generations.

As discussed earlier, the classic STR DNA test used in CODIS can compare what the FBI defines as "close relatives." STR DNA can also be useful beyond that—for instance, the NIJ notes that "STRs are extremely useful in applications such as the construction of genetic maps, gene location, genetic linkage analysis, identification of individuals, paternity testing, as well as disease diagnosis [. . .] STR analysis has also been employed in population genetics."[1] But the reach of SNP DNA tests is what attracted genealogists—this technology can draw a line between you and, say, your sixth cousin once removed. With that increased power, it's easy to see how they could be used to help solve crimes and identify John and Jane Does.

CeCe Moore, known as the "DNA Detective," is one of the most famous investigative genetic genealogists in the United States, and her work is known worldwide. Moore now heads Parabon NanoLabs' genetic genealogy department, and she is the genetic genealogist on PBS's *Finding Your Roots* with Henry Louis Gates Jr. She has also consulted on a number of other television shows and media projects, like an ABC docuseries about her own work, *The Genetic Detective*.[2] CeCe talked with me about the inception of investigative genetic genealogy—then mostly called forensic genealogy—and how she and her colleagues saw the potential to use this new technology to solve crimes. The shift to "investigative" over the past few years has been made to differentiate investigative genetic genealogy from both traditional genealogy and from the established field of forensic genealogy, which predates DNA-based work and focuses on tracing heirs in legal cases.

Like every investigative genetic genealogist I met, CeCe was first drawn to non-forensic uses of DNA, such as the ability to improve family-tree and adoptee searches. But she soon saw the potential for more. In the winter of 2021, while I was still waiting for Ina Jane Doe's extraction results to come back from Astrea, we sat down to talk over Zoom.

"Very early on," CeCe told me, "I realized that the techniques that I had developed to resolve unknown parentage for adoption, donor conception, and unknown or misattributed paternity were fully applicable to

Jane and John Doe cases. I followed Websleuths and cold cases, so when I was working as a genetic genealogist, in my free time, which I didn't have much of—I actually followed true crime. So, I was well aware of many of the Jane and John Doe cases. I knew way back in 2010 that genetic genealogy could be used in the same way for those types of cases as in unknown parentage cases, and I started trying to find a way to make that happen from very early days. My idea was that we needed to start a separate database that was specifically for law enforcement's use rather than using the existing databases. From the very beginning, I was asking: *How about we have a database that's fully consented, specifically for this type of work?* I brought it up many times in our community."

I asked where these conversations were happening, and she explained, "Genetic genealogy, as you may know, is a very active online community. It started with mailing lists, RootsWeb mailing lists and Yahoo groups, and then largely moved to Facebook. And now, most of the activity is there. So when I first got very involved in the genetic genealogy community, I was advocating for and trying to organize different efforts. For example, I thought we should create a certification program specifically for genetic genealogy, but no one else seemed to be interested in that idea. I thought we should explore using genetic genealogy to identify Jane and John Does, but I didn't find a lot of enthusiasm or support for it in the early days."

CeCe also recognized some essential ethical issues that we're still discussing today. "Very quickly, it became clear there was a slippery slope . . . that if you identify a victim of a violent crime, very likely, it could lead to an arrest since most people, especially women, are murdered by someone close to them. And so, if a woman disappears and her husband doesn't report her missing, and then we identify her, that's going to make the husband a suspect very quickly. It became clear there was no black and white between suspect cases and Jane and John Doe cases. On the other hand, I felt very strongly that Jane and John Doe cases, or unidentified remains cases, were very similar and in line with adoption and unknown parentage cases. It's giving someone their biological identity, providing answers and resolution to families, so I didn't see it as very different ethically. It's different in that it is just not as joyful, because you're reuniting families in death instead of life, although we did run into that in adoptions as well. Plenty of times we found the birth parents deceased, or we *just* missed somebody."

One of the other early and important figures in investigative genetic genealogy was Dr. Margaret Press. Margaret is one of the co-founders of DNA Doe Project. The other co-founder, Dr. Colleen Fitzpatrick, has moved on from the organization to focus on her private IGG business, Identifinders; before she left, I had the chance to interview her about Julie Doe's case, and feature her on the podcast. Colleen's name should be familiar, as she was the investigative genetic genealogist who worked with Dr. Derek Abbott to identify the Somerton Man.

Since Margaret and Colleen began DNA Doe Project in 2017, it's grown from a two-person project to a nonprofit with eighty-odd volunteers and several employees who take on jobs like media, education, and finances. DDP's mission is simple: use IGG to solve unidentified-persons cases. They help departments fundraise for testing funds, and as a nonprofit, they provide the genealogy itself for free.

Though Margaret considered herself a hobby genealogist since her teens, she started working with DNA kits as early as the mid-'00s; at that point, public interest was in building family trees and identifying relatives. She spent most of her time helping individuals—even some of her own relatives—track down their biological fathers and other family members.

But in early 2017, Margaret made a life-changing decision: She decided to read a Sue Grafton novel. As Margaret later explained to me, "She mentioned that her story, which was fictional, was based on a real Jane Doe from Lompoc, California. And she actually appealed to her readers for any help, any tips that they might have. She included a sketch. She had paid to exhume the skeleton so that a sketch could be made, and DNA could be obtained from the body in about 2003 or so. I suddenly had an epiphany that identifying a John or Jane Doe, if there's DNA, why can't they be sent to Ancestry and treated like an adoptee? You just need to find the parents. I'd never heard of John or Jane Does, never on my radar, never thought about them. So I messaged Sue Grafton and asked her if this Jane Doe was still unidentified and if anyone had approached her about using genetic genealogy to try to identify the body. And within a day or so, she actually responded and said, 'Nope, had not been tried. Nope, not been identified.'"

Margaret wasn't the only person thinking along those lines—though she didn't know it then. CeCe Moore had long been working to puzzle out how genetic genealogy could be used in forensic cases, and Dr. Barbara Rae-Venter, an experienced genealogist who would go on to identify the Golden State Killer, was exploring similar terrain. It's almost as if an electric current ran through the world of genealogy, prickling with possibility. Margaret told me that after Sue Grafton said she'd be tied up working on a book for close to a year, Margaret decided to see if there were other cases she could assist on. But she'd need access to DNA profiles: lots of them.

"I started reaching out to Ancestry and FTDNA and all the companies, saying, 'If I can get DNA for a dead body, can I send it to you?' And they all said, 'No, no, you can't. We don't deal with dead bodies, don't deal with law enforcement,'" Margaret recalled. "And then I reached out to CeCe and to Colleen separately in Messenger and approached them about the idea. And basically the answer I got everywhere was it cannot be done because they will not let you in. So all those doors were closed."

But Margaret wasn't willing to stop there. She remembers continuing to speak with Colleen as they brainstormed alternatives: "In my internet searching, I came across a guy, just a random genealogist, who had the same question, but for his dead father, which is how does he get his dead father's DNA into these databases? And he discovered he could circumvent Ancestry.com and FTDNA and actually get a DNA file from an independent company, an independent lab, and go directly to GEDmatch, which is not a testing company at all, but a sandbox where anyone could upload their file from anywhere. So the guy that I found on the internet, his father was dead, but he found that the hospitals all retained biological samples from the patients for 10 years.

"So this guy got a tumor biopsy from the hospital lab. Whole genome sequencing had suddenly come way down from tens of millions of dollars down to about a thousand dollars. I had never known this. I always thought it was way out of sight of your average consumer. But people were doing this for themselves, getting their whole genome sequenced. He also found a guy in Germany, Thomas Cron, who had written an open-source script, a program that would take that whole genome file and reduce it to something that looked like it came from Ancestry or 23andMe. That was the key. Those were the three ingredients that we needed because then I went to Colleen and said, 'Bingo, I found how we can do it. We get DNA extracted from a body. We go to the whole genome lab. We get Thomas to run his script for us or help us run his script. We create a 23andMe-like file. We upload it to GEDmatch and that's our answer.'"

At the time, Margaret and Colleen had no idea that CeCe Moore, Dr. Barbara Rae-Venter, and others were working out the same problem: how to get DNA from a decedent into a file that GEDmatch could support. She'd soon learn as genetic genealogists across the United States began to communicate in online discussion forums dedicated to the topic. But initially, Margaret and Colleen used their own savings and Colleen's law-enforcement connections to begin doing their work. It so happened that one of the first unidentified decedent cases they received was a famous one: a man who'd died in 2002 under the alias Joseph Chandler Newton. It was discovered after his cremation that he'd been living under the assumed identity of a deceased child who'd been killed in a car wreck in 1945.

Although the man calling himself "Joseph" had been cremated, Margaret and Colleen had a very small sample to work with: a biopsy from a malignant tumor the man had removed before his death. As Margaret remembered, "All that was left was just a tiny amount and it was 99 percent bacteria. So it took a lot of work to get sufficient data out of that sample. We didn't know what effect the formaldehyde would have." But luckily, they were able to get a match and quickly began their work.

Margaret says that she and Colleen then procured a usable file, which took twenty-four hours to "batch" into GEDmatch's system—that is, to fully process so that it could be compared with other results. One of their volunteers—there were very few back then—spotted a low match, at 48 cM, and a few other possible leads. The match 48 cM signaled a distant relative, maybe a third or fourth cousin a few times removed. The higher the cM, or centimorgans, a match shows, the more DNA shared and, thus, the closer to an identity. The match 48 cM was a far ways off.

They worked on those leads for months until a volunteer found something promising in a family tree: a couple that might be the answer. Margaret told me that they spent all night examining a winding family tree that led them, in twisting branches, toward the man's true identity. When she finally went to bed, exhausted, she heard her answering machine click on: "Colleen called me and left a message. I could hear her on the phone machine while I was drifting into sleep. 'Margaret, wake up, wake up, wake up, Margaret. We got them. We got them. We got them Margaret. We got them.'"

Them is the union couple: two people who tie a branch together and lead directly to the identity of a Doe. I've heard this magic couple described to me in different ways by different investigative genetic genealogists, but to my understanding, they are the key: the two people whose union ultimately led to the birth of the unidentified deceased. Margaret's team had identified them; that led them to a name: Robert Ivan Nichols. It was March 2018. The identification had to be verified, so local law enforcement tracked down Robert Nichols's son and had him submit a DNA sample.

It was a match.

On June 21, 2018, police announced that they'd solved the case. But questions remained. Per the *News Herald*: "Nichols, who received a Purple Heart in World War II, divorced his wife in 1964, telling her 'in due time you will know why.' [. . .] He was reported missing by his family in 1965, and numerous attempts by authorities to locate him were unsuccessful. The family never heard from Nichols again after 1965."[3] Nichols had no criminal record, and investigators found no obvious reason why he had assumed a new identity. He died with over $80,000 in the bank—which he could have left to the son he'd abandoned in the 1960s. He did not. Nichols, who died by suicide, left no explanation regarding his assumed identity.

Just a few weeks later, Margaret, Colleen, and the few volunteers who'd gathered with them—who would become DNA Doe Project— solved another famous unidentified persons case. "Buckskin Girl" was a young woman whose body was recovered from a ditch along a roadway in Troy, Ohio, in April 1981. She was nicknamed "Buckskin Girl" because she wore "a fringed buckskin jacket."[4] Investigators suspected she'd died shortly before she was found, but they had no leads as to who her killer might be, or her identity. But Margaret, Colleen, and the volunteers were able to work with a lab to develop a profile from a blood sample that had been retained from the 1981 autopsy, and they solved her case only weeks after they identified Nichols. "Buckskin Girl" turned out to be Marcia King, a twenty-one-year-old from Arkansas. The announcement of Marcia's identification was originally scheduled in late April, on the thirty-seventh anniversary of her discovery, but the press release had to be moved up because the story had leaked: "A half sibling started posting about it on Facebook. It got out, and then it went all over, and people said, 'Really, really? That's your half-sister? Prove it. Show us a photo.' They're so cruel . . . cruel."

How Marcia's family was treated informed Margaret's approach to helping future families prepare for the onslaught following a case, or in giving law enforcement information to pass on: lock down social media.

And the solves just kept coming. Less than two weeks later, the identity of the Golden State Killer was announced: Through use of familial DNA, investigative genetic genealogist Dr. Barbara Rae-Venter's work led to the identity of the serial murderer and rapist Joseph DeAngelo.[5] The fact that Michelle McNamara's posthumous and best-selling book on the case, *I'll Be Gone in the Dark*, was released just a few months before DeAngelo was caught raised the case profile even more. Just a year later, Dr. Rae-Venter was involved in the identification of three of the four Bear Brook victims. A citizen detective and librarian, Becky Heath, was also involved;

she and Dr. Barbara Rae-Venter "each discovered the victims' identities independently within just a few weeks of each other."[6] The victims were three children and a woman found in fifty-five-gallon metal drums in Bear Brook State Park, thought to have died somewhere between 1977 and 1981. The identified victims included Marlyse Honeychurch and her children, Sarah McWaters and Marie Vaughn; Marlyse was dating serial killer Terry Rasmussen shortly before the time of her death.[7]

The fourth victim, a child between two and four years of age, remains unidentified, but investigators know that she is the child of Terry Rasmussen, and think she has genetic relatives living in the Mississippi region.[8] And so 2018 marked the beginning, at least in the public's awareness, of the investigative genetic genealogy revolution. But it also generated a whole new conversation about privacy, inequity, and forensic use.

———•———

There is no public, wholly forensic database in existence today that all investigative genetic genealogists may access. That's not to say companies aren't working on versions of this: Othram Inc. maintains a database for use in their work, called DNASolves, which the public can contribute to, but it's dedicated to Othram's casework in cooperation with law enforcement. And NamUs has begun to fund IGG work, which means they will support IGG testing via partnership with Othram Inc. But the public can't upload their own kits to NamUs (and there isn't a function that would make that feasible). GEDmatch, founded in 2010,[9] is the closest thing we have to what CeCe envisioned: a database of non-forensic samples—meaning, collected by private citizens and uploaded voluntarily, which any IGG company working with law enforcement can access, and can then be compared against forensic cases. It's not a dedicated forensic database, but it's in the realm. FamilyTreeDNA (FTDNA) offers law enforcement the same basic comparison ability as GEDmatch.

Despite what many people think, private DNA banks like Ancestry .com and 23andMe aren't open to forensic casework, and many cold cases don't have any DNA on file at all. Those that do may have the wrong kind of sample. In Doe cases, the deceased may have been cremated, with no samples held back for future testing. Or someone may have saved something small: like a hair sample, or a classic blood card, which archives a very small blood sample.

In other cases, the decedent has been buried and must be exhumed for a sample to be retrieved; that in and of itself is another costly procedure. Depending on the state, there can be a *lot* of red tape. And even then, there's no guarantee that a sample will be viable. When an unknown decedent is buried, they are usually interred at the expense of the county, in areas of local cemeteries known as potter's fields or indigent burial sites. That might mean interment in a simple plastic or canvas bag, a pine box, a metal box—it just depends on the decade and laws of the community. Water often seeps in when it comes to these kinds of burials, though, and water is the enemy of DNA collection.

The labs that prepare kits for genetic genealogy may prefer different remains for sampling than those that work with the more classic DNA samples, like those submitted to CODIS or prior to 2022, NamUs; I've seen sampling in those cases focused on long bones. In the best-case scenario, a lab like Astrea would want a tooth, or a hair, or bone from the temporal lobe to help them create a SNP profile, though they can work with just about anything. What they can't do is take an old DNA profile, an STR profile that was prepared for CODIS or NamUs, and turn that into something suitable for genetic genealogy. That's the bit that's never explained to reading audiences who comment on articles: *There's DNA on file—why hasn't this been solved?* If a case can be solved via CODIS, it will be. But the samples are not synonymous, or interchangeable.

It's no wonder people are confused by this; it's also no wonder people still have privacy concerns regarding the use of DNA. That territory has been brought up dozens of times since the first investigative genetic genealogy, or IGG, solves. Concerns over use and which crimes should fall under law enforcement use of public DNA databases prompted GEDmatch to enact a policy in spring 2019: Users had to actively "opt in" to law enforcement use of their DNA for law-enforcement cases. Users who had uploaded prior to that were automatically opted out, and had to manually log back into the site and opt in.[10]

I knew genealogists who were worried when this change came, because they suspected, rightly so, that a significant number of users never would do that. Even companies that did have regulations in place struggled to maintain a balance between helping the police and protecting their users' privacy. As BuzzFeed reported earlier that same year, GEDmatch had violated its own terms of service in allowing a Utah law-enforcement agency to search for an offender that fell outside its then-standing limitations of use in cases of murder or sexual assault. In 2018, investigators in Centerville, Utah, "wanted to catch the assailant who broke into a Mormon church on Nov. 17, 2018, and put a 71-year-old woman who was playing the organ in a chokehold. She passed out several times, according to a police press release, but survived the attack."[11]

They contacted GEDmatch for help; though this attack did not meet the criteria users had agreed to when they submitted their DNA to the database, the database's co-founder, Curtis Rogers, was eventually convinced it would be the right thing to allow the search. The assailant was arrested, but major privacy concerns unfolded.[12] Cases that had been in process suddenly lost access to any potential matches that weren't "opted in."

I can still remember the investigative genetic genealogists in my social circle posting pleas that we all log back into the site and opt in. But Rogers believed it was necessary to protect users, telling CNN that "certainly there was a short-term loss but I think this is going to make us stronger. Stronger ethically (and) stronger for support among people who put their information on our site. I think it's the right step to make."[13]

Since then, the IGG community has actively encouraged everyday citizens to upload their data to GEDmatch and to FTDNA, which also began requiring an opt-in (but automatically grandfathered in previous kits). Private companies and nonprofits alike rely on the databases for both perpetrator and unidentified persons cases—and for close to two years, there was worry that Doe kits would not be solved. GEDmatch addressed that concern in January 2021, with yet another TOS update, which the DNA

Doe Project posted about on their social media accounts. From January 11 of that year on, choosing "Public + OPT OUT" (i.e., making your DNA publicly available for comparison but opting out of law-enforcement use) did *not* preclude a kit's application in unidentified-decedent cases. DDP explained what making the "Public + OPT OUT" choice would mean from that point on:

> Public + opt-out: DNA data is available for comparison to any Raw Data in the GEDmatch database, except DNA kits identified as being uploaded for Law Enforcement investigation of a Violent Crime. John and Jane Does are uploaded for Law Enforcement purposes, but for the purpose of identification only. So this change is intended to exclude Does from the consequences of customers opting out (or of being opted out). Assailant kits will still only be compared to those who opted in. If you are concerned about having your results used for identifying Does, you should remove your kit from GEDmatch or mark it private or research. Opting out will no longer prevent that.

That doesn't mean that law enforcement or IGG companies or contractors can upload Doe kits as if they are private citizens' results; there's a special portal, GEDmatch PRO, which is "designed to support police and forensic teams with investigative comparisons to GEDmatch data. The portal separates police comparisons of GEDmatch data from standard genealogy activities and offers a range of tools most relevant to help further investigations."[14] That portal has a cost to use, and the cases uploaded through it do not publicly display to non-LE users. So, though I may match with a Doe case, I won't see that kit in what GEDmatch terms my "one to many matches." However, I will see all non-forensic matches: my relatives, listed from the highest centimorgan (cM) match to the lowest.

Since my parents have uploaded to GEDmatch, my top matches are in the 3000+ cM range; the next highest matches are 100 to 200 cM, which are much more distant relations—probably something along the lines of a second cousin once-removed, or a very confusing relationship like a half-first cousin twice-removed. Of course, there's a range, and DNA doesn't behave in a neat manner, with precise, regular measurements that indicate an exact relationship. My husband discovered an aunt later in life, but their cM overlap range indicated they might be half-siblings versus nephew and aunt. Genealogy work was needed to refine their connection.

That's because some very different relationships can look similar, at least from a cM perspective. I worked with a family who uploaded their kits to a private DNA database. When their results came in, the private company—which doesn't display actual measurements, but rather relationships—suggested the siblings, who had different fathers, were likely first cousins. We had to manually make adjustments in their "relationship" field to sort it out. On GEDmatch, no relationship is assigned; you just see that number and have to use genealogy to help you interpret it. Hopefully, users have also uploaded their family trees—which they can gather from private sites and share to GEDmatch as well. But Dr. Margaret Press told me that people are much less likely to upload family trees than DNA profiles.

Though many people *have* uploaded since 2018, there's still an uneven population representation on GEDmatch and on FTDNA. That's because the private sites are also uneven: Based on population, white people are well-represented, but there is far less data available on every other racial group. Specifically, there is plenty of data on white people of Western European descent, or so two DNA Doe Project volunteers told me during a 2022 podcast interview.[15] That's true in larger genetics studies, too, which has been a real issue in health research and the development of treatment and medicine meant for all populations. In forensic work, this means that a Black or Indigenous decedent, for instance, would (on average) be more difficult to identify than a white decedent of Western European ancestry. I highlight "Western" here because the DNA Doe Project has told me before that some Eastern European populations are also underrepresented in the databases. Exceptions are Eastern European Ashkenazi Jewish uploaders, who are well-represented in most databases.

But that's not the only disparity in data. In an article published in the *California Law Review,* "The Racial Composition of Forensic DNA

Databases," authors Erin Murphy and Jun H. Tong pointed out that official forensic databases, like CODIS, show a very different kind of imbal-
ance. "First, we obtained data from states in response to our requests
under freedom of information laws. Second, we devised an original
estimate based on public information about each state's DNA collection policies and the demographic data that matches those policies. In
other words, we reverse-engineered the national DNA database. Both
approaches revealed dramatic disparities in the racial composition of
DNA databases, including that DNA profiles from Black persons are
collected at two to three times the rate of White persons." They found
higher collection rates for other populations, too, such as Indigenous
Americans.[16]

When it comes to voluntary DNA uploads, there are myriad reasons
people hesitate to contribute, but a low level of trust in law enforcement
use is certainly one of them. That hesitancy isn't limited to a single community, but the more investigative genetic genealogists understand about
why people don't take or upload tests—like distrust of law enforcement,
fear of data tracking, or the discussions of blood quantum within Tribal
Nations, where enrollment governance varies from one people to another
but is certainly not decided by a random home DNA test[17]—the better
they can answer questions of people who are considering sharing their
information.

Factors like recent immigration can make a decedent's identification
more difficult, too; this comes down not only to genetic matches in the
database, but access to archival records, language barriers, and methods
of recordkeeping that vary from country to country. Even a lack of familiarity with how certain religious records are kept—say, Catholic birth and
marriage records—can hinder a researcher who is unused to working
with them. If those records are kept in a language the researcher doesn't
speak, then translation takes even longer. And even in families that have
been in North America for generations—or forever—the lasting legacy
of chattel slavery, the boarding school programs of the United States and
Canada that removed Native children from their homes, the '60s scoop in
Canada that fractured Native families and put children into foster care

or closed adoptions, war, forced and crisis relocation, and even natural disasters—can all affect researchers' quests to track their family trees through the generations.

I've only personally observed investigative genetic genealogy done on cases where victims were presumed to have been born in the United States or Canada, but I have friends who work on cases of victims who are suspected to have originated in Mexico, Central America, or South America; this work is desperately needed, not least because so many unidentified decedents are recovered at the Southern border. Investigative genetic genealogists have told me that Hispanic and Central / South American Indigenous decedents are much less likely to have a three-digit cM match in the databases. According to my previous conversations with volunteers at DNA Doe Project, the lowest threshold they can work with is a distant relation—a 20- to 30-cM match, which might be a sixth to eighth cousin, or some equally far-flung connection. But that is slow work; while they can solve cases with numbers that low, seeing 100, 200, 300, or more, that's when an investigative genealogist can count a case solve in days or weeks, not months or years.

That's one of the reasons DNA Doe Project has begun using social media to encourage uploads to GEDmatch, starting with their booth at an annual true crime convention, Crime Con 2022, where attendees had the chance to "match" with twelve Doe cases presented at the DDP booth. Since then, DDP has spotlighted a new case each month—or several cases, depending—to which users can have their kits compared. The match numbers are announced at the end of the month. This has proven to be a popular tactic, encouraging a substantial number of new uploads to GEDmatch. For the 2022 National Hispanic Heritage Month, DNA Doe Project featured Does described as Latino, Hispanic, and/or Indigenous—twelve cases in all. According to the infographic they published October 31, 2022, 116 new DNA kits had been uploaded to GEDmatch as a result of these "Doe Spotlight" drives; that accounts for 22 percent of total GEDmatch uploads during the period. Twelve percent of those uploads were a result of the Hispanic Heritage Month campaign[18]— which specifically sought out Hispanic/Latino/Indigenous uploaders.

Those new kits included one of the highest matches that DDP's new initiative had brought in.

The United States and Canada aren't the only countries interested in investigative genetic genealogy and other DNA technology. GCLAITH—that's the Grupo Científico Latino-Americano de Trabajo Sobre Identificación Humana, or Latin American Scientific Working Group on Human Identification—has met regularly at the International Symposium on Human Identification (ISHI) conference, which is held in the United States. Over the past thirteen years, representatives from countries and regions like Mexico, Brazil, Ecuador, Guatemala, and the Caribbean have formed networks to discuss how to organize and expand forensic DNA databases and begin to use the burgeoning private DNA test market to serve the cases of unidentified decedents.

For now, the United States remains the primary country where investigative genetic genealogy is most often used to close cases and identify decedents. The identification of the famous Somerton Man in Australia—using IGG—was more exception than rule; IGG isn't as regularly employed in Australian cases, and the public doesn't have the same database access we have in the United States. The same is true for the UK and Ireland. While there are solves to be cited in a growing number of countries—for instance, a cold-case Swedish double murder solved in 2021[19]—there are continuing issues of lack of access that prevent researchers across the globe from engaging in IGG: whether it be accessible ancestry records, affordable consumer DNA tests, or networks to support both.

One thing people ask me, when they find out I research unidentified-persons cases, is why IGG isn't used to solve them all. After all, the technology is there, and the people with the skills are waiting; there are both for-profit companies and nonprofits offering lab services, genealogy, or both. Even with the challenges faced by uneven representation in databases, couldn't each case still be attempted?

Unfortunately, it comes down to money.

———•———

In Ina's case, we were lucky. With hair and teeth, and no exhumation necessary, the costs were lower than they might have been. Still, without Dr. Harkins Kincaid's work and the aid of a grant, it would have been very difficult for Amy and me to manage the funding for her full DNA extraction and profile and the genetic genealogy that would lead to her identity. We could have used another lab, but the total cost would still have come in around $7,000 or more. And where was that money coming from? My personal funds and Amy's lab.

That's the other bit that isn't explained to the public: allocation of budgets. We read quite a lot about how money is spent in law enforcement, but not so much about the freedom departments have to re-allocate that spending to other things. Cold cases are not given the budget of fresher cases—and that's in both money and time. I've interviewed dozens of detectives, officers, and agents, and rarely found one who operated within a unit dedicated only to cold cases. More often, it's something they take on along with active investigations, and work they have to pause every time a new missing-persons or homicide or unidentified-persons case comes across their desks. That means a *lot* of pauses.

There are always detectives or medicolegal officials who are focused on the unidentified, or they have a case they've worked for decades that they are absolutely devoted to solving. I've met them. But for every case that has a dedicated investigator attached to it, there are countless others that simply gather dust. Consider, too, that *so* many of the unidentified are people who were marginalized in life: found at camps for the unhoused, or along the Southern border, or died of drug overdoses, or in other circumstances that push them beneath society's radar. The funding isn't there for them when they're alive, let alone after they've passed. Plus, there are always homicides of known people, with families demanding answers and headlines that will stick around longer in the news cycle. And there's the question of resolution, too: When you close an unidentified-persons case, you're often still left with an open homicide investigation. If IGG funding was to be offered to departments, it's likely it would, in many cases, first be allocated to perpetrator cases.

But if a lab or genetic genealogist or nonprofit like the DNA Doe Project is connected with a department or a coroner's office, then avenues could open. Some companies actively seek out their own new cases and crowdfund for them, or apply for grants in partnership with the medico-legal offices. Others, like the mostly volunteer-staffed DNA Doe Project, don't actively contact law enforcement; it usually works the other way around. They are able to offer the IGG for free and help departments without the money for the lab tests raise donations for the rest.

More recently, a number of true-crime celebrities—podcasters and writers and YouTube and TikTok stars—had gotten interested in funding cases. In 2018, the arrest of Joseph DeAngelo, the Golden State Killer, knocked over a genetic domino and ushered in a fresh wave of interest from the public. The true-crime community, whether it was active participants in forums or lone donors who followed the news—they were ready to watch it complete its path. Some, like Ashley Flowers of Audiochuck or the YouTuber MrBallen, have even formed their own nonprofits and foundations to aid in casework. Twitch streamers can now play with these true-crime nonprofits as beneficiaries.

Where will investigative genetic genealogy take us in the future? The leading voices in the field are pushing for regulation and certification in the field, so that it is treated like other forensic work. There was an announcement made about official certification initiatives in the summer of 2022, so that eventually agencies seeking IGG services could seek out genetic genealogists who are certified via a governing body. The main drive behind that, according to my conversations with Dr. Margaret Press, is to make sure that basic standards are followed across the field—so all are trained to properly upload kits to GEDmatch and FTDNA, to use the correct portals and law-enforcement limitations, and to follow ethics standards that ensure genealogists will maintain access to these essential databases that help them solve crimes and identify decedents.

Of the forensic-science avenues I've had the chance to learn about, investigative genetic genealogy is the newest, but it's perhaps the most exciting because of the sheer possibility. The public is just as enamored. How that will affect budget allocations, though, remains to be seen. More often than not, departments have limited funding for expensive lab tests. Despite what TV tells us, law-enforcement agencies aren't equipped with touchscreen simulators that conjure up strands of 3-D DNA for detectives to scowl over before they say *Run it*, and have the case solved in forty minutes. Wouldn't that be nice?

Generally speaking, departments and medical examiners don't have Hollywood budgets.

Perhaps an exhumation would be needed, and multiple rounds of testing are expected due to the poor state of the remains. Accessing the deceased for testing might cost thousands. This isn't to say medicolegal professionals fail to pursue identification; many have worked hard to be sure as many resources as possible go toward their Doe cases. And there are private citizens funding cases on a much larger scale than Amy or I could do, and then there are the foundations and nonprofits, but I haven't seen a lot of organized discussion about how law-enforcement budget allocations might permanently change. With the proof of concept in front of us, headline after headline, perhaps that's on the horizon.

CHAPTER THIRTEEN

THE CASE: ASTREA

November 2021—Santa Cruz, California

S o far, Ina Jane Doe's story has moved neatly down the timeline, with our work on her case lining up with each day, week, month that passed as we worked: June, July, August, and on. But the DNA work is trickier. It takes weeks or months, depending on the tests themselves and how busy the lab is. While each process, well, processed, other things moved forward, like Carl's forensic art and the case announcement. So, a little backtracking is in order, to follow Ina's hair, and her tooth, as they made their way from New Hampshire to Santa Cruz, and how that raw material became a file that Redgrave Research could upload to GEDmatch, and key to solving a case. It's a journey I'd thought about before, in bits and pieces, but never broken down into steps, not past the forensic Monopoly markers of "go to lab" and "now solve this case." In real life, things were a little more complicated.

So, let's go back—temporarily—to November 2021: That's when all the paperwork was completed. Ina's samples had been ready at Amy's lab in New Hampshire for more than a month, but there was still electronic paperwork to sign between Astrea and the Jefferson County Sheriff's Office, and a round of phone calls to make to explain what to fill out where, and all the extremely boring and necessary tasks that are never shown on television but that keep track of important things like chain of evidence and who did what when.

I wanted to see how a DNA lab like Astrea actually did their work. I'd interviewed CEO Dr. Kelly Harkins Kincaid before but having someone explain a process is quite different than actually watching it happen. Normally, I'd be able to pull off an interview like this on my own, but I knew I'd be touring a clean lab and carrying around recording equipment inside a hazmat-type suit while remembering questions; it seemed like a tall order. So, I booked two flights to Santa Cruz. The producer of *The Fall Line*, Maura Currie, agreed to come along: How often do you get the chance to visit a state-of-the-art DNA lab? She only lived a state away from Santa Cruz, and she'd been doing field recording since her days as a public-radio intern. I also promised that she could pick out the hotel. As a twenty-five-year-old with a love for spreadsheets, she was made for this duty. She eagerly started googling boutique bed-and-breakfasts.

———•———

Maura lived in Northern California for a chunk of her childhood and was used to its highways and redwoods and hilly terrain. But I'd only ever been to Los Angeles and Orange County; my experiences had been limited to business meetings and that time my high-school best friend had taken me to Goth Day at Disneyland. I'd seen a lot of people on acid riding in teacups but not a lot of otherwise notable scenery.

We both flew in on Delta and rented a car so I could drive us the forty-five minutes or so to our destination. I wasn't sure what I was expecting out of Santa Cruz, but it certainly wasn't that it would remind me so much of Oregon . . . although, that might have been more about the tourist memorabilia than the actual setting. Maybe I'd been misinformed, but I had no idea Bigfoot was such a big selling point. But the merch for the cryptid started hot and heavy, even at the airport; I took pictures for my other podcast, *One Strange Thing*. Maura and I called it our supernatural pandemic baby. We'd started it as a home for all the strange news stories I came across when researching cold cases: the mysterious blobs in Texas, the demon-like creature that roamed Dover, Massachusetts, the house that had dripped human blood in my hometown of Atlanta. Ever see that chart that helps you figure out whether you should start a new project based on how much spare time you have?

I never pay attention to that chart.

What I saw of Santa Cruz in our forty-hour stay was beautiful. Maura chose a tiny hotel that sat on a main thoroughfare, well within walking distance of Seabright Beach. There was a steep rockface to the west, dotted with expensive-looking homes that had an amazing view of everything below. The hotelier showed us how to make pour-over coffee in the communal kitchen and advised he would not be available in the morning; I advised Maura that we would be DoorDashing coffee to the room. Across the street was a business that we couldn't quite figure out: Was it a restaurant? An apartment complex? We took pictures anyway, because out front they'd placed a carved statue of a very sad-looking sasquatch flanked by an equally forlorn wooden alien.

Bigfoot was clearly a big a retail theme, though—that and the redwoods. We managed to duck into a bookstore before we grabbed dinner and I had my pick of cryptid-related souvenirs to carry home. This time, I also found a grow-your-own redwood kit packed in a neat little cylinder. My son could take his best shot at fostering it in the Georgia red clay. Maura and I went to a restaurant along the Seabright Pier and ordered food that was dressed better than we were; I took a picture of her taking a picture of me and posted it to my Instagram stories. Our mothers both "liked" it. We ended up sharing a king-size bed at the little hotel—no doubles left—and I fell asleep to the sound of a little fountain outside and absolute clouds of pungent smoke seeping under the door. Someone, somewhere was taking advantage of California's relaxed marijuana laws.

We woke up early and got our coffee. Maura figured we'd better dress for ease; she pinned back her chin-length hair and decided on a romper and sneakers.

"Can I wear glasses with a hazmat suit?" she asked me, draining the last of her coffee. "Guess we'll find out." She stopped by the bathroom door and gave me a look as I squinted into the mirror. "You're going to end up with eyeliner all over your face, I can tell you that right now."

"It will be just like Goth Day at Disneyland, then." I put the eyeliner back.

We headed out to Astrea's offices in West Santa Cruz. They were located in a business park with a set of wide, geometric pillars bracing the front door. Dr. Kelly Harkins Kincaid met us outside to guide us through the maze of hallways and stairwells to the office and lab areas where we'd be shadowing senior scientist Dr. Cristina Verdugo. She and I had spoken many times before, and had had a video call or two, so I knew who to look for: She was around my age, though she looked younger—California life, maybe?—with light hair. Kelly was dressed in the kind of layers I'd gotten used to seeing on lab scientists: a fleece vest zipped over a lightweight long-sleeved shirt. Labs tended to be chilly. Kelly had charge of more than one lab, but the work done for Astrea had to be kept completely separate. They specialized in degraded DNA, after all, and the samples had to be protected at all costs.

Kelly was especially suited to design that environment—her doctoral work had combined paleopathology, bioarchaeology, and genetics—so she understood the work she was doing from the perspective of several scientific positions and could speak anthropology with Amy, genetics with the genealogists, and devise her own boutique solutions to difficult sample quandaries. Whenever I described her specialty areas to other scientists, they all made impressed noises, so I figured it was pretty intense stuff.

She led us to an area where we could safely leave our belongings.

"Cristina's just in here," Kelly said over her shoulder. I gazed into a glassed-off room, white-on-white, full of hooded stations, centrifuges, and much more I didn't recognize. We dropped our things off so that we could begin our project: following Cristina and a sample. She had dark, curly hair and was just finishing up at a computer near the door when we arrived. After introductions, she walked us toward the area where'd we need to put on protective clothing.

Another scientist stood at what Cristina called the "accession bench"—where she logged in newly arrived samples into the system and assigned them QR codes. She pointed out a few different items that were key in her line of work: a thermal cycler, fireproof cabinets for storing active case files, a dead-air hood for hair and bone sampling where airflow wouldn't disrupt delicate work. The list went on. The equipment was standard, though perhaps not all labs had to worry about wildfire like Santa Cruz did. It was more about what Astrea was able to accomplish: Because they were trained in extracting and sequencing ancient DNA, they'd have several approaches and solutions in mind for any given situation.

Simply put: Astrea knew what to do if things didn't go to plan. They didn't need to stop at *failed extraction*. They could often avoid it all together.

As we walked past several whiteboards used to track cases, Cristina told us, "The stuff that we're working on now—they're all unidentified cases that have gone to labs between three and fourteen times, is what we've heard. And they're just never able to get enough DNA to do anything with." But with the kind of expertise she and Kelly had, from their background in ancient DNA, they often had success.

We paused in front of a stretch of black flooring that looked just like the padded floor mats at my high-school deli job. I assumed we wouldn't be making sandwiches.

Cristina gestured with her chin. "We have sticky mats down. Just to make sure that whatever's on your shoe is going to come off before you cross into the space." We'd be covering our street clothes with white cleanroom suits and booties and changing out the KN95 masks we'd worn into the building for fresh, lab-supplied surgical ones. But first, we crossed the sticky mat with a Velcro-like ripping noise—leaving behind what, I didn't want to know—and then took turns with multiple sets of gloves, hair coverings, the suits, everything I'd seen in the movies. By the end of it, Maura looked like she'd walked off the set of *Contagion*. I saw myself reflected in her glasses and decided I'd make a good extra myself. Before we put our phones away, we took several photos. I told Maura she should use hers on "the apps." To my surprise, she eventually did. Those were some *interesting* first dates.

After we got Maura's recording equipment situated and we crossed into the clean area, I asked Cristina to start at the *beginning*, and she was kind enough to do so. She explained that whether you're looking at an STR or a SNP profile, the basic extraction steps for DNA science are the same: lysis, which is a disruption or breaking of the cell to release DNA; separating the DNA from the cell debris and any other material; using a binding agent to collect the DNA; purification to wash away all the unbound material; and finally elution, to release the purified DNA into solution so that it can be analyzed or inspected. Eventually, the scientists will be able to examine the sample and its quality: How much usable DNA is present? How high is the bacterial contamination?

Consider the exposure a sample might have had. If skeletal remains were found in the woods, exposed to the elements for forty years, a tooth would be a much more protected sample to send to a lab; predators would have been less likely to break it open and expose the inner tissue to bacteria. But if the victim had serious cavities and active dental decay at the time of their death, much of that protection might be broken down.

Cristina showed us a set of samples that she said had been "incubating" and explained what they'd do with them. She gestured to a table of equipment. "One of the steps requires us to centrifuge the DNA that's currently incubating through these columns. Once I add the binding buffer and spin the sample, that's what binds the DNA to a silica pellet in the column, and lets the liquid pass through. So I'm just setting up my columns right now. And then I'm going to set up my binding buffer."

She had a checklist laid out neatly on the counter and tapped it with a gloved finger.

"What's the centrifuge doing?" I asked. "I mean, I know what it's doing, it's spinning, but what state do you want the material inside to be in?"

I was pretty sure my son, who had recently asked for a centrifuge after seeing one on YouTube, would have found this to be the highlight of the tour. He'd explained to me that a centrifuge could separate a substance into its components by high-speed spinning—like cream from milk—but I wasn't sure what Cristina was up to. Probably not making butter.

She explained, "Basically, that's centrifuging down, the first of two steps. At first it's to get all of the bone as compacted as possible. We spin it at a certain speed and then we spin it again at a faster speed. The idea is that you want it as compact as possible so that you don't pipette any bone powder when you're putting the DNA solution into the column, because that will clog the column. And then, I'll aliquot out binding buffer into each of these 15 mL tubes. There's another buffer that goes in with that, and then the sample goes in. I'll invert the tube, mix it really well, and then that is what goes into the column to be centrifuged down. We're trying to get everything really homogenized so that it is efficient when it's being spun."

One of the most interesting things she showed us were the incredibly precise procedures and methods for pipetting reagents from one thing to another—not just order, but rules about pipettes in gloved hands being held near open tubes, or the vital nature structure and lists and training and the multiple lines of defense in place played to avoid human error in testing and in introducing contamination. Since they weren't breaking open prefabricated kits and following another manufacturer's instructions, there was a lot to remember. That's why Cristina liked her list. You memorize it, but it's still there. The pipettes looked a lot like what came in my son's science kits: thin plastic tubes that suck up and dispense liquid in drops. We'd used them at home for everything from growing our own mold to writing in invisible ink.

It seemed that everything at Astrea was about checking lists, and procedure—which made perfect sense when you consider how bad contamination could be for a sample. *Take the lids off the samples. Put the lids back on. Follow the process.* After all, as Cristina said, "It's part of what is protocol for working in ancient DNA. If I were to sneeze in the hood at this moment, when all of these samples, like if I had the lids off of these, my DNA, even if it was just from a sneeze aspirating out to the air is enough that all of these samples' signals would probably be even lower or totally gone."

She explained the "eluting process" as well, where the DNA that had been bound to the silica pellet was released via elution in a warm solution. That was when they'd be able to see what they were working with. Cristina patiently explained that, yes, the DNA stayed on the silica "for a hot minute," as I'd inquired—about a hot fifteen minutes to be exact.

As we were finishing up, another Astrea employee brought in the day's mail. There was good news: Amy's overnight package had arrived. Ina Jane Doe's samples were officially in the lab. Since the paperwork with Jefferson County was finished, Amy had been able to send the samples that she and Sam had taken back in September, and she had paid an obscene amount of money to get them there as quickly and safely as possible. We hurried out of the layers of sci-fi gear and untangled Maura from the cords we'd strapped inside her clothing to record the tour.

Since hair and a tooth had been sent, Astrea would examine and extract DNA from both samples and decide which yielded the best return. Cristina seemed pleased with the hair strands and tooth that Amy had packaged up. "We'll get these logged in and get started."

We met back up with Kelly, and Maura and I took the scientists out to lunch. It seemed like a fair trade, considering we had loitered in their lab for at least two hours. It was a beautiful day in Santa Cruz, so we ate somewhere with patio seating and QR code menus, and the French-press coffee was good enough that I didn't notice until halfway through the meal that my extremely expensive lunch salad didn't have any dressing. I was willing to overlook a lot of dry lettuce for quality caffeine.

Maura had set up another, much smaller mic at the table, which the waitress was polite enough to ignore. I wanted to talk a little more with the scientists about what made Astrea unique. I knew their training in bioarchaeology and paleopathology were essential in terms of their skill set developed around ancient DNA, but how did anthropology come in? And how did that combination of skills set them apart?

Cristina considered my questions, and replied, "What we've realized in talking with law-enforcement agencies is, because their understanding of this new tech is limited, they tend to take certain aspects of it, like the haplotype or the haplogroup information, and they want to translate that into a race, which is not something that we do as anthropologists. We're not just putting people in a box and then moving forward. What we've tried to do, because we have the knowledge that we have, is explain it."

Kelly nodded. "Another aspect that sets us apart is that, as anthropologists, I think a lot about being good stewards of genetic data, being caretakers of this very private information and thinking about ways to keep it secure and protect privacy. And so, I don't know if that sets us apart, but it's something I spend a lot of time thinking about. How do we be good stewards of this data in this era of genome privacy?"

Cristina swallowed a bite of her sandwich, then gestured with her water glass. "Or even just handling the actual material itself. I think I'm very careful with that. I take the time to look at what I'm going to do before I do it, with the understanding that this isn't just a hair or a bone sample, but this was a person."

I paused and looked at Maura. She mistook it as a silent request for a French fry and dropped one on my plate. "That's interesting. It sounds just like what I hear Amy tell students during lab at her school, about treating human remains with respect and dignity and empathy."

Kelly laughed. "Yeah. You can't take the anthropologist out of the geneticist once it's in there."

"Do you feel like that's affected the creative approach to your techniques?" I remembered the whiteboard of cases they'd had up in their lab. Kelly had told me that some had failed in other labs as many as a dozen times or more.

Kelly shrugged. "For better or worse, we don't like to give up because we have a pretty broad knowledge of what is methodologically possible. We know that there's not just one single technique or one single path. For better or worse, we want to keep trying when something doesn't work the first time."

With that, we moved on to discussing lunch, the free popcorn the waitress kept bringing—no complaints there—and our flights home. Maura and I dropped the scientists back off at the lab an hour later, and twelve hours after that, I was flying back to Atlanta. My husband and son were so used to picking me up at the airport that the stop-and-start traffic at the hellish terminal curve put my kid to sleep. He woke up when we pulled into our driveway, and we had to talk him out of planting his new redwood at nine p.m. Just as well: When we read the fine print, we discovered that it could only be planted after two weeks of rain, and that it had to germinate in the refrigerator for at least that long before. This was not going to happen in Georgia, in November. On the bright side, his new Bigfoot foot cast kit was ready to go. He planned on telling his grandparents that he'd discovered a sasquatch print by the back gate, near the swing set.

As for Ina Jane Doe: Her case wouldn't be waiting more than a season. I sent an email to thank Astrea for hosting us, and then in early December, I heard back: Ina's extractions looked amazing, meaning it had been a success. There was not only enough usable DNA in the package Amy had so carefully assembled, but it was some of the best samples they'd seen in their lab. Kelly wrote that they'd let us know as soon as her sequencing was finished, and a file prepared for the genealogists.

That was my cue to introduce the two parties: Astrea Forensics, meet Redgrave Research. Lots of CCs, listing of initials after names, cases solved, shared colleagues. The drill we run through to say, in so many words, *I can be trusted, and so can the person I am copying here.* Formal emails aren't particularly exciting on their face, but there was absolute electricity running underneath these exchanges. Because we all knew what this meant: So long as there were workable matches in GEDmatch for Ina, her case was well on the way to being solved.

CHAPTER FOURTEEN

THE CASE: REDGRAVE RESEARCH

September 2021—Orange, Massachusetts

The fall of 2021 was also when I made my first and only trip to Orange, Massachusetts, a town I can honestly say I didn't even know existed prior to my arrival. This is not a knock on Orange; I'm from a region where we have towns the size of a busy QuikTrip. After all, my grandparents spent decades living near a lake in a place called Ninety Six, South Carolina, population 2,000-ish. It's not Orange's fault that Boston and Salem are taking up all the attention on the map.

I traveled to Orange when I was in New Hampshire, on my visit to Amy's; it was about a two-hour drive from the university, so Amy, Sam, and I headed down there to check out the Redgraves' new office space. Lee and Anthony Redgrave operated the Trans Doe Task Force, their law enforcement and student-training program, and all other projects from their home, so it was exciting that they finally had some separate working space. It was the kind of real estate that made my Atlanta heart jealous: a mixed-use loft converted from some sort of old factory, with a gym, a coffee bar, a tattoo studio, and even a laundromat. The rent would have been *insane* in a bigger town. Railroad tracks ran behind the building, giving the whole space a more urban feel than I'd been expecting.

237

There weren't many married couples in investigative genetic genealogy—or forensic genetic genealogy, as Lee and Anthony preferred, though Anthony told me that if he got to pick, he'd have gone with "genealogical human identification." I had to admit, it was a good option. Lee and Anthony had been some of the very first volunteers at DNA Doe Project. They'd eventually gone on to focus on their own business, Redgrave Research Forensic Services, and their nonprofit, the Trans Doe Task Force.

As trans men, both Lee and Anthony had been keenly aware of the disturbing lack of care in treatment of trans and gender-expansive cases: There were decedents whose identity in life was misinterpreted or missed altogether by medicolegal professionals. The Trans Doe Task Force had started with a simple question. Anthony, who is both trans and intersex, wondered: *How would I be identified if my body was found?* Anthony had developed an interest in genealogy early in life and used it to learn more about his own family and origins. Lee, who is an adoptee, also learned about genealogy, at least originally, to trace his family of origin. But then, they wanted to do more. Even as they helped to identify the dead with DDP, they were left with growing concerns of the way the cases of trans and gender nonconforming individuals were handled, or even recognized. The disturbing descriptions written up on databases—the same kind Taylor Flaherty described, terse entries of "man found in women's clothing" (*What clothing? How would this person's loved ones recognize them without an actual detailed description of the items?*), lack of choices for "sex" or for pronouns in missing-persons bulletins. The list went on.

Lee and Anthony pointed this out to me soon after we met, showing me how to spot context within descriptions of victims' clothing, physical description, or even the crime scene that helped me flag cases that might fall under their purview. Homophobic and transphobic language surrounding anything from gender-affirming surgery and care to labels like "transvestite" or "cross-dresser" could obscure the cases of decedents, which meant their families and chosen families were less likely to recognize descriptions in police bulletins or forensic art.

Anthony also taught me to think about the intricacies of DNA testing: the kind of profiles that gave a *sex* result for decedents didn't carry the nuanced information that could indicate, for instance, an intersex condition. Anthony pointed out that a decedent's skeletal remains might come back as, say, XY, but that might not tell their whole story. It was one of the many issues Lee and Anthony considered when they searched through databases and scoured NamUs, looking for cold cases that might have been misinterpreted or mishandled.

By November 2021, I'd been working with the Redgraves, on and off, for a couple of years; this was, however, the first time we'd gotten to meet in person. They preferred Facebook Instant Messenger to texting, and to phone calls, so almost all our communication took place online. They were also night owls who stayed up late, working on genealogy projects, and were usually getting to bed about the time I woke up. Sometimes, we passed, ships in the internet seas, in late afternoon.

When we drove up to their office in Orange, Sam and Amy and I weren't the only visitors in town. Viktor Veltstra, a member of the Trans Doe Task Force's nonprofit board, had arrived a few weeks earlier. He had charge of TDTF's first-of-its-kind database, LAMMP: *LGBT+ Accountability for Missing and Murdered Persons.* It was designed to address the failings of other reporting systems and databases that mishandled, underreported, misreported, and in some cases even slowed down the progress of cases in the LGBTQ+ community.

The database, which was private—meaning that users had to request access and prove their credentials as professionals—did take submissions of information from the missing or murdered individuals' chosen friends and family. That way, more accurate information regarding gender presentation, name, and much more could be included, and Viktor, Lee, and Anthony had a real chance of matching them up with an unidentified person who they'd manually entered into their database.

This warehouse office served multiple purposes, and today we were there for Redgrave Research Forensic Services; Amy and I hired them to handle Ina Jane Doe's genetic genealogy. But this wasn't the first time for me. When my husband decided he wanted to find his birth father, we went to the Redgraves. It had taken them a day or so to complete the work. We'd discovered that his birth father had died at eighteen in a car accident. We weren't sure if he'd even known my husband existed. But there was a younger sister, that aunt from 23andMe, who had become a treasured connection. So, I knew what they could do.

We got out of Amy's RAV4 and wandered into the building. There were several floors, and we ended up at an empty coffee bar and in a giant industrial laundromat before we finally found Redgrave Research's office tucked into a corner, its door decorated with stickers and postcards. We posed for a picture outside their office. Then we sent it to them. That worked; Anthony and Lee appeared, along with Viktor, and ushered us in.

"Dr. Amy! Sam! Laurah!" Anthony greeted us. He'd gotten in the habit of calling Amy *Dr. Amy* when talking about her to his genealogy students; Sam also did some work with them, but she didn't engage much with the students, so she was *Dr. Blatt* when need arose. I'd gotten into the *Dr. Amy* habit with my son. He called all my other friends "Auntie": Auntie Brooke, Auntie Maura. Amy wasn't exactly the auntie type. But she sent him presents, like a book on the cryptids of West Virginia or bugs she fixed up in paraffin, frozen like amber. So, she became Dr. Amy, whose mail was superior.

Everyone hugged; we were gentle with Lee, as he was recovering from surgery. Lee, Anthony, and Viktor were all around my age, and showed signs of a counterculture youth that were familiar to me: tattoos, band pins stuck onto their jackets, and broken-in boots. I'd brought Viktor a few *Fall Line* pins for his coat; I'd had them printed up in the one-inch punk style because they fit so nicely onto a motorcycle jacket lapel. I gave Anthony a bag of gummy worms we'd bought at a gas station on the way, because I knew he liked to eat candy when he was up late, looking at DNA or building family trees. He paid me back with several sets of googly-eye stickers to take home for my son. Or, Anthony said, to stick on anything that struck my fancy on the way.

"Do you want to go on a tour of the building?" Viktor asked. We did indeed. He walked us through the whole place, including the back, to show us the lonely train tracks running behind. The most interesting part was a large, shared art space where various craftspeople came to make their work: fabric art, boots, 3-D printing, and more. Actually, we met a man who was still sorting out the 3-D plastic garlic bulbs he'd printed for the annual festival—which celebrated garlic. He let us all pick one to take home.

When we walked back into the office, I noticed they'd hung up Anthony's forensic art—that was something he was teaching himself—along with sketches from other cases. I recognized two drawings: one was of Joseph Henry Loveless, whose torso had been discovered in a cave in Idaho. The Redgraves had been on that case with DNA Doe Project, Amy, and Sam. It was a fascinating story. When Loveless's remains were recovered, in the late 1970s, experts thought he'd been in that cave for a relatively short time. But it turned out the environment of the cave had preserved what was left of him—what was found in 1979 and 1991. When the genetic genealogists began to work on his case, however, they realized he was much older, and had been in the cave much longer. The tree showed that Loveless was from a lineage dating back to the polygamist days of the Church of Jesus Christ of Latter-Day Saints. Loveless had been a bootlegger who'd murdered his own wife before going on the run; he'd been killed himself, by parties unknown, around 1916.

I looked up at the unfamiliar art pinned up over their double desktop screens.

"Who is this?" I pointed to a reconstruction of a young white male with shaggy, light hair.

"Jasper County John Doe," Lee replied. "Anthony just finished that one."

I remembered the case; my research assistant, Bryan, had been working on his identification as well. The Jasper County John Doe was a known victim of serial killer Larry Eyler—one of several unidentified victims that remained, long after Eyler's death. Though Eyler's exact victim count is unknown, it's estimated that he murdered at least twenty-one young men between 1982 and 1984. In a few months' time, the Redgraves successfully identified this particular John Doe as nineteen-year-old William "Bill" Joseph Lewis.

Another case they were working on was considered Canada's most famous unidentified-persons case, the Babes in the Woods: two children, siblings, who were found murdered in a public park in 1953. Redgrave Research was actively working on that case with the Vancouver Police. I'd tried and failed to set up an interview with the lead detective. Even after Redgrave Research solved the case, months later, the press had a difficult time gathering information on the little boys, Derek and David D'Alton, and Canadian law enforcement was close-lipped.

I sat on the edge of a futon couch and thumbed through the TDTF pins and stickers Anthony had made. My students had eagerly grabbed up the first round he'd sent me in the spring, so I needed to restock. The visit wasn't formal; we were there to see our friends and take a break amidst our research work for Ina. The Redgraves talked with Amy and Sam about their genetic genealogy certification program while I studied the highly decorated walls. They were proponents of collaborative case solving, just like Margaret and the volunteers of the DNA Doe Project, and I'd get to know some of the Redgraves' students as I observed their casework over the next few months. Some students were seasoned genealogists who'd been handling adoption cases for years. Others were moderators of Reddit forums, or professionals in research or archival fields, or volunteers for the Trans Doe Task Force, or college students interested in missing-person cases. There was a lot of variety.

But they all learned to build family trees in ways that made my head spin.

Lee and Anthony had worked as a team for a while, but it was only in the past two years that they'd been collaborating with students and with Viktor, who had graduated from the certification program, on TDTF and Redgrave Research cases. Lee told me that their relationship was part of what made it all work so well; they'd been a couple for a very long time, and married for years, and raised a child together. But even before that, they bonded on what he described as "a symbiotic level." He said, "I can't say that I think that we would be doing any of this without the relationship that we have."

Sam and Amy casually started flipping through a forensic dentistry book—something really old and terrifying—that was sitting on the desk. Viktor was on his phone; he was helping track a missing child on social media. That was a big focus of Viktor's: on-the-ground missing-persons work. Lee and Anthony had set up something on the computer for a project they'd be working on with their students that evening, so I decided it was a good time to ask them more about the program. I knew about their students, because they'd worked on my husband's case as well. But I wouldn't understand the full organizational approach until I got to watch them work on Ina's case.

"Okay, questions for my notes," I said, pulling out my phone for that purpose. "You train your students on forensic cases, which is an incredible experience for them, but also something that could be potentially sensitive—police files, people's DNA information, family information. I know there's an NDA as a matter of course, but how else do you approach teaching students to use best practices when approaching this work?"

Lee leaned back in his chair. With all of us in the room, space was scarce; I could almost have touched his computer's keyboard. "A lot of it is set up on the front end. A lot of people do not realize all the moving parts that are behind the scenes. So, we try to show our students all of those steps, from start to finish. We show them communications that we have with agencies. We show them how we respond. We even sometimes say, 'oh wow, we've gotten this communication, we haven't responded yet. How do you think you would respond?' What we're trying to do is set people up for their own successes. When they move on from us, they're going to go and do whatever they're going to do, but we want them to be more equipped to do it when they leave. One of those things is setting them up to know how to ethically run an operation and then we're modeling that to them."

I'd given up and started recording with my voice memo app. "And is that all teamwork? Do people work alone, too?"

Lee wiggled his hand in the "semi-sometimes" gesture. "When we bring on a new person, we have our own conversation with them. They have to sign the NDA, but then also they're thrown into a group of people who are having this active, ongoing conversation about what is the best way that we can treat these cases? What's the best we can do, and how can we support each other in doing that team effort. I think that for some people they prefer to work individually, and that's fine for them, but we prefer to work in a team for a number of reasons. One of the reasons is just that it works better when you have multiple people trying to solve the problem. But also in an educational setting, I really like that the team is the asset. Everyone's holding each other accountable. You want to do your best, not just for the cases or for the clients, but you want to do your best for the team as well. And that's going to make an intrinsic motivation for their students because it's a social experience for them as well, being a team member."

It sounded interesting, but it was hard for me to imagine, in practice. Viktor told us how the student teams worked in Discord, on voice chat and text chat at the same time, with each team member pulling in information on different branches of a family tree, or looking up news clippings, or searching yearbooks. Organized chaos, maybe? I'd see it in action soon enough.

On February 3, 2022, I was sitting in my closet when my phone screen lit up. Although hiding from my problems in a closet would have been an appealing option on most afternoons, on this particular day, I was recording podcast narration. I'd put my cell on silent, because my producer, Maura, would annihilate me if she heard buzzing in the background of the tape, and she was on the line while I read. But I needed to stay alert in case something happened with my son at school, so this was a good compromise. I almost always remembered to turn down the volume. When I didn't, I'd hear her mute button come off, and disapproving noises swell up.

This time, I'd remembered. When I took a second to sip water and flip script pages—unlike most of my friends, I didn't record off a computer screen or tablet, because it gave me a migraine—I took the chance to look at my phone. It was a text from Amy: *Check your email.* But I knew I'd have to wait until Maura and I were done. Maura was far more frightening than Amy. She'd once sent me an audio track consisting only of my spitty mouth noises and heavy breathing to show me what she took out of each track. I learned that day: You don't cross an engineer-producer.

As soon as I was freed from the closet, I ran downstairs to let the dogs into the backyard, because I'd heard faint barking for the last hour or so. There was clearly a squirrel that needed chasing. I checked the time; I had an hour before I needed to go pick up my son from his second-grade class. All responsibilities managed, I could sit down and see what this email was about. I hoped Ina's results were in, but knowing Amy and the work we did, it could be just about anything. We were trying for an exhumation order in another Illinois case. They'd said the ground was too hard in winter, but maybe something was planned for spring?

I'd been right the first time. There it was: I was CC'd on the email from Astrea. Kelly had copied me, Amy, the Redgraves, and Jefferson County to tell us that Ina Jane Doe's file was complete. Everything had been a success: Once the Redgraves got the data, or kit, as they called it, they could upload it to GEDmatch. Then her kit would take twenty-four hours or so—usually less, at least with my own kits—to batch.

Anthony had shown me that process when he let me sit in on a student tutorial for uploading; when they got the file, they'd put out a call so that interested students could log onto a Zoom call and watch him go through the upload in real time. Anthony would use GEDmatch Pro, of course, as required, so that Ina's kit was uploaded through the forensic portal. Though she could be compared with all GEDmatch kits, her case still needed to be processed as a forensic case, and through the proper channels.

By the time I'd driven to my son's school, picked him up, and gotten him to karate class, the call had gone out: It was time to join the Zoom. I couldn't exactly participate while Shihan was shouting about katas, but I listened in via AirPods and phone. I followed along as Anthony went through the portal process, and I heard him answering questions: No, they'd only upload to FTDNA if there weren't high enough matches on GEDmatch. Yes, they were hoping for a relative of at least 100 cMs. Two or more at 100 cM or greater would be ideal. He wasn't sure how long it would take the kit to batch: There were some tools we could look at right away while Ina's file processed so it could be run through GEDmatch's major function, the "one to many" comparison. Then we'd be able to look at all her matches, from the highest to the lowest, and any family trees those members had been kind enough to upload. But for now, there were a few things we could do: Look at Ina's ancestry estimate with a tool so complex that I couldn't make heads or tails of it. And we could do one-to-one comparisons, too. That meant that Anthony could run our personal kits—because we knew the numbers—against Ina's.

They tried Amy's first, since she was from the Midwest. No segments shared. Viktor Veltstra's kit was next; in addition to his LAMMP and TDTF duties, he was a teaching assistant in the training program, having completed it himself and become an investigative genetic genealogist. He'd been run against plenty of Doe cases. This time, no segments shared. That was to be expected—more common than not—though Lee Redgrave told me he'd once found that he shared a segment with an unidentified person whose case he was working on. It was the thinnest connection, a most distant cousin, a single spot of color variation on the program Anthony liked to use to visualize DNA.

Then they ran my kit against Ina's. We shared a segment: a tiny, bright link between our histories, so many generations back or cousins removed that I wouldn't have claimed to call her any relation. But the thread was there. Not nearly enough centimorgans to be useful. But we were connected, through some little strand of stories, across the regions. My mother's side of the family were mostly Swiss-German, so I imagined the connection might be somewhere else, stretched out in the expanse of my father's family tree. But really, it could be anyone. I'd matched to Julie Doe, too, the case that first introduced me to the Redgraves, Trans Doe Task Force, to DNA Doe Project; again, not enough to be of any help—8 cM. But I felt the same way each time: We are connected to cold cases in ways that may not seem apparent. Maybe we share a single slice of DNA;

maybe we can relate on a different level. As parents, or children, or brothers or sisters, or people who want better for the ones they love. That's a beginning, to shorten the distance.

Right before Ina's kit dropped, I'd sat in on a Zoom session with the Redgrave students, watching Anthony use DNA Painter for another case; it's software that allows for the visualization of DNA data. It shows genetic genealogists which specific segments of DNA are shared across matches, and not just *that* a pair is related, but *how* they are related: which segments connect them. Once the kit dropped, Anthony would be able to compare Ina Jane Doe's kit to others via DNA Painter, too. It could help him when looking at relatives and trying to discern their particular relationships.

It took less than a day for the kit to finish batching, and everyone was irritable, excited, texting, and messaging on Discord and Facebook. I was on a deadline for the podcast but didn't want to miss anything, so I carried my laptop around the house with me in case I needed to get on a Zoom call: into the kitchen, stuck on the back of the counter while I chopped carrots, or into the dining room to stand guard while I helped my son with three-digit subtraction. I tried not to drain my AirPods; last time we'd been on a genealogy call, they'd died, and I'd had to use my computer speakers. My son kept interrupting to quiz the Redgraves about Minecraft. It was not an ideal work environment.

Finally, on the evening of February 4, I got the text:

It's ready.

I logged into their private Discord channel devoted to the case, and onto Zoom, hoping I'd be able to keep up with both at once. Watching them work was dizzying; listening at the same time reminded me of the times I'd drank Everclear back in college. They'd offered to teach me the genealogy. But the first time I'd seen trees expand, one after another, like some kind of unending game of unfolding tiles . . . it felt like the first time I'd read a story by Jorge Luis Borges, about the maddening nature of the infinite.

I didn't think I'd get past the first step or two before my brain collapsed. I could follow the DNA part a bit better, at least in its elementary stages—this amount means one of these relationships, this amount another level of closeness, this another, until you're a sibling, or parent, or child. But honestly, I was happiest staying in my lane: watching them work, and pulling newspaper articles, census records, or yearbook photos, anything else they might need from me. All I needed were some starting names.

I had to minimize the Discord chat so I could concentrate on Anthony's Zoom presentation: too much information all at once. I'd met a few of their students before, in person—Chelsea, for instance, had come up to UNH for the podcast panel—but I couldn't pick out one voice from another in the excited chatter. Things settled down, though, when Anthony shared his screen with the rest of us. He'd checked Ina's ancestry composition before—she was of European descent, though the countries suggested by the Oracle tool on GEDmatch didn't always jibe with what the genealogists found in their family trees. Anthony and Viktor had told me, for instance, that Italy had a habit of just kind of . . . popping up in Oracle ancestry results. Were there Italians in the family trees? Sometimes. Sometimes, not so much. I assumed that there was an explanation for this that I didn't fully understand; when I ran my own, I understood even less. My ancestry showed a bewildering array of combos, but the top listing indicated my forebearers had possibly originated from the Orkney Islands off the coast of Scotland, France, North Germany, and England. I imagined some combination of German and French might come out as Swiss, but otherwise? I couldn't follow the threads like I might on Ancestry or 23andMe, where the software sorted everything out for me with kindergarten simplicity.

For Ina, that bit wasn't important for now; her results just confirmed what had been presumed at the time of her discovery. But if her family tree got twisty or confusing, the suggestions made by the program, limited as it might be, could be helpful in the genealogists' research. They might use DNA, but they did plenty the old-fashioned way: painstaking building out of generations, scouring census lists, and searching for clues.

Anthony was talking; I settled on my bed so I could concentrate. I could hear my husband and son struggling with another math assignment downstairs. Well, fair enough, because I had my own.

"I'm now running Ina Jane Doe's kit through the 'one to many' tool," Anthony said over my AirPods. He clicked on Ina's kit—a combination of letters and numbers assigned by the system—and hit Submit. I knew what would pop up after the slight lag: all her matches, the people who had taken the time to download their own raw DNA data from other sites and upload it on GEDmatch, ranked from highest cM to lowest. Those lowest numbers . . . the scroll was nearly endless. But at the top, that's where we'd be focused, fingers crossed for a number in the hundreds.

Who were the people who'd bothered to submit? Many were likely genealogy buffs who'd uploaded kits for themselves and other family members. I'd found one of my own second cousins on every single possible genealogy site; he'd written to me to ask about some gaps in the family tree I had no idea how to fill. I'd sent him on to my dad. Those were probably the bulk of users. But plenty had uploaded for other reasons. Some were probably looking for something more: missing relatives. Birth parents, or siblings, families that they'd never met. The truth regarding questions they'd never received satisfactory answers to.

We all waited for that half second, hoping that a match of at least a hundred would appear at the top of the screen. They'd descend from there, down to the lowest matches.

"This *is* good." Anthony sounded jubilant as I focused in. Number one: 432.1 cM. Number two: 168.2 cM. Number three: 159 cM. Three numbers over a hundred. And that 432.1 cM? It was the highest I'd ever seen during observation of a case . . . which amounted to three sessions. Still, I knew that was a big deal.

Essentially, this meant Ina's case would be solved quickly. Perhaps in a day, or even less. My eyes burned at the thought. That meant that within a week, Jefferson County would probably be in contact with her family. And then, if they wanted, I might be, too.

The genealogists worked in a fashion I found both highly efficient and confusing: Each claimed a person on the list of top matches—the top twenty or so—and said they'd start working on their family trees. If the uploaders had included their trees, it made it all the easier, but if not, they could hop over to Ancestry.com and work back and forth, pulling information from one place to another. Sometimes, these twists took much longer to solve, at least fully; I knew of one time a Canadian student had to go to a local library and dug through out-of-print phonebooks for leads. But based on what we had, I didn't think it would come to that. Actually . . . wait, what did we have, precisely?

I didn't want to interrupt their work; I went back to watching the Discord and muted voice chat so I could follow all the links they were posting to this tree or that. I had access to the main tree Anthony was overseeing—a master tree, you might say—on his account, but I wasn't sure exactly how all the branches would eventually connect. From what I understood, it's almost as if they were building a wall, and every genealogist took a different section and set of bricks. Eventually, they'd run into one another and create links.

Basically, they'd build out each match until they found the connective tissue between the branches. They were looking for a few key things: the MRCA, or most recent common ancestor, shared between each match and Ina Jane Doe, and what they called the XCA, or crossover common ancestors. This tied into the phenomenon that the DNA Doe Project previously explained to me as the union couple: basically, the grandparents, or even parents, that drew together the lines of the tree and ended at the Doe. In the final stages, Anthony would run a probability calculator that showed the various family members—say, a group of siblings, or sets of cousins in a family—and how likely they were to be Ina Jane Doe. But we'd need to do research, too. That's where social media came in handy, and news stories: When people went missing, their families talked about them. The news may have covered their cases. But even if they didn't, we could see something else: when they stopped appearing in the family. Did mentions disappear? That was a clue in and of itself.

While they worked on the connecting trees and happily posted memes and stickers in their Discord chat, I paused to look into the possible familial relationships. Ina's top match, 432.1 cM, might be a great-great aunt or uncle, or half great aunt or uncle, a half first cousin, a first cousin once removed, a half great niece or nephew, or a great-great niece or nephew. There were other options, but those were by far the likeliest. By 10:30 p.m. or so, the Redgraves and their students narrowed the relative down to a first cousin once removed. This individual had been adopted, which always added a layer of research difficulty, but still, it was a strong, strong lead.

The genealogists would stay up on this all night; they were talking in the Discord and chat about making coffee and drinking soda. I was not so stalwart. I usually went to bed around nine p.m., prime granny time, because I got up at five or so to drink coffee and work out before anyone bothered me. An hour of quiet time is something to be treasured. But it also meant that I couldn't hang. By eleven p.m. that night, my eyes were aching, and the chat was blurring into a chorus of numbers and names I couldn't follow.

They were hot on a dozen trails all at once, but circling that first cousin once removed in tighter, concentric circles. They were researching on Newspapers.com, checking yearbooks on Ancestry, looking up birth and death records. I thought for a second, and then typed in the Discord: *Anthony, you're recording this, right? I'm not going to make it. I've got to go to sleep.*

He answered me back over my AirPods. "I am. Get some sleep."

I'd be able to read the chat back in Discord, and see all the things people found: photos, census records, even photographs.

"Okay . . . well . . . don't solve it while I'm gone." I'd actually be happy if they did, though it would be most exciting to watch it in real time. But needs must be met: I went off to brush my teeth, peek in my son's room to make sure he was breathing—normal behavior when your child is seven, I'm sure—and found my husband downstairs watching one of his dopey supernatural melodramas. I kissed him good night, packed my son's lunch, and figured I could sleep for six hours or so; they'd probably be close to solving it when I woke up, but I'd have time to catch up.

I would not have time to catch up.

I slept—no dreams since we'd seen the park in Illinois, so that was a good thing, but maybe also a bad one because I slept right through my alarm. I didn't get up until seven, and then it was a rush to get everyone out of the house, and dogs fed. I didn't have a text from Amy, but she went to bed even earlier than I did. And Lee and Anthony weren't texters.

When I finally got to sit down and check Discord, my fingers were tingling with pins and needles, like they'd fallen asleep. That happened sometimes when I was really nervous. I opened Ina's forum, and there it was—a photo.

In six hours, start to finish, they'd begun with a 432.1 cM match on GEDmatch, and ended at a woman who'd last been seen in Tennessee. I followed Anthony's notes: The team had collaboratively solved this case, that was certain. And they'd known Ina's real name for hours while I was asleep.

No more Ina Jane Doe. That had been the hope. And here we were.

———•———

Her name was Susan Minard Lund. She was only twenty-five years old when she disappeared on December 24, 1992. She had three small children. Her case had been closed by the Tennessee authorities. They'd said she'd been found, in Alabama, in August 1993. But that couldn't be the case. Susan had been dead for at least seven months before that.

It looked like a yearbook photo had been posted in the Discord. Junior year of high school? Senior, maybe? The image was black-and-white, but I could tell she was a redhead. It was something about the depth of the tone in the gray. Her shoulder-length hair was cut in a sort of shag, just like Kyana had guessed. I loved her expression: serious, not quite a smile, with no teeth showing, looking directly at the photographer as if she saw something in them and wasn't sure what she thought of it.

There was just the faintest asymmetry to that smile; if I didn't know to look for it, I wouldn't have spotted it. Amy had been right, too.

OMG! What is happening??!? I typed.

But really, the answer was obvious: *everything.*

CHAPTER FIFTEEN

THE ANSWER: SUSAN MINARD LUND

We hadn't come upon the missing-persons report of Susan Minard Lund in our research. We might have, eventually. But maybe not. It mostly comes down to the news archives and the exact right string of search prompts to summon up the stories that would match. Even then, it's a long drive, if a fairly straight one, from western Tennessee to southern Illinois. But we didn't find her early on because there was no trace of her in the missing-persons databases. And that wasn't a mistake; her case was closed around August 1993.

You can't find someone who isn't there.

But with investigative genetic genealogy, the path to Sue was a short one. It's not always that way, but thankfully in this case, things had fallen into place with a dizzying speed. After Redgrave Research identified the branches of Sue's family and found the "union couple"—her parents—it was down to figuring out who was missing. With some families, that can take quite a while; I do the same work, so I know. You go through phone listing records and addresses and census registrations to see when names suddenly cease activity. You check marriage certificates.

But you also go to social media. Never underestimate that; it's a treasure trove of information. Facebook is the best if you're looking into an older case: Gen X and the Baby Boomers are holding fast on that website. Some families keep themselves to themselves, and I don't blame them.

I've always been that way. Some are willing to keep their posts public, maybe in hopes someone sees them. Maybe just because they haven't thought about how much is available if someone decides to look. All it takes is one photo to connect the dots.

In Susan's case, the pattern was clear: Everyone in the family discussed her disappearance. There was no question who was missing; her name kept coming up again and again across their social media. Her sisters had been looking for her for a long time. Two of her sisters, Ann Marie and Pam, had been posting back and forth about her for years. The comments could be followed on their own pages, like a timeline. They had even shared forensic sketches of Jane Does from Tennessee. After all, that's where their sister had gone missing. As recently as November 2021, when we had been watching for the DNA, they were asking each other: *Does this look like Susie?* Though the Redgraves looked back through months' worth, years' worth, of Facebook posts, they didn't see any mention of Ina Jane Doe. I didn't, either.

On Ancestry.com, the Redgraves tracked down the black-and-white photo of Susan; she was Susan Minard back then. That's the face I woke up to. I made coffee and sat down to read through what the team had discovered about Susan over the past several hours. She was from Highland, Indiana, originally. She'd married Paul Lund right out of high school. Their marriage certificate told us he was nineteen, and she was eighteen, when they married in April 1986. His occupation was listed as *service attendant*; Susan's was listed as *none*. They were both Catholic; religion wasn't always included on the certificates, but apparently Lake County, Indiana, found that information worth something.

Highland, Indiana. That's where I wanted to start. Within thirty minutes, I'd found the color version of the black-and-white photo the genealogists had discovered on Ancestry. It was Susan's senior portrait. The local library in her small Indiana hometown of Highland had scanned all the yearbooks. Her hair was a beautiful, bright, true red. She had such dark eyes: almost black, at least in the photo's light. Nearly all the students on the page, surrounding her, were smiling. But Susan looked so serious. I wondered if she'd had trouble with her teeth, even back then. Then again, I never smiled, either, in pictures. Never knew what to do with my mouth. My senior picture had looked something like hers.

I only found one other mention of Susan in the yearbook—in an index, where each student's club affiliations were listed: *Susan Minard, Aide; Booster Club, FHA.* I had to google the last one, though I had a guess. I was right: Future Homemakers of America. They'd rebranded to Family, Career, and Community Leaders of America. I went through previous years and found her pictures, but no other clubs or listings. But she was called "Sue" in some of the listings; she must have gone by that. Her brother Charles—Chuck, in the yearbook—showed up, too. He played football. I didn't see Pam or Ann Marie. Those were the names we knew for sure, the sisters who'd been posting about her. Family trees had various levels of privacy, and we couldn't always determine age gaps in public records.

But I'd eventually speak to most of Sue's siblings and find out that she was the youngest. I'd find out they called her Susie. I'd find out that she played softball, but that had fallen off by high school, and that she was a little shy, and kind, and loved animals more than anything. She'd climb under a porch to rescue a kitten or try to befriend a chained and growling dog through a metal fence. I'd learn that she'd met her husband, Paul, when she was still a teenager, playing video games at the arcade. That she was married by eighteen and missing by twenty-five.

———•———

There are so many ways to tell the story of Susan Minard Lund, and all of them are important. But each way paints a very different picture and leads down a different road. The path we discovered in those first few days, after we found her, among the 1990s news coverage of her disappearance in Tennessee? That's one narrative. But the views of two of her sisters, Ann Marie and Pam, gave me further insights that never made it to the papers. And the memories of her middle child, Crystal, who was only four years old when her mother disappeared. Well, they were colored by the belief her mother had run away and left her behind. When she found out that wasn't true, everything had to be reconsidered.

But let's start with the papers, because for almost thirty years, that's all the public really knew.

On December 24, 1992, twenty-five-year-old Sue Lund left her Clarksville, Tennessee, home for the last time. The story that appeared in the newspapers went something like this: The young mother decided she wanted to make a pumpkin pie for Christmas dinner, and left her three children—five-year-old Paul Jr., four-year-old Crystal, and the baby, Angel—with her husband, Paul. Paul was in the army, in military intelligence, and stationed at the nearby Fort Campbell. The family had only recently relocated to Tennessee; Paul had been stationed in Germany for years while Sue and the kids lived back in her home state of Indiana. They'd found a little rental on Harrier Court, not far from the base. But "not far" is relative; Paul and Sue didn't have a car. They didn't have a phone, either, though one was supposed to be installed after the holidays. If Sue, a stay-at-home mom, wanted to call her sisters or parents, which she did several times a week, she had to walk to a pay phone. Pam would later tell me she thought the pay phone was about a mile's walk away from Sue's house, at a convenience store.

Sue had to go on foot if she wanted to accomplish any last-minute errands, too. *The Clarksville Leaf-Chronicle* reported that on December 24, at 7:30 p.m., Sue left "to buy groceries at the Tradewinds Shopping Center."[1] That might sound odd, shopping on Christmas Eve, but several outlets reported that Sue wanted to stop in at the Winn Dixie to get ingredients for a pumpkin pie—a last-minute Christmas dessert. The store had closed early, but Sue wouldn't have known that.[2] It's not as if she could've googled that to find out. The weather forecast for Thursday, December 24, was frigid for the South; highs in the upper twenties, and lows in the teens.[3] The Tradewinds Shopping Center is about three-and-a-half miles from Harrier Court. On foot, that would be a one-way walk of over an hour, at a normal pace. Would Sue have walked at a normal pace? Maybe. But Paul told reporters that his wife was about three months pregnant when she disappeared—barely edging out of the first trimester. When I was three months pregnant, I was pushing down nausea and falling asleep at eight p.m. every night. A frigid, three-and-a-half-hour nighttime walk for an expectant mother doesn't sound like a pleasant trip.

The Clarksville Leaf-Chronicle reported that Sue didn't return from her walk, and that Paul reported her missing soon after. The paper notes that he called police that evening. When the search for her actually began is unclear—but there was one; the Leaf-Chronicle's continued coverage noted that, by January 3, Clarksville Police had spent "more than $5,000 dollars" looking for Sue Lund. In today's money, that's roughly $10,500. Those efforts included helicopter sweeps and "polygraph tests of Mrs. Lund's husband."[4] For his part, Paul told the press that he took leave from the army—two weeks, which seemed to be what he was allowed—to search for his wife. As he explained to Leaf-Chronicle, "If you sit around, it seems like you're not doing anything but waiting, and that's hard for the whole family. We try to keep occupied." He also informed the paper that the family, including Sue's siblings and parents, who'd rushed into town, were passing out flyers. In that particular January 8 article, Paul is pictured with his daughter, Crystal, and a portrait of Sue in the background. It's hard to say for sure, but it seems to be her senior photo.[5] The flyers featured the same photo, with the handwritten words:

MISSING PERSON
COME HOME
WE LOVE YOU
WE MISS YOU
MOMMY WE
LOVE YOU
NAME: LUND, SUSAN
HEIGHT: 5 FEET/60 IN
WT: 120 LBS
EYES: BROWN

There's a line cut off that I can't quite read, but I think it's *Hair: Red.*

Fort Campbell authorities also investigated Sue's disappearance, although they maintained a lower profile in the press than the Clarksville Police. Early on in the investigation, Clarksville law enforcement expressed the theory that Sue had left the area of her own volition. Their evidence for this were multiple sightings of her, or someone who looked like her, that they told the media had been called in: first in Nashville, and then in Kentucky, where police claimed she was "spotted frequently."[6] Then-Captain Doug Pectol said that "at least four" people had seen her in Hopkinsville, Kentucky, and that Tennessee authorities would be working with Kentucky to do "spot checks."[7] Within a week of her disappearance, the narrative had slowly shifted to *runaway mother.*

Paul wasn't convinced that Sue was in Kentucky, sightings or not.[8] As he told the local paper, "I'm hopeful. You've got to be as hopeful as you possibly can be in a situation like this. You also have to be prepared for the worst because if it happens you have to be prepared. I hope she comes home real soon. If I were to come back home and she was sitting on the couch, there would be no questions. I would hug her."[9]

After January, there was a lull in news coverage; Sue's case wasn't mentioned often, except to say there were no developments. But in April 1993, her story drifted back up into the headlines: NO GRAVE DISCOVERED IN SEARCH FOR LUND. Apparently, Clarksville authorities had gotten a tip that Sue's body had been hidden away in a clandestine grave not so far from her own home on Harrier Court. But there was nothing to be found, and law enforcement said that though Sue's was an active missing-persons case, "there is no investigation of foul play."[10]

In July 1993, there was strange news: Sue's case was going to be closed. According to Clarksville authorities, she had been located in Alabama; precisely how or why she'd gotten there was never detailed—in fact, the name of the town was never released to the media, because, as law enforcement told reporters, "she'd committed no crime."[11] Investigators merely said that a TBI (Tennessee Bureau of Investigations) agent had been in phone contact with the woman who said she was Sue; she'd also spoken to an Alabama State Trooper and said that "she didn't want to be bothered." That, as far as the media coverage went, was that. More than six months after a highly publicized disappearance, the missing woman, who was said to be pregnant, was found and wasn't coming home. Nothing was said of a baby. No charges were to be filed. No one in Sue's family was quoted as to how they felt about this; if they were, I couldn't find the articles. No one quoted Paul or asked if he'd had a chance to speak to his wife. Susan Lund was declared "found," and that was that. Clarksville seemed to move on.

That's one version of the story. What the Clarksville Police Department thinks about Sue now, I can't say. Could she have somehow been in Alabama at some point? Possibly. There was a month between her disappearance and the time her remains were discovered in Wayne Fitzgerrell Park, and her head hadn't lain in the park all that time. Even in that cold weather, there would have been more decomposition, more insect activity. Animal predation. Sue could have been alive for some of that time. Her remains might have been stored in such a way that decomposition was halted. Perhaps in a freezer. But because her remains had been placed in just such an environment by the coroner—it was noted in her file— prior to autopsy, studying preexam pictures wouldn't tell us one way or another. There were plenty of possibilities, but no clear path to a single truth. Not without knowing who had killed Sue, and that would be an entirely new investigation.

Would Clarksville have any information about who might have been involved? What about who had convinced them that Sue was alive and well in Alabama, so long after she was dead? They didn't respond to my request for an interview. But I know what her sisters think about that, and what they say her parents knew. Their parents drove down to Alabama, all the way from Indiana, to see about this woman who claimed to be Sue. Why Clarksville authorities didn't believe them and instead took the woman at her word, I can't say. But I do know that Susan Minard Lund had been dead since winter, her remains abandoned in an Illinois State Park. And without an open missing-persons case, her family would have—did have—a much harder time looking for her. And her children grew up believing she wanted to be gone.

———— • ————

In early February 2022, I drove to the UPS Store a mile or so from my house. I needed to make it there before 5 p.m., and I was cutting it close; my ancient Scion XB slid into a spot in front just in time. I had to overnight a home DNA kit to Sue Lund's sister Pam.

The Redgraves, their students, and I had spent time tracking down information to finish out their file, like news clippings and official records, and then we'd contacted Jefferson County to let them know that there was a tentative match for Ina Jane Doe. One of the quickest ways to confirm that was for one of Sue's siblings to take an at-home DNA test. When she got the results, the Redgraves would help her download the raw file and upload it to GEDmatch Pro. We'd have confirmation in a day.

We got word that Detective Captain Bobby Wallace had spoken with Pam and Ann Marie at around 3 p.m. He called Amy; she got me on the line, which involved a call-waiting-and-merging feat we didn't know we were capable of, and we listened to his summary. I was told Pam had been in the car when he called. She'd had to pull over to the side of the road to process the news: Her baby sister, Sue, had finally been found. But confirmation was still needed. There was a second call, with Pam and her older sister, Ann Marie, and Pam's husband, who asked most of the questions. Pam and Ann Marie were in shock. They were scrolling through Jefferson County's Facebook posts about Ina Jane Doe, looking at Carl's art, looking at the description of the crime, and how their sister had been discovered. They saw the word *decapitation*. They saw *homicide*.

Pam agreed to submit her DNA. The Redgraves had plenty of kits at their house; so did I. I sent them out to families who'd been on the podcast who wanted to get their DNA into GEDmatch, and I tried to stock up during sales. After messaging Viktor, I determined that the Redgraves weren't home—they'd gone to the next town over for a dentist appointment, and because Anthony didn't drive, both he and Lee were there.

They wouldn't be back in time to get a test to her overnight. Why did it have to be overnight? It didn't, not after nearly thirty years. But because it had been thirty years, none of us could wait. So, I gathered my son into the car and we went to UPS and paid something like sixty dollars to get Pam that test by the next afternoon. I had spent that much money on much worse things in my life.

We'd spent close to a year trying to identify Ina Jane Doe. It was nothing compared with what Sue Lund's family had faced. There had been rumors swirling that she had left her children, that she'd been on drugs, even that she had run off with a boyfriend to start a new life. Her sisters had never believed that. But they didn't have proof. And proof was what they'd needed all those years that Sue's case was closed. That's what they told me, and a lot more, after we met.

And it wasn't long until we did meet. Pam's kit was processed in a few weeks, and then Lee and Anthony had it uploaded to GEDmatch in a flash. After it batched, the kit told us what we already knew: Susan Hope Lund, born Susan Minard, was Ina Jane Doe. That was March 6, 2022; we could officially declare the match with Pam's additional data to back it. No surprise to any of us; I'd been certain as soon as I saw Sue's photo.

The Jefferson County Sheriff's Office announced that there would be a press conference on March 11, 2022, at the Mount Vernon Courthouse. Amy planned to fly out early—the date fell during her university's spring break—and see her sister and nephews, and then drive into Mount Vernon with her dad. I'd fly into St. Louis and rent a car, and meet Kyana, who'd just started working for me on *The Fall Line* as a research assistant. She'd never been to a press conference before, and she'd worked with us since the beginning; it seemed fitting she should come.

In the week between Sue's identification and the press conference, we were all busy. The Redgraves and Jefferson County had plenty of preparation to do. After the Jefferson County Sheriff's Office made announcements regarding Sue's identification and case, Anthony would give a presentation for the media via Zoom from Massachusetts to explain the investigative genetic genealogical process. Tennessee authorities would not be participating; her case file was going to officially be transferred to

Illinois sometime that spring. Amy and I both spoke with Sue's sisters, and I began correspondence with her daughter, Crystal, too. We—the Redgraves and I—knew we needed to tell Sue's family to get ready for the onslaught.

There would be many wonderful people coming forward to wish them well. But social media is ugly, too. Everyone knows that. And they'd better lock down before the official announcement came. Her name might leak a day or two early. That happened pretty often, usually accidentally, when a family member might say, on their own social media, something about their family member being found. But there were people with alerts set, or who checked and searched as a matter of course. They'd have that information posted to Reddit or Websleuths in hours. It was better to be ready: Hide pictures of your children. Delete identifying details.

It would be hard enough for Sue's family members to watch the discussions occur without more fuel for dissection, and based on my experience, they *would* track the activity; it was nearly impossible to restrain yourself when your family's tragedy was splashed everywhere, with commenters weighing in on every decision that they thought a family might have made. There's so much that can go wrong there: so little we really know about cases when we're caught up in conjecture and online speculation. So many assumptions, so few facts. It would be hours or days before anyone knew that Sue's missing-persons case had been closed in Tennessee, that her siblings and parents, despite their best efforts, couldn't pursue. Sue's husband, Paul, had moved on after the case closure—he'd left the army and relocated his children to Virginia because his family still lived there, and they could help. Eventually, the kids would move in with their paternal grandmother, Paul's mother, though their father remained nearby and involved. Paul later remarried. He died in February 2020, two years before Sue was identified.

But his children—Sue's children—and most of her family were alive to process the news.

I'd never know what it was like to be the child or the sister of a woman who went for a walk one night and never came home. But I did learn that

Pam and Ann Marie's version of the story included much more than what was released in the papers. And that's another mystery altogether.

———•———

Getting into the St. Louis Airport and on to Mount Vernon was a *bit* of a journey. Kyana's flight was delayed, twice, and then canceled. She was coming from Boston, and by the time she got a new flight sorted, she was going to arrive sometime around eleven p.m. I'd arrived at one p.m. from Atlanta. I couldn't wait for her in St. Louis because I had plans to take Ann Marie and Pam out to dinner. I didn't want Kyana trying to take a rideshare to Mount Vernon; it was over an hour's drive, and the rideshare area of the airport was in a far-flung corner. Eventually, I arranged for Kyana to be met by a driver from a limousine service that would shepherd her in safety from St. Louis to Mount Vernon, or so they assured me.

I checked into a Drury Inn and Suites and texted Ann Marie at around four; she and Pam were in the same hotel, and even on the same floor. I made plans to meet up with them and offered to take them anywhere they wanted for dinner. They said they'd seen a Cracker Barrel across the road. I didn't know they had those in Illinois, but I was game. I hadn't been to one since I was in kindergarten. They'd had some kind of peg game I'd played while my grandparents took a break from selling tin art at a South Carolina craft show.

I took a shower to get the travel off me. Planes were like that; I always felt greasy, even if it had been a short flight. My son called me on Face-Time to explain something absolutely mystifying about Roblox; I was an hour behind in Illinois, and he was already in his pajamas. He told me they'd ordered a pizza and were going to eat it in front of the television. Classic *Mom's-out-of-town* fun. I told him I missed them, and I did—even though I'd just left. I'd been gone so much. But this would be one of the last trips . . . for the moment.

I brushed my hair and put on lipstick and still looked tired, in the bright light of the hotel bathroom, but then again, I knew that Pam and Ann Marie wouldn't care. When I knocked, just a few doors down from my own, there they were: one tall, close to my height—Pam—and one small and slight—Ann Marie—both looking a little like Sue.

But they didn't call her that.

"This is Susie," Ann Marie said. She and Pam sat across from me at the restaurant. She pushed a small stack of pictures toward me just as the waitress brought our drinks: iced tea for them, Coke Zero for me. "We lost a lot of pictures when my parents' house flooded. And then there was a fire. But we still have a few."

We paused to order. I got some kind of salad, which may have been a waste of a Cracker Barrel trip, but I was too nervous to be hungry. Families didn't make me nervous, not usually. But I had been thinking about Ina Jane Doe for so long: who she might be, and who missed her, and what happened to her before her killer had driven down that lonely road at the park. I was used to working on cold cases of the unidentified with experts or with families and law enforcement on the stories of the missing and murdered. But sitting at a table set with ketchup and sugar packets and dishwasher-pitted silverware, looking into the eyes of two women who had just gotten the news they'd wanted, but not wanted, about their sister. This wasn't the first time I had seen a case I'd worked on solved. But it was the first time I'd played such a direct part. And now there was a stack of photographs, saved from fire and flood, to tell a little piece of the story. I hoped I'd hear it all. But we'd start here.

I looked at the top photo: Sue in middle school, or high school, wearing glasses—the only photo I'd see of her in glasses, big 1980s frames with the pink-tinged lenses—and a rainbow-striped sweater. Sue, a little younger, and smiling, dressed mostly in white: an athletic jacket. Maybe from when she played softball? It was the only time I'd seen her with such a short haircut. It was also one of the only clear photos I'd noticed of her smiling, wide, with teeth. She looked happy. She looked happy in all the photos. Happy at her wedding reception, which Pam said they'd had at their parents' house, when Sue was just eighteen. Pleased to be looking tough posing in a camo T-shirt next to a rifle—maybe it was her brother Chuck's, or her own? Laughing with her best friend at her reception, and then with her sisters, all of them, and her mother. Sue, one of the shortest in the family, was in the back. She had to be standing on something to be seen. Throughout her teens and twenties, she wore variations on the same haircut from her high school senior picture: fluffy and with the bangs I'd observed on nearly everyone else in her yearbook, big and full. She looked like one of my students. She'd been so young.

There were pictures of Sue up on Facebook, too, but none of these had made it there. I thought Ann Marie must have gotten them out of safe-keeping to bring to the press conference, or to show me, or both. We went through each, and Pam and Ann Marie told me everything they could remember about her.

I didn't take notes on our conversation at dinner. You don't, at a meal with a grieving family. But we talked a lot about Sue. And they had questions for me, too. I answered everything I could: about why Amy and I had asked to work on her case, and how we met, and the parts each person played, piece by piece, to get us to this, the night before a press conference. They asked things I didn't have the answers for, though I wish I did: What did Tennessee have to say about this? How would Jefferson County pursue the case? How had the genetic genealogy worked? I could explain some of that, but Anthony would do a better job the next day, during the press conference. But what I didn't have was the information Pam and Ann Marie needed most: What happened to Sue on December 24, 1992?

We spent a quiet evening together and, on the way to pay the bill, browsed in that strange front area that Cracker Barrel has—part tourist trap, part country store. I was looking for some things to take home to my kid, of course: some horrible flavor of Peeps (was it even time for Peeps?) that he would love, and some kind of card game that involved cats. Pam was looking at gifts for her daughter. She leaned over the display, and from the angle, with her hair falling across her face, she did look a little like Sue.

Ann Marie got caught up looking at mugs and key chains.

"Unicorns," she said, showing me the cup she'd picked up. "I love them. They're my thing." When she turned it in the light, the glitter caught everything around us.

Ann Marie and Pam let me come to their room to scan the photos of Sue. There was hotel bedspread in the background of some of them, but I could crop that out later. I wanted to remember Sue's face. Amy needed to see these pictures, too. I got Pam and Ann Marie's permission to show them to her—she'd want to see Sue from different angles. The only pictures likely to run in the paper would be her senior portrait, and perhaps the one or two I'd seen on family members' social media. These were different. They further supported Amy's original thoughts about Sue's case: that any asymmetry would have been so mild, or fully unnoticeable. That her friends and family wouldn't have recognized her in the original forensic descriptions.

When I got back to my room and collapsed across the burnt-orange bed runner, I realized I'd missed a text from Kyana. Had her car not showed up? I got the tense feeling that hit me when my son's school called; that was always followed up with information about a fever, or a playground injury. I opened my messages.

> This man has on a driver's hat and he is playing light jazz for me.
> He offered to stop for snacks. I'll be there at 11.
>
> What kind of car is it?
>
> I don't know, but it's fancy.
>
> I left a key card for you at the front desk. I'm going to wait until you get here to go to sleep but I might be in the bathroom when you get here.

I had a fairly complex skin routine that I might have skipped that night, but I didn't think I could go to bed until Kyana was safely in the room. Was this what it was like to have a teenager? Worried about a young person, free-range in the world? If so, I wasn't looking forward to it. I'd always disliked that many people described their interest in true crime as preparing them for all possible dangers—when, really, most of its avid consumers were the safest people in the nation. But spend enough time actually involved in the cases, and maybe paranoia started to seem sensible. I sat up, working on a script, until I heard the hotel door click.

Kyana breezed in with her backpack and stories of the day and night of airport hell, and I knew I could finally go to sleep. Pam and Ann Marie, down the hall? I hoped they'd be able, too.

CHAPTER SIXTEEN

THE ANNOUNCEMENT

A my was almost late to the press conference. She and her dad had to drive through a real snowstorm to make it to Mount Vernon, and she was a little shaky by the time she walked into the basement of the court building. They were both wrapped in layers of winter gear and clutching fresh Starbucks cups. Kyana and I had driven all of two miles, and it was simply cold and damp, but I'd been worried enough about ice that I'd taken my time, too. The snow was supposed to start in Mount Vernon around two or three; hopefully, Kyana and I would be safely back in St. Louis by then, returning our car and catching the shuttle back to the airport.

I shook hands with Amy's dad—he had her smile, exactly, and an excellent Midwestern accent—and was introduced to the law-enforcement officials I hadn't met yet. One was the sheriff: He was going over his remarks as the local TV crews set up cameras. Bobby Wallace was there, and so was the retired Scott Burge, who'd been on Sue's case for so long.

"Amy? No, Laurah," Bobby corrected himself. We shook hands. He'd only met us once in person, and for a few minutes. We'd talked plenty on the phone, though.

"She's the little one," I told him. I pointed to Amy, who was speaking to Scott Burge. She clutched her coffee through a layer of mittens.

I glanced into the main room, where the press conference would be held. There were twenty or thirty folding chairs arranged in a semicircle, a projection screen, some computers, and a podium. One of the Redgraves' senior students, an experienced genealogist named Kaycee who lived in-state, was there, too; she was in charge of running the live feed. Anthony would speak about Sue's genetic genealogy and identification, and Kaycee's job was to make sure the feed worked. I was relieved as I did not want to be responsible for any technology. Kaycee was fiddling with some cords and her phone, which she'd set on a skinny tripod. I wasn't sure how this played into the livestream that Anthony had told me was going to Twitch, and would be eventually posted to YouTube, but how one even accessed Twitch was above my generational pay grade.

Just then, Pam and Ann Marie walked in, accompanied by a tall, burly man with a beard and glasses—their brother Chuck—and Chuck's wife. Ann Marie had brought some of the pictures of Sue that I'd seen the night before; she'd hold one of the photos up during the entire presser. She sat on one side of Pam, and Chuck on the other, in his flat cap and glasses. Pam's long, red hair was the brightest spot, another reminder.

Right before we were set to begin, the sheriff, Jeff Bullard, motioned me over. He was reviewing his remarks regarding the order of operations in Sue's identification.

"How should I refer to you?" he asked me. It took me a second, but then I realized: Professionally speaking, Amy was a doctor of anthropology and a professor. The Redgraves were forensic genetic genealogists. I was . . . a more abstract member of the team.

"Writer? Researcher?" I offered. "I'll still be a principal senior lecturer at Georgia State University in Atlanta through the summer. Department of English."

He made a note on the paper. "Professor. We'll go with that one."

Amy walked up beside me, looking a little pale.

"Are you cold?"

"I'm going to be, uhm, giving some remarks," she said, with the enthusiasm of someone announcing an IRS audit. "I'll speak sometime after the sheriff and Anthony. Maybe during Anthony's presentation. I'm not sure." Amy loathed public speaking. She could get in front of a group of students and lecture on anything, but stick a podium and a microphone at the front of a room, and remove the students? Her worst nightmare.

"I'd do it for you, but I assume they want you to discuss skeletal analysis." I squeezed her shoulder. "Just pretend the cameras are students."

I introduced Amy to Pam and Ann Marie; they'd talked on the phone and emailed, but this was their first time seeing each in person. Sue's sisters thanked Amy for all her work on Sue's case. I knew they had more questions, but some would be answered during the presser, by Anthony. Amy would speak more with them afterward, too, and I'd spend the next few months interviewing Pam and Ann Marie and Sue's middle child, Crystal. I'd text Amy during those conversations to help explain anything they wanted to know. Anything we *could* answer, anyway; there was still so much none of us knew.

As the press conference began, I sat against a back wall, next to Chuck's wife. She smiled, shyly, and we both turned to watch the sheriff begin his remarks. I held my field recorder in my lap so it wouldn't get in anyone's way. Television crews and journalists gathered in the closer seats, and Pam, Ann Marie, and Chuck sat off to the side of the podium, in their row.

Sheriff Bullard shuffled his notes and began. I could see him twice: once right in front of me, and once through the scope of Kaycee's phone, locked in on its tripod.

"I am pleased to report that investigators of the Jefferson County Sheriff's Office and specialists of Redgrave Research Forensic Services have confirmed the identity of Ina Jane Doe, an unidentified woman whose remains were discovered twenty-nine years ago in Jefferson County. The identity of that woman is Susan Lund of Clarksville, Tennessee. . . ." The sheriff went on to mention the names of the people who'd joined him today for the presser, and to thank people who'd worked on the case over the years, and to acknowledge Sue's family.

"After several attempts to try to generate leads to identify the victim, which is crucial in any homicide investigation, the case went cold for many years. In February 2021, Dr. Amy Michael approached investigators with the Sheriff's Office, and offered to reexamine the case using new and updated forensic methods. At that time the Sheriff's Office turned the evidence over to Dr. Michael and researchers and scientists with the Redgrave Research Forensic Services group and they began their work. And it was impressive work that led to breaking open the case. And at this time, I would like to turn this conference over to Anthony Redgrave, who I advised will be online with us to explain the process of how this identification was made."

Anthony's PowerPoint filled the screen behind Sheriff Bullard, and I saw Anthony himself in the upper-right corner of the screen. He looked serious in his black button-up shirt, with his long, red beard neatly styled. Anthony began his presentation with a review of the timeline of the case: when Redgrave Research had made their announcement of involvement, when Sue's DNA had finished processing at Astrea, how long it had taken to identify Sue, and how Pam's DNA had been used to confirm Sue's identification. Then Anthony cued Amy.

"I'm going to pass this slide over to Dr. Amy Michael if she wishes to speak."

Kyana, who was a few seats away, glanced at me. Amy did *not* wish to speak. But she would, because she took her job seriously. Amy had to adjust the microphone down—Sheriff Bullard was a tall man—and she cleared her throat before she began.

"Okay, thanks, Anthony. I'll be brief. My name's Amy Michael. I'm an anthropology professor at the University of New Hampshire, though I am an Illinois native and I'm from right around Peoria, so I knew of this case for many years. A reanalysis of the skeletal and dental remains took place at my secure lab at the University of New Hampshire with assistance from Dr. Samantha Blatt from Idaho State University, who is a friend and a colleague. Updated forensic methods were applied to estimate the age, sex, and ancestry. All of these were generally confirmed, though I believe that Ina Jane Doe, who we now know as Susan Lund, was a little bit younger than what was originally reported.

"I determined the facial asymmetry that Ina Jane Doe expressed was milder than originally thought, and so that new forensic art that you'll see reflected here, reflects my reanalysis. So concurrent to my anthropological research, Laurah Norton, a writer and researcher based in Georgia who is also here today, began to comb through possible missing-persons matches in the immediate region and actually throughout the Midwest. So all of our national databases have improved a lot since 1993, and Ms. Norton was able to search for potential matches as well as similar crimes locally and throughout the region. She also continued to research the recovery scene and utilize digitized newspaper databases to provide additional context."

Amy said that Anthony would explain the genealogy portion of the presentation, and walked to a chair next to her dad. She didn't even hurry.

Anthony picked up where Amy left off. "Thank you, Amy. I would like to say that Amy and everyone who's ever worked on this case has really set us up for success. Whereas the forensic genetic genealogists, we tend to be the closers on cases, and it's really the investigative process that laid a good foundation for us. So, one of the first things that we look at when we've uploaded a DNA data file to GEDmatch is the admixture or estimate of the ethnicities present in an individual's ancestry." Anthony clicked over to a slide that showed a pie chart; I recognized it from GEDmatch as an ancestry breakdown.

Anthony explained that Sue's ancestry results indicated her family had been in the United States for several generations or more. "After evaluating the genetic admixture we look at the list of matches in the database that from most to least genetic materials shared. Logically we'll look at those that are potentially the most closely related first, but we may need to look at more distant relatives depending on how the research goes. The total shared between Jane Doe and her DNA matches can be used to make an estimate of their actual relationship to each other. But that relationship has to be confirmed with genealogical research, as there are a number of different relationships two people can have depending on how much genetic material they share."

He shifted to a slide he'd made himself; I recognized the numbers. They were an anonymized version of Sue's top matches in GEDmatch.

"In this case," Anthony continued, "the closest relative shared 432.10 centimorgans with Jane Doe, centimorgan being a unit measurement in autosomal DNA. Making their relationship most likely to be a half first cousin or first cousin once removed. There are a number of other potential relationships that are less likely but still possible, making identification take a little longer than a direct one-to-one comparison. But we won't know the actual relationship between the two until we get closer to making identification. We'll usually look at dozens of DNA matches and build their family trees as we work on the case."

Anthony then clicked to a chart that I'd seen before; it was a kind of mock-up of a family tree that focused on MCRA—Most Common Recent Ancestors. "The DNA matches in the database are not only likely relatives of Jane Doe, but some are relatives of each other. Through a process called triangulation, we assume that if we can determine how the DNA matches are related to each other, Jane Doe probably descends from the same family since she shares DNA with them. So, we look for the most recent common ancestor first or MRCAs, a couple or individual who are in the direct pedigree of two or more DNA matches. We will find several MRCA couples during research that will cluster together, often indicating that there are two sides of a Doe's family tree."

Anthony pointed to two "clusters" of matches the genealogists had found early on—two separate groups of ancestor-couples that tied the tree together. He explained that they'd used a tool called What Are the Odds, or WATO, to create "conditional probability hypotheses" based on these MCRA clusters and showed a screen that illustrated that. "By using the combined probabilities of Jane Doe's potential relationships with the DNA matches and their relationship to each other through a common ancestor, the WATO tool can be used to rank hypothetical individuals in the probability tree by likelihood."

Anthony explained that the point of this tool is to help genetic genealogists narrow down possibilities: In this particular case, they had two paths, cluster one or cluster two. The tool lets them know which is more probable to be Sue's direct line of ancestry and, thus, the place to direct their energy first. They wouldn't ever use it to eliminate a line without research, but it made their work much more efficient.

Anthony then started walking the audience through the key to identification: finding the union couple. "Since there's two different groups of DNA matches, there's one that's likely to be on Jane Doe's maternal side, and the other is likely to be on her paternal side. Though now we're looking for a crossover common ancestor, or a couple consisting of one individual descended from one MRCA group, and one individual descended from a different MRCA group, representing a place where the DNA of both could combine in their descendants." He pointed out Sue's grandparents and parents, and how they led straight to Sue and her siblings—and explained how we'd researched their family and confirmed one sibling was missing. Then he pulled up the information regarding Pam's matching kit, which had confirmed Sue's identity.

"This is the really satisfying part that I like and the part that we always hope to see when we're getting close to an identification. So, adding these numbers to the WATO probability trees that we showed you earlier, rendered all other high hypotheses no longer possible except for as a full sibling of the target tester. When the other distant relatives in the database were included, this makes none of the other relationships possible."

Anthony went through some numbers on the case—including how many matches they'd found—and then expressed the condolences of his entire team to Sue's family. Afterward, he thanked the genealogy team, including Viktor and the students—Samantha Dunne, Kaycee Connelly, Chelsea Hanrahan, Andrea McCarthy, Elizabeth Marshall, Pam Stigsen—and everyone else who'd aided in our work, from Astrea Forensics and the Hubbard Center at UNH to Dr. Albee at Suncook Dental.

Finally, Sheriff Bullard reiterated the department's collective condolences to Sue's family and reassured them that the investigation wasn't finished yet: Sue's killer still needed to be identified. Because of that fact, he told the audience, "There's not going to be any other specific details released about the case at this time, due to the fact that we are just going to roll up our sleeves and start digging into it again. And we want to make sure what's proper to be released and what needs to remain confidential."

And with that, Susan Lund's identity was announced to the world. Reporters came to the sheriff, and to Pam and Ann Marie and Chuck, and asked them all the questions journalists do. Amy was interviewed, too. Kyana and I waited by Chuck's wife, listening to them speak. I hugged Ann Marie and Pam goodbye before we left.

Fortunately for us, Kyana and I made it back to St. Louis without encountering the threatened snow. We ate lunch at a Mexican restaurant, mostly in silence, because we both scrolled through our phones, watching the posts appear, one by one, about Sue. I'd had a Google Alert for Ina Jane Doe. Now, I added Susan Lund. There would be a lot to keep up with, at least for the next month.

One thing Pam said, that was quoted in multiple newspapers, was what I remembered most.

"I'm just speaking on behalf of her three children," Pam said. "They just really want people to know that they're grateful to find out that they weren't abandoned by their mother. She didn't leave her kids, not willingly. For her six-year-old, her only son, it was really important for him to come to grips that his mom didn't abandon him."

Pam had worried about that so much over the years. Ann Marie, too. Neither of them believed that Sue would have ever left her children, but with the Alabama story, and the case closed, there wasn't much else they could say. But they thought about the events of the winter of 1992 and early 1993 a lot. When technology caught up, they began to do all the research on the case that they could. They saved news clippings and scoured for any and all signs of Sue—or an unnamed Doe who might be Sue. They never believed the official story. And they'd been right.

When Pam and I talked later, during a recorded phone interview, she told me all the things she remembered that differed from the news reports. Ann Marie did as well. Some of what they said seemed possibly important to their sister's homicide case, so I made a call to Jefferson County to relay those potential leads, and told them to be sure to mention the information when they spoke with detectives. I knew, even then, that I couldn't write about all the new details I'd learned; it could harm a future homicide case. The same thing went for what Sue's daughter, Crystal, had to say. But what I could record, and share, was plenty.

I had questions that only Sue's family could answer. Pam and Ann Marie told me that Sue didn't have torticollis—not anything like that. No back problems, no spinal issues that they knew of. Of course, that didn't preclude internal irregularities that no one would be aware of, such as the beginnings of arthritis that Dr. Klepinger had noted. I'd had an MRI when I was thirty and been told my shoulder was in the beginning stages, something I wouldn't have otherwise known. Amy hadn't been able to reexamine Sue's vertebrae, so I didn't have additional information to go on.

Ann Marie herself had issues with scoliosis later in life, but Sue hadn't had any problems they'd known of at all. She did, however, have issues with her eyes; she'd had a surgery when she was little, and then worn glasses with different-colored lenses. And then there were her teeth. Pam and Ann Marie had no recollection that Sue was having serious dental issues around the time of her disappearance. The advanced decay we'd seen would have developed over time and been quite painful at some point. Pam couldn't speak to that specifically, but she had some ideas.

My official interview with Pam took place in the late spring of 2022. I sat in my recording closet—every house should come with one—so I could capture my phone call with Pam and get it transcribed. It was always deadly hot in there from April until November, but the sound was excellent. Lawn mowers, barking dogs, UPS—nothing could penetrate all the padding. Pam and I talked a little, and then I asked her about Sue's dental history. Amy and I had wondered if so many pregnancies, so close together, had been hard on her enamel. Pam said that the whole family had issues with thin enamel as far back as she could remember.

"We all used to have that. I remember as a kid getting treatment, enamel treatment. I remember them always telling us that we had no enamel and needed some kind of coating on our teeth."

"You got them sealed, maybe? They did that to my kid's molars when he turned seven."

"Yeah, a couple times when we were kids, you know. Sealed, something like that. So we wouldn't get more cavities."

I remembered what Amy and I had discussed. "When I was pregnant, I got two cavities. I have thin enamel, too. Baby just seemed to leach the calcium right out of me. Was it like that for Sue?"

Pam couldn't remember, or maybe Sue hadn't said. But she did know this: As far as she knew, Sue hadn't actually had dental care through most of her pregnancies. Pam knew that because Sue hadn't had health insurance, either. There had been issues with the army benefits, but when Paul was back from Germany, before their move to Tennessee, she and the children were finally covered—that was the rough timeline that Pam recalled.

I wondered when Sue had gotten that particular dental work that the dentists were convinced would be an identifying feature. Pam wasn't sure, and neither was Ann Marie. But with the state of decay she was dealing with at the time of her death, I'd have to imagine before. Wouldn't an army dentist have treated her other teeth, too? Or maybe she'd had the root canal done right after her marriage. Maybe she'd planned on having dental work in Tennessee and simply hadn't gotten a chance. A lot can happen in seven years. I thought that four pregnancies must have been especially hard so close together.

But no. Maybe not four. *Three pregnancies.* That's what Pam knew of. There had been no fourth as far as she was aware. Obviously, she couldn't say for sure, but Sue and Pam had spoken every week, and sometimes every day. Pam and Sue weren't just sisters; Pam had been one of Sue's best friends. Before Paul came back from Germany, they'd lived together, and even for a little while after, before Paul moved his family a few states away to his new assignment at Fort Campbell. Pam and Sue had been close in age, and longtime confidants. But Pam had never heard anything about a fourth baby. There hadn't been anything said about Sue being pregnant, as far as Pam knew, until after her sister disappeared. When I spoke to Ann Marie, she said the same thing.

"I'm pretty sure she would've said, because she still had a baby in the high chair," Ann Marie told me.

"When did you first hear about her maybe being pregnant?"

"I would say while we were there that week. We were there because we stayed with them and we went and ate at different places. And we put up flyers and then he said, 'She was pregnant.'"

This was the part that caught me up. On one hand, mentioning a pregnancy could suggest that Sue had a reason to run off. A pregnancy she hadn't told her sisters about could hint at a pregnancy outside the marriage. It could give an excuse, a reason. Then again . . .

"One thing I wonder about . . ." I paused, staring at the swaths of black soundproofing my husband had installed in our spare room closet. "If the police were declining to search. If I was desperate, I might say somebody was pregnant just to get them to look for her. I might gamble on authorities searching harder for a pregnant woman."

When I checked Sue's police file, there was nothing in her bloodwork to indicate a pregnancy test was run on her blood sample. I hadn't seen pregnancy tests run as a matter of course in most of the 1980s and '90s cases I'd worked on for the podcast—ones where they still had blood or bile that could be tested—but then again, in those cases, an autopsy would have likely revealed pregnancy. Either way, I didn't see any mention of HCG (often called the pregnancy hormone) in Sue's blood tests. There had been a tox screen, which had come back clean of everything but nicotine.

I talked about that with Pam during our call. I remembered what my mom had said about smoking: She'd quit during her pregnancy with me and then taken it back up.

"Did Sue smoke when she was pregnant?"

"Susie always quit when she was pregnant," Pam told me.

With Paul deceased, there was no way to know for sure. But Crystal, Sue's daughter, and I walked through the possible scenarios anyway when we spoke. There were only so many options: Paul thought Sue was pregnant or had reason to say she was, or Sue *had* been and hadn't told her sisters. This time she had kept smoking during pregnancy. Or it was a sign she hadn't been pregnant. All were possibilities. Delaying dental work could have been a signal, too. Or it could simply be they weren't able to afford it. Or they'd gotten health insurance through the army but hadn't signed up for dental yet. It was a separate cost for each dependent.

What I'd learned from five years of crime research was that this was the point where you stopped. Or where I stopped, anyway. Without actual evidence—not theories that get squeezed into the shape of facts, but real proof, the kind that could be taken to court—that's where speculation can sidle into conspiracy. Sue's children and sisters and brother could speak with Jefferson County and help them begin to unravel some of the confusion. Detective Captain Bobby Wallace was the person who would be able to request access to Fort Campbell's records, and then review them. He'd have Tennessee's files. He'd be able to put together the information. And the things I'd learned in interviews that might be pertinent to his homicide investigation? I passed those on. But he'd want to discuss those points on his own, too, when he interviewed the family.

And there was one other important detail. Pam remembered when she talked to Sue on the phone that day, they'd discussed Christmas dinner. She couldn't recall the exact time, but she knew that Sue hadn't planned on a pie. This, despite what had been reported in the papers—that her whole trip had revolved around that chore. Apparently, Paul had gotten the groceries earlier in the week; since they didn't have a car, one of his Army buddies had driven him to the store to get groceries for the family.

Pam told me, "I asked her, I said, 'Well, what did he buy?' She goes, 'Just the regular food, but it's okay . . . The kids don't eat all that stuff anyway, they eat simple food, like what I make them.' I said, 'No, I get it. I get it.'"

Pam said Paul usually ran that errand unless Sue's best friend was in town, visiting; she was dating a soldier at Fort Campbell and would drive Sue on errands if she was around. But no, as far as Pam knew, Sue hadn't planned on going to the store that evening.

And this opened up a whole *new* line of questions. If she wasn't going to the store on December 24, 1992, at around 7:30 p.m. . . . . where had Sue been going? It had already been strange that she was heading out to a grocery store that was already closed, in the freezing weather. Could it have been that she was simply walking to the pay phone again? Had she needed a break, made up an excuse? Or could she have just decided to make a pie after she spoke to Pam, and decided on that long, late, cold walk? Maybe she planned on trying the convenience store for ingredients?

During her interview, Ann Marie told me that when she and her parents had come in from Indiana after Sue went missing, the police sat them down and questioned them. On the whole, this made sense, considering the multiple rounds of questioning that Paul had experienced, but Ann Marie noted that it had been intense, particularly considering they lived out of state and hadn't been anywhere near Tennessee when Sue disappeared.

"We went to the Army base there and got interrogated," Ann Marie recalled. "But I want to say it was the FBI from Tennessee that investigated us because while we were in the office, we were in separate rooms. They were asking, I would assume the same questions because my parents and I, we collaborated afterward. But they asked me, where was I? Did I fight with her? I'm like, 'We're siblings. I'm sure we have fights. But did I ever want her dead? No.' And so they asked for my employer. So while I was in the office, they went and called my employer to make sure that I was where I was."

Ann Marie continued, "I tried to get it on *America's Most Wanted*, but they never returned my call. We put up flyers. My parents put one up on their front door. They talked to everybody about it, all the time. It was always on their mind, always, it never left. And I said, 'Mom, sometime we'll find her.'"

Pam was close in age to Sue—their birth order was Ann Marie, then Mary (the sister I hadn't met), and then Pam, Chuck, and Sue in quick succession. I hadn't seen Pam in the yearbooks because she'd dropped out of high school when she got pregnant, and quickly got her own place; she said Sue used to come there to hang out all the time, before she met Paul. Pam had gone on to finish school later and become a nurse.

Ann Marie could remember a lot of Sue's childhood from a more adult perspective. "Well, me being the oldest, we got to change her diaper and we all thought it was fun. Like she was a live baby doll. I mean, we got to pretty much take care of her. And I mean, my mom did, but we got to, too.

And it was more or less, we watched her being born, she was born like right as my mom got to the ambulance outside. So we all got to watch it. We have this big glass door and we got to see it and we heard her cry."

"What was Sue like as a kid?" I'd asked Pam the same question. I could hear the smile in Ann Marie's voice, which sounds like an untrue thing that people tell you, until you've done a lot of phone interviews. You really can begin to discern expressions just from sound.

"She loved animals, oh my God. She brought home every stray. And my dad finally had to say, 'Susie, it's enough.' I mean, she would bring home any animal, any animal. And when she lived with me for a while, she would bring animals all the time."

Ann Marie thought that Sue might have become a vet if she'd gone on to college. She'd certainly kept up her love of animals. Crystal, Sue's daughter, told me that one of her clear memories of her mother involved them discovering a stranded kitten when they were on a walk. She said Sue would take the kids on long walks to entertain them, often stopping for ice cream for the way back. On one of those occasions, they'd heard a kitten crying from underneath someone's porch. Sue had crawled down into the darkness and spiderwebs to bring the kitten out. They'd taken it home with them.

Pam stressed that when they were kids, Sue would choose animals over almost anything else. "We used to do these family reunion trips up to Michigan a couple years in a row near where my cousin's grand-parents owned a farm, a dairy farm. And by that [time], we were maybe preteens or something, and you know how many people like to get up at five o'clock in the morning? Not many, but my sister would get up at five o'clock in the morning to go with my uncle to the farm. So she could hang out with these cows and the other animals on the farm. It is some hard work, but my sister loved it. She was out there every day that they went instead of being at the beach and swimming and you know, stuff like that, even though she loved to fish."

I asked Pam and Ann Marie if they knew of Sue having any serious injuries, and Pam remembered two: a blow to the head when Sue was little—she'd run straight into an iron clothing pole in their yard—and

Sue falling off some bleachers when they were teens. "We were all klutzy. But she was running off the bleachers and fell into a fence. And then from the fence she fell onto the ground. But I can't remember if she hit her head that day because her stomach was bleeding from hitting the fence. She probably did, but we were so focused on the blood, on that injury."

I thought of that old, healed injury Amy had noted on Sue's cranium. It could have come from either event.

I also asked Ann Marie about Sue's friends and life in high school, but she'd been out of the house and starting her own life by then. Pam, however, remembered it well. "I wouldn't say she had a whole lot of friends, but she had like a really close group of friends that she hung out with all the time. A lot of people liked her. Susie wasn't like a girly girl though; you know what I mean? She was more, more tomboyish in some ways. She did like to dress up if she was going somewhere, but she didn't dress up to go to the high school. Jeans and a T-shirt."

Pam said she and Sue both weren't particularly focused in school, but she thought that might have changed, for Sue, if she'd gotten the chance to grow older, along with her sister. It had for Pam, after all.

"She could have been anything by now," Pam emphasized. "Because I bloomed late in life. Susie and I were just kind of go with the flow kind of people. We weren't really serious about doing something in life in the beginning, but I finally went to school and got my nursing degree and I always told Susie, I said, 'I'm most likely going to end up being a nurse when I'm older.' And she always would say, she goes, 'Well, I'll probably be working in a veterinary clinic.' I said, 'Most likely, or choose to be a farm hand.' And we would laugh. She goes, 'Yeah, I'll be a farm hand.' And I said, 'Yeah.' We could actually see each other doing that. And I always just thought eventually, especially out when I started nursing school, I'm like, oh my God, Susie, probably would've been [like] 'Hey, I'm going to school with you.' We probably would've gone to school together. Probably would've been something silly we would've done to motivate each other."

I asked Pam to describe Sue's personality, and she told me many of the same things that Ann Marie did; Sue was sweet, and honest, and uninterested in intrigue. "She was just a very down-to-earth person. She's not the type of person that people would pick on or anything like that. Because she was just so friendly and nice. People met her, they liked her. It was just pretty much that simple because what you see is what you get. She didn't have any hidden agendas; she either liked you or she didn't like you. And if you were nice to her, she liked you, it was just pretty much that simple. You're good to her, she's good to you."

That attitude had gotten Sue through a lot in life. She had issues in her marriage at various points, but by the time Paul was back from Germany, Pam said they'd agreed to make a go of it in Tennessee—a fresh start for the family, at his new station. They hadn't had much time living together over the previous three years, except when Paul was on leave, and some of that time had been at Pam's house, where Pam and Sue had shared caregiving duties for all their children. When Sue was in Tennessee, she was lonely. Her best friend was sometimes in town, but otherwise, she didn't know anyone. Those long phone calls to her sisters and parents were some of her only forms of socialization.

On the night Sue disappeared, Pam remembers that her sister called her at five or six p.m. It was dinnertime; she recalls that vividly because a pizza delivery interrupted their conversation. Pam had gotten it as a treat for the kids, and the delivery driver was someone from their high school—an old friend of both sisters. She'd even put him on the phone to say hello to Sue. So, the memory was locked in place by that event when she thought back on it. Dinnertime, on Christmas Eve.

"She was telling me how she liked [Tennessee], because it was in the country and she really realized that this is where she belongs in the country. She goes, 'I'm not a city person . . . I love this out here.'"

Pam added that Sue was feeling overwhelmed with Paul gone much of the time, and without a car and phone; she was used to sharing childcare with Pam, and having that daily companionship. But she also told Pam how much she loved being with her kids, for those long, uninterrupted stretches—she was getting to watch them change and grow every day, without work or outside obligations to interrupt.

And then they'd talked about Christmas dinner. That's when Sue said she had all her groceries. That she knew what she was making.

There was one final thing Pam mentioned about that call that I found interesting. Sue had told her she was thinking about getting a job, if she could manage it with the kids, to bring in more money for the family. Finances were tight; she was already worried about the number of presents the children were getting that year. Sue's best friend had brought some gifts down, but Sue was still worried about the future. And it struck us both: If she was pregnant, would she be looking for a job? Another mark in the mystery column. It kept growing.

There were so many strange things about that Christmas Eve, and the days that followed. Sue's daughter, Crystal, has recollections that are hard for her to separate: What does she remember for sure, and what has been told to her that has shifted into memory? That's how it is for everyone when we think back to childhood: Family stories are part experience and part rote repetition. But Crystal can recall some things. She remembers Christmas Eve because it was the last time she saw her mother. And she's sure Sue left the house that night.

"I knew she was going to the store," Crystal explained. "And I was begging to go with her and she was like, 'No, not this time. You got to stay home.' And now that I know what happened to her, I'm like, 'Jesus. Maybe if I went with her, she wouldn't have been kidnapped or I might've been kidnapped, too.' Kind of crazy thinking about it."

Crystal wasn't sure of what time this exchange happened; she'd only been four years old, and it was nearly thirty years ago. But it was dark out. Of course, at the height of December, it gets dark early. "I know my dad wanted to get us down for bed. So I'm thinking it was pretty late."

I asked her if there was a reason her father wouldn't have gone, instead of her mother, if Sue had been going to the store.

Crystal thought about it. "I think it's because she wanted to call my Aunt Pam." She paused, then added, "And she didn't have her dog with her. I actually talked to one of her friends. She said she always had Sheba with her. She loved walking Sheba, her white husky. I remember Sheba."

Would Sue have taken Sheba on a walk to call Pam? What about a walk so much farther, to the store, where she couldn't bring her inside?

Crystal remembered waking up on Christmas morning and opening presents with her brother and sister. She was worried they'd be in trouble; they hadn't waited for their parents. But then her dad came downstairs alone. She remembers him being dressed. She has the sense that he'd been up all night. No car, no phone.

Crystal told me that as far as she could recall, it took her days to realize her mother was missing, and not just on her way home. That seems reflected in the newspapers at the time; in a *Leaf-Chronicle* article published a week after Sue's disappearance, Crystal is described as showing the reporter a portrait photo of Sue and "proudly saying, 'That's my mama.'"

"I was a mama's girl according to everyone," Crystal said. "I would always cuddle with her. She would always sing a song to me . . . 'You Are My Sunshine.' The same song I sing. My son loves that song, too. For the first five years of his life, I had to sing it to him every night, to get him to go to sleep. Now, he sings it with me."

It was confusing for Crystal to grow up with those memories, of a mother who had loved her, and the story that the same person had left her behind.

"That's why everything was always weird. My mother's family, they're like, 'Oh, she loved you. You were her little princess.' Where my dad's mom was nothing but negative about her. Except my dad's dad, my grandpa on his side, he loved my mom. He thought she was the greatest thing ever. He had a picture of her until he passed away."

"He didn't believe she ran away?"

"No."

"How do you think your dad would feel getting this news?"

"I think he would be shocked. I'm not sure how he would . . . he would never really want to talk about her. Finding out has made me wonder how my life would turn out differently if she hadn't gone missing. I used to go to the pool a lot. And I would ask every redheaded woman I saw if she was my mom."

"How old were you?"

"This stopped when I was like eight . . . I didn't realize how big the country was. So any redheaded woman, I'm like, 'Hey, that could be my mom.'"

Crystal grew angrier at the lack as she moved into adolescence. She needed her mother more than ever. "At one point I hated her, I will admit that. At one point, I hated her, especially when I was in my teens. Because I thought she just up and left. And then, now that I know what happened to her, I feel guilty for being angry and having hatred towards her."

Crystal had been particularly relieved to hear about the results of Sue's toxicology testing. One thing she'd feared was that her mother was using drugs, and that had something to do with her disappearance. At least as far as her autopsy went, there was no evidence. Forensic toxicology has developed a great deal since 1993, and the samples in Sue's case were limited, but there were no indications in her bloodwork from that era. Her sisters had no prior knowledge of drug addiction, so they couldn't comment beyond being unsurprised by her clean results.

It was only when Crystal hit her early twenties and began to investigate her mother on the internet that she realized that she could find no trace of the right Susan Lund, or Susan Minard—though she found people with the same names—that she began to believe her mother was missing not by choice but because of foul play. No addresses. No social media. No phone numbers. She began to visit missing-persons websites and look at UID forensic sketches and photos. And when she found a website that allowed users to leave messages for missing relatives, she wrote a long post to Sue. She doesn't remember the name of the website. But it felt good to write the message.

She dreamed of her mother. Crystal told me of one that stuck with her. Like my own, it took place in the forest. But she knew who was waiting there. "I know this sounds crazy. My aunt Pam loved it because she had similar dreams about my mother. For a long time, I kept having the same dream. It was like it was real. We were in the woods and I was talking to her and I asked, 'When are you coming home?' And she would get real serious and sad and say, 'I live here now.' It was by a hill in the woods."

Ann Marie had dreams, too, in the years Sue was missing, but of Sue's disembodied head, talking to her. It's one of the reasons the call from Jefferson County, about the discovery of Sue's identity, had been so shocking.

"It was hard hearing [that news], especially that they just found a head and that they've had the head for all these years," Ann Marie explained. "And it's just now them getting to us. It was kind of like, *Well, why couldn't you have found us earlier?* You have all these questions, but we didn't ask them. We were just shocked that they found a head. It was like our validation that what we suspected the whole time was true. That she was gone. When somebody's missing, you swear you can hear them in a crowd say, 'Hey,' calling us. Or you swear you saw her, so you turn around and you follow this car to some place and it wasn't them. You just catch yourself doing that stuff. But after the phone call, Pam and I just cried and we were hugging. It was a validation. And it was a shock that it was just a head, not the whole body. Because then we had a whole different set of questions."

It was even harder for Ann Marie to think of their parents. They would have taken the circumstances of Sue's death very, very hard. What parent wouldn't? To know your child was murdered, and then dismembered? But they would have at least *known.*

"When my mom was actually physically dying in their front room, because my dad let her die at home. We tried everything to save her, but she died. She goes, 'Annie, Annie.' I said, 'What mom?' She goes, 'I see Susie.' I said, 'Go with her mom, go with her.' And within an hour or so she was gone."

Ann Marie's voice broke. "Both of my parents died wanting to know what happened to her. And I did promise them that I would try my hardest to find out. And I will go to their grave and I will personally tell them everything that I found out when I know beyond a shadow of a doubt, everything. I will personally go. And it will be one of the hardest things I've ever had to do."

EPILOGUE
WHAT COMES AFTER

Eight months after the press conference that announced Sue's identity, we still couldn't name her killer. I'd spoken with Detective Captain Bobby Wallace on a number of occasions and given him what information I had, but I wasn't privy to an open homicide investigation. Sue's family wasn't, either. All they knew was that detectives from Illinois would be the ones interviewing them, not officials from Tennessee. Amy had returned Sue's remains to Jefferson County; the coroner there would have to go through some official paperwork and death certification, with Sue's real name, to allow for the release to her family.

Amy told me that a coroner couldn't directly hand human remains over to a loved one. Instead, they'd release the deceased to a funeral home, one picked out by the family, and then the family would work from there to make whatever arrangements they wanted. I hoped it wouldn't take too long. Everything had been slowed down by the pandemic, and then Ann Marie had been sick, and then the worst thing of all: Pam's son had been killed in a car crash. When Ann Marie called to tell me, I was in the parking lot of the grocery store. I'd stopped in to buy my own son his favorite muffins for his school lunches. Amy and I sent flowers to Pam, but it didn't feel like enough. Nothing ever would.

Bobby had delayed his trip to Indiana because of the tragedy and Ann Marie's illness. Then a major case hit Jefferson County, and it took up much of his attention; he told me he'd be in and out of town, working. I wasn't sure when he'd be able to head back to Indiana, or Tennessee. Sooner rather than later, I hoped. But that's the thing with old cases. Sue had been identified, but the leads on her murder were thirty years cold. New cases would always come in, disrupting the work. There was no dedicated cold-case squad. Most departments didn't have one. We were hoping to begin our work on the second Jefferson County case: the man who'd been found in 1995 in the sleeping bag. It was his file I'd climbed the desk to retrieve. It was just a matter of time, literally.

Crystal and I talked on and off. She'd run through her childhood, again and again, trying to separate stories and memories. She'd had to tell her son what happened to his grandmother. She'd sent me a picture of him and texted that he had Sue's eyes. She was right.

Ann Marie and I still kept in touch, too. She texted me throughout the summer for updates on the arm I'd found out about through that article, the one that was stored in Indiana, in formalin, and for which there was no paper trail. That Sue had been dismembered, the postmortem violence of it . . . Ann Marie couldn't get it out of her mind. If that arm was Sue's, she wanted to know, so it could be laid to rest, too.

For months, I had nothing to tell her. The results from the Hubbard Center, at UNH, had been inconclusive. They'd offered to run the test for us, for Amy, really, as part of their foray into forensic DNA research. Astrea had sent them a special boutique kit for formalin-tainted testing, but the results pulled from the arm still showed mostly bacterial DNA. They believed they could possibly rule Sue out, but it wasn't concrete. Dr. Kelly Harkins Kincaid still had a few ideas of things she might try, and offered to do so. After all, Astrea had her information on file.

In November 2022, I picked up my son from school and drove him to an indoor trampoline park so that he could bounce out the energy that had bottled itself up through a few days of intensive schoolwork. Whenever he couldn't go on the playground as much as he liked, he'd thump around the house, doing what he alleged was "parkour" off furniture and nearly colliding with the dogs. This was a much better alternative.

I plugged my laptop into the sad little alcove set aside for parents and watched his blond head bounce away into a sea of other children. He'd run into a few friends from his old school—I recognized them by their new private school's polo shirts—and I could settle in to work with the knowledge that he'd be springing onto things for a few hours, at least.

I put in my AirPods to drown out the noise. A podcast would have been pointless, so I chose one of the Spotify playlists I'd made when I had writer's block—a good time to organize everything—and took a sip of the already-flat Diet Coke I'd bought at the snack bar. I opened Twitter, which was not what I was supposed to be working on. There, I saw a timeline peppered by retweets of the same announcement: one of the most famous Jane Doe cases in the United States had been solved. The woman known only as the "Lady of the Dunes" had finally been identified as Ruth Marie Terry. I had to go through a few browsers to read the *New York Times* article on the case, but finally discovered that Ruth had been from Tennessee and was thirty-seven years old when she'd gone missing. Apparently, she'd gotten married shortly before her disappearance. The man was Guy Muldavin. This was back in 1974. Guy had been married before; he'd also been convicted in connection with the disappearance of that first wife and of their daughter.

The *Times* reported that "mutilated human remains" had been found on his property after his first wife and daughter's disappearance. Somehow, though, Guy had received a "suspended sentence" and was free two years after their disappearance. Then, in 1974, his second wife, Ruth, was gone. No one had ever connected her to the partially dismembered Jane Doe found in Provincetown—not until now. The FBI had confirmed her identity by comparing the DNA of a son she'd given up for adoption in the 1960s.[1] Othram Inc. had done the IGG and DNA testing in Ruth's case; now the Massachusetts State Police would investigate her murder. They hadn't directly named Guy as the suspect during a press conference on her case, but it tracked.

I texted Amy. She'd be home from classes by now, probably outside with Lucy in the garden.

Lady of the Dunes is IDed.

I sent the link.

No way!

I'd always connected her case to Ina Jane Doe's, to Sue, in my head. Not that I thought there was any criminal link. Just the red hair, and the violent postmortem treatment of their remains. Ruth had been found with her hands removed, her head nearly decapitated. And now there was a fairly clear line to the man who probably killed her if we went by what he'd done before. He'd been dead for some time. So, sadly, had Ruth's sister. According to the *Times*, she'd used sites like Ancestry.com and 23andMe to try to find Ruth, right up until her own passing.

Another famous case was solved. Or partially so. Hopefully, Ruth's family would have more answers coming. But it wasn't always how things worked. Often, the wheels stopped turning after identification. In these older cases, witnesses were often dead and suspects, too. It wasn't a satisfying ending, but it was the truth.

My laptop had gone to sleep; I'd spent too much time staring off into the distance, thinking about Ruth. I could see my own smeary reflection through the fingerprints on the screen. I had alarming dark circles ringing each eye. Was that age, or work, or just a trick of the light? The night before, I'd been up too late, again, reading through an old news article. There was a case in Florida I'd wanted to work on for years. "Japanese Gardens Girl," the decedent was called. I'd gotten nowhere with the department for the podcast, but maybe if we could offer more than just coverage—if we could offer funding—they'd respond.

She was thought to be a teen or young adult, possibly of Caribbean descent, who'd been killed in Miami-Dade County back in 1981. It had been a vehicular homicide, and police suspected she'd been intentionally hit; whatever vehicle it had been, it ran over her twice. I'd unsuccessfully filed FOIA twice, only to see on Unidentified Wiki a note that her case file had been lost at some point. But I also noticed that there were two fairly recent reconstructions, so I knew there must be *something* left, somewhere. Maybe her remains were available, and Amy and I could offer to work on her case, and fund testing if it was needed. I opened the Google Doc file we shared, where we listed the cases we most wanted to work on, and made a note next to "Japanese Gardens Girl": *case file lost??*

Amy's notes were in the Doc, too. Cases that she thought needed skeletal reanalysis. Cases from resource-poor areas of the country. Cases where it was clear no anthropologist had ever consulted, or where she thought my research could be helpful. We were awaiting exhumation approval on another Illinois John Doe, a more well-known case than we'd usually be interested in. We figured those were the cases that other people would pick up. But this was a special exception.

Amy and I were both interested in trying to identify decedents who'd passed away at asylums and institutions. Her parents had both worked in mental health care and were familiar with the care facility where this particular man had lived and died. By then, there were better names for hospitals and facilities. But when this particular man had begun his tenure as a forced ward of the state, the language—and the setting— had been much harsher. "John Doe No. 24," later known as John Doe Boyd—a name he was given so he could collect social security—had been a living Doe. That meant that he'd been unidentified in life as well as death—a person not connected to his identity during his life span. Those cases were rare and usually tied to amnesia, or an inability to communicate or to communicate in a way that authorities understood. In the 1940s, he'd been discovered as a nonverbal Deaf teen on the streets in Jacksonville, Illinois. He was only partially clothed, and police described his behavior as "aggressive."[2] Although there was a school for the deaf in Jacksonville, the young man wouldn't be taken there. Authorities didn't even check at the school. Based on nothing more than behavior in custody, authorities decided he was cognitively disabled, which in that time and place would have precluded his admission to the school. The fact that he was Black was a deciding factor, too.

Instead of being placed in an educational track, he entered the state institutional system and would live until 1993 without a known identity. He was able to write down the name "Lewis," but no one was ever able to follow that clue to its conclusion.[3]

In 2000, local Illinois reporter David Bakke, who had covered John Doe Boyd's story, wrote a book about his case. Amy had read it and had me read it, too. She told me that folk singer-songwriter Mary Chapin Carpenter had written a song about the unknown man titled "John Doe No. 24," and paid for his headstone. Its inscription read:

> life's a mystery
> But so too is the human heart

It was a line from Carpenter's song. I thought about that while I updated my notes in our file, by his entry. I'd found something I thought might be important, in the historical records. It was information that hadn't been digitized when David Bakke wrote his book. When John Doe Boyd had been found, a name was written on the inside of his vest: *George Dunkley*. As Bakke noted, that had been a dead end for authorities. But I'd spent days in ancestry and census records, chasing down two family lines. One was a family who'd immigrated from the Caribbean a few decades before John Doe Boyd was found in the alley.

But the other . . . A George Dunkley had died in Illinois, at a nearby institution, just a few months before John Doe Boyd was found in that alley. And based on my research, when a patient died, their clothing would be retained—unless there had been a communicable disease that could be passed. Could John Doe Boyd have been at the same institution as George Dunkley and somehow left or escaped during intake? That process took weeks if David Bakke's description of John Doe Boyd's own experience was any indication. It was a lead, at least. And Amy and I could go to Jacksonville and learn so much more. There were still people alive who'd worked with John Doe Boyd in his last years. There were records and archives and libraries. The exhumation order in Peoria, where John Doe Boyd had been buried, was taking a long time to go through. Maybe we could discover his identity without it.

I texted Amy.

> I just updated the doc. I'm going to email South Carolina. And we'll talk to your New Hampshire people. And we need to get back in contact with ISP.

There were three dozen other cases on our list. We could fund two or three. More, if we worked with a nonprofit like DNA Doe Project, or if an agency got a grant, or we got one ourselves. I could think of another dozen we should add.

My son's sweaty face appeared before me, pressed up against the railings that separated the trampoline area from the parents' holding tank. He said something I couldn't hear. I realized my AirPods were still in. I hadn't heard the last five songs.

"I need my water. Also, I made a new friend."

I passed him the bottle through the tight slot, like we were spies exchanging messages at some rendezvous point. "Oh, really? What's their name?"

He looked baffled. "I don't know. He didn't tell me. Thanks, Mom!" He shoved the bottle back through, and I caught it the moment before it crashed into my laptop. I saw him take off with a short boy in the same private school polo shirt that my son's other friends were wearing. He never asked their names, the children he met at parks or pools or camps. It didn't seem important.

When I looked back down, I had another message from Amy.

> I'll take care of that on Monday. Saw your new notes. I have some thoughts. Adding to the doc.

I scrolled down through the document, past each person whose identities we didn't know, past the hyperlinks and NamUs case numbers and Doe Network summaries, to look for what Amy had come up with. Laughing children and pounding feet made it hard to concentrate, so I slipped my headphones back in.

Names *were* important, after all. They were the key to everything.

An hour later, I was ready to stop working, maybe stare at TikTok for a while until my son was totally dehydrated, but then another email alert popped up. They always do pop up, don't they? I would have ignored this one, but it was from Dr. Kelly Harkins Kincaid. It was the tenth or eleventh in a thread that we'd titled *Possible Susan Lund Arm?*

Kelly finally had an answer for us. Though the sample was not good enough to be used for investigative genetic genealogy, they'd been able to pull enough data to discover one thing: this was not Sue's arm. I knew that Ann Marie and Crystal would be disappointed. They didn't like the idea of Sue's body, still out there, scattered where they might not ever find her. They wanted to lay to rest as much of her as they could. We'd need to call Jefferson County and let them know. Amy would do that. I would call the family. I texted Amy to let her know what Kelly had discovered. Kelly said that maybe some advanced techniques used by her colleagues in the ancient DNA world could get a better sample. She knew people we could talk to. Kelly didn't like to give up; it was why we all got along.

But we'd need a lot of money to afford something like that. A grant. New samples, maybe bone. The trampoline park noise seemed to grow louder, bouncing off the walls around my little alcove.

Amy wrote back.

But whose arm is this?

I responded.

I have no idea.

And I didn't. There's a dead end as often as there's a satisfying answer—even one that brings more questions—in this work. We'd need to return the sample to the coroner in Indiana, and report the findings there, as well. We were probably at an impasse. But still . . .

I opened the Google Doc back up to add "Indiana Arm Doe" to our case list. But I was too late. Amy had already completed the entry herself.

Because there's always a chance.

And because we don't like to give up. Not without a lot of fight.

ACKNOWLEDGMENTS

Without the help of a number of people, the completion of this book would have been impossible.

First, my greatest thanks and appreciation to Ann Marie, Pam, and Crystal for sharing their memories of Sue and their willingness to participate in this story.

Thanks to Bryan Worters for serious assistance in fact-checking and background research. Thanks to Dr. Amy Michael for repeated explanations that, no, bones don't actually connect that way, eternal friendship, and a hundred other kinds of help. Without Dr. Kelly Harkins Kincaid, I'd still be googling "elution." Thanks to Dr. Samantha Blatt and Dr. Jen Bengtson for all the on-the-fly lessons, Maura Currie and Brooke Hargrove for working around my writing schedule and keeping me going, Sarah Turney for the endless pep talks, and all the wonderful scientists and experts who were generous with their time.

Special thanks to Redgrave Research, the Jefferson County Sheriff's Office, Astrea Forensics, the GBI, Suncook Dental, the Tilton School, DNA Doe Project, Parabon, UNH, and SEMO. Thanks to Dr. Steffen Poltak, Dr. Anthony Redgrave (achieved after the events of this book!), and Carl Koppelman for the art included here. Much appreciation to Todd Matthews for connecting me to so many experts, to Kyana Burgess for research assistance, and to Audrey Waterman.

Thank you to Meredith Miller and Lily Dolin at UTA for being the best literary agents on the planet, and to Carrie Napolitano at Hachette for being the kind of editor who will get attic dust on her favorite Buffy T-shirt in the name of science. Thanks to Georgia State University's

Department of English—especially Dr. Lynée Lewis Gaillet—for eternal encouragement.

And finally, thank you to my husband and son, who are always willing to pick me up at the airport, and to my parents, for never telling me to major in something practical.

NOTES

Prologue

1. Nancy Ritter, "Missing Persons and Unidentified Remains: The Nation's Silent Mass Disaster," *National Institute of Justice Journal*, no. 256 (2007): 2–7.

2. Hayley Guenther, "Q6 Cold Case: Thousands of Human Remains Yet to Be Identified Throughout the U.S.," KHQ Right Now, February 13, 2022; Nancy Ritter, "Missing Persons and Unidentified Remains: The Nation's Silent Mass Disaster," National Institute of Justice, February 1, 2007.

Chapter 1

1. "Wayne Fitzgerrell State Recreation Area," State of Illinois Main Site (Department of Natural Resources, n.d.), www2.illinois.gov/dnr/Parks/Pages/WayneFitzgerrell.aspx.

2. "Wayne Fitzgerrell Sra Resort Rebid," State of Illinois Main Site (Illinois State, August 2017).

3. Illinois Digest of Hunting and Trapping Regulations 2021–2022 § (n.d.).

4. Associated Press, "Two Girls Find Human Head," *Herald and Review*, Decatur, Illinois, January 31, 1993, 8.

5. Associated Press, "Two Girls Find Human Head," *Herald and Review*, Decatur, Illinois, January 31, 1993, 8.

6. "Marion, IL Historical Weather," Weather Underground, https://www.wunderground.com/history/daily/us/il/marion.

7. Associated Press, "Expert Called to Help Identify Headless Body," *Pantagraph*, Carbondale, Illinois, May 11, 1993, 2.

8. Robert Kelly, "Dental Work May Help Identify Decapitated Woman," *St. Louis Post-Dispatch* (Missouri), February 2, 1993, 5A.

9. "Police History: How a Magazine Ad Helped Convict a Rapist," Police1 (LEXIPOL, August 28, 2018), www.police1.com/police-products/investigation/dna-forensics/articles/police-history-how-a-magazine-ad-helped-convict-a-rapist-wEnPKjpf6S3brBpF/.

10. "VICAP: Fighting Crime for 25 Years," FBI (FBI, August 27, 2010).

11. "Lake profile—Rend Lake," Department of Natural Resources (I Fish Illinois, 2022).

12. "1990 Census of Population General Population Characteristics Illinois," www2.census.gov/. U.S. Department of Commerce Economics and Statistics Administration, April 17, 2009.

13. Diane Fanning, *Through the Window* (New York: St. Martin's Paperbacks, 2007).

14. Thomas Beaumont, "Resendiz-Ramirez Link to Dardeen Killings Explored," *Southern Illinoisan*, July 5, 1999, 3.

15. "Angel Maturino Resendiz: The 'Railroad Killer,'" CBS News, CBS Interactive, September 3, 2017.

16. Dianne Fanning, *Through the Window* (New York: St. Martin's Paperbacks, 2007).

17. Bob Cyphers and Sara Bannoura, "Gruesome Murder of an Illinois Family Remains Unsolved as the Main Suspect Is Executed" (KMOV, January 21, 2022).

18. Associated Press, "Expert Called to Help Identify Headless Body," *Pantagraph*, Carbondale, Illinois, May 11, 1993, 2.

19. Charles Bosworth Jr., "Headless 'Jane Doe' Burial Set: Body Afire at Litchfield Unidentified Since May," *St. Louis Post-Dispatch*, August 7, 1993, 1B.

20. Associated Press, "Expert Called to Help Identify Headless Body," *Pantagraph*, Carbondale, Illinois, May 11, 1993, 2.

21. Charles Bosworth Jr., "Headless 'Jane Doe' Burial Set: Body Afire at Litchfield Unidentified Since May," *St. Louis Post-Dispatch*, August 7, 1993, 1B.

22. Wes Smith, "A Community Seeks Justice for Murdered Woman Dumped in Park," *Chicago Tribune*, January 22, 1996.

Chapter 2

1. Leonard J. Paulozzi et al., "John and Jane Doe: The Epidemiology of Unidentified Decedents," *Journal of Forensic Sciences* 53, no. 4 (2008): 922–927.

2. "Missing Persons Statistics 2021 (Infographic): Black and Missing," BAMFI, November 3, 2022, www.blackandmissinginc.com/statistics.

3. Amna Nawaz and Talesha Reynolds, "New Documentary Highlights Plight of Missing Black Women and Why Their Cases Go Ignored," PBS (Public Broadcasting Service, November 23, 2021), www.pbs.org/newshour/show/new-documentary-highlights -plight-of-missing-black-women-and-why-their-cases-go-ignored.

4. "Frequently Asked Questions," NamUs (National Institute of Justice, March 26, 2021).

5. "RTI Awarded National Missing and Unidentified Persons System Contract," RTI International, May 5, 2021.

6. "What Is Rapid DNA?," ANDE Rapid DNA, June 6, 2018, www.ande.com /what-is-rapid-dna/.

7. Anne Bridgman, "Missing-Children Phenomenon Fuels School-Fingerprinting Programs," *Education Week*, February 25, 2019.

8. Anne Bridgman, "Missing-Children Phenomenon Fuels School-Fingerprinting Programs," *Education Week*, February 25, 2019.

9. "Next Generation Identification (NGI)," FBI (FBI, June 24, 2022), https://le.fbi .gov/science-and-lab-resources/biometrics-and-fingerprints/biometrics/next-generation -identification-ngi.

10. "Next Generation Identification (NGI)," FBI (FBI, June 24, 2022), https://le.fbi .gov/science-and-lab-resources/biometrics-and-fingerprints/biometrics/next-generation -identification-ngi.

11. "Next Generation Identification (NGI)," FBI (FBI, June 24, 2022), https://le.fbi.gov/science-and-lab-resources/biometrics-and-fingerprints/biometrics/next-generation-identification-ngi.

12. Sonali Kohli, "After 27 Years of Hoping, a Family's Worst Fear Is Confirmed," *Los Angeles Times* (Los Angeles Times, May 12, 2017), www.latimes.com/local/lanow/la-me-ln-andrea-kuiper-identification-20170512-htmlstory.html.

13. "Andrea Kuiper," Unidentified Wiki, accessed December 14, 2022, https://unidentified-awareness.fandom.com/wiki/Andrea_Kuiper.

14. Sonali Kohli, "After 27 Years of Hoping, a Family's Worst Fear Is Confirmed," *Los Angeles Times* (Los Angeles Times, May 12, 2017), www.latimes.com/local/lanow/la-me-ln-andrea-kuiper-identification-20170512-htmlstory.html.

15. "Woman in California Vehicle Crash Identified 27 Years Later," BBC News (BBC, May 12, 2017), www.bbc.com/news/world-us-canada-39901639.

16. Sonali Kohli, "After 27 Years of Hoping, a Family's Worst Fear Is Confirmed," *Los Angeles Times* (Los Angeles Times, May 12, 2017), www.latimes.com/local/lanow/la-me-ln-andrea-kuiper-identification-20170512-htmlstory.html.

17. Mike Dash, "Body on Somerton Beach," *Smithsonian*, 2011.

18. Ben Chesire and Susan Chenery, "Marriage and a Mystery," ABC Australia, 2019.

19. Derek Abbott, "Timeline of the Taman Shud Case," Timeline of the Taman Shud Case—Derek, n.d., www.eleceng.adelaide.edu.au/personal/dabbott/wiki/index.php/Timeline_of_the_Taman_Shud_Case.

20. Lisa Zyga, "After Years of Forensic Investigation, Somerton Man's Identity Remains a Mystery (Part 2: DNA, Isotopes, and Autopsy)," Phys.org, June 3, 2015.

21. Ben Cheshire, "'Did He Marry Me for My DNA?': How One Woman Could Crack the Somerton Man Mystery," ABC News (ABC News, November 4, 2019), www.abc.net.au/news/2019-10-15/a-marriage-and-a-mystery-somerton-man-romantic-twist/11377458.

22. "Plastic Surgery Statistics," American Society of Plastic Surgeons, 2020, www.plasticsurgery.org/news/plastic-surgery-statistics.

23. Brian Palmer, "How Much Could the Police Learn from Jasmine Fiore's Fake Breasts?," *Slate Magazine* (Slate, August 24, 2009), https://slate.com/news-and-politics/2009/08/how-much-could-the-police-learn-from-jasmine-fiore-s-fake-breasts.html.

24. "Unidentified Male," 2752UMFL, n.d., https://doenetwork.org/cases/2752umfl.html.

25. Brian Palmer, "How Much Could the Police Learn from Jasmine Fiore's Fake Breasts?," *Slate Magazine* (Slate, August 24, 2009), https://slate.com/news-and-politics/2009/08/how-much-could-the-police-learn-from-jasmine-fiore-s-fake-breasts.html.

26. Matthew Taylor, "King's Cross Fire: The Story of Body 115," *The Guardian* (Guardian News and Media, January 22, 2004), www.theguardian.com/world/2004/jan/22/transport.uk.

Chapter 3

1. Peter Vronsky, in *American Serial Killers: The Epidemic Years 1950–2000* (New York: Berkley, 2020), 8.

2. Associated Press, "Lawmen from 5-States Probe Redhead Murders," *Schenectady Gazette*, April 25, 1985.

3. Steve Huff, "The Forgotten Redhead Murders: Coincidence or Serial Killer?," *InsideHook*, January 3, 2018, www.insidehook.com/article/crime/cold-case-redhead-murders.

Chapter 4

1. Joseph Caputo, "Solving a 17th-Century Crime," Smithsonian.com (Smithsonian Institution, March 1, 2009), www.smithsonianmag.com/arts-culture/solving -a-17th-century-crime-50842762/.

2. Joseph Caputo, "Solving a 17th-Century Crime," Smithsonian.com (Smithsonian Institution, March 1, 2009), www.smithsonianmag.com/arts-culture/solving -a-17th-century-crime-50842762/.

3. C. Soanes, A. Stevenson, and S. Hawker, "Forensic," in *Oxford English Dictionary Online* (Oxford: Oxford University Press, n.d.).

4. "Anthropology," *Oxford Advanced Learner's Dictionary* at OxfordLearnersDic tionaries.com, https://www.oxfordlearnersdictionaries.com/us/definition/english /anthropology.

5. "What Is Carbon-14 (14c) Dating? Carbon Dating Definition," Carbon Dating Service, AMS Miami—Beta Analytic, July 5, 2021.

6. Graham Brewer, "Search for Missing Native Artifacts Led to the Discovery of Bodies Stored in 'the Most Inhumane Way Possible,'" NBCNews.com (NBCUniversal News Group, September 4, 2022), www.nbcnews.com/news/us-news/search -missing-native-artifacts-led-discovery-bodies-stored-inhumane-w-rcna46151.

7. "Compliance," National Parks Service (U.S. Department of the Interior, accessed March 27, 2022), www.nps.gov/subjects/nagpra/compliance.htm.

8. Ash Ngu, "How to Report on the Repatriation of Native American Remains," *ProPublica*, February 3, 2023.

9. Ash Ngu and Andrea Suozzo, "Does Your Local Museum or University Still Have Native American Remains?," *ProPublica*, January 11, 2023, https://projects.propublica .org/repatriation-nagpra-database/.

10. Logan Jaffe, "The Museum Built on Native American Burial Mounds," *ProPublica*, January 27, 2023, www.propublica.org/article/repatriation-nagpra-museums -dickson-mounds-museum.

11. "NAGPRA Grants," National Parks Service (U.S. Department of the Interior, November 18, 2022), www.nps.gov/subjects/nagpra/grants.htm.

Chapter 6

1. M. Katherine Spradley and Kyra E. Stull, "Chapter 3—Advancements in Sex and Ancestry Estimation," in *New Perspectives in Forensic Human Skeletal Identification*, ed., Krista E. Latham, Eric J. Bartelink, and Michael Finnegan (Academic Press, 2018), 13–21.

2. D. Freid, Martha Spradley, Richard Jantz, and Stephen Ousley, "The Truth Is out There: How NOT to Use FORDISC," *American Journal of Physical Anthropology* S40, no. 103 (2005).

3. S. Longato, C. Wöss, P. Hatzer-Grubwieser, C. Bauer, W. Parson, S. H. Unterberger, V. Kuhn, N. Pemberger, A. K. Pallua, W. Recheis, R. Lackner, R. Stalder, and J. D. Pallua,

"Post-mortem Interval Estimation of Human Skeletal Remains by Micro-computed Tomography, Mid-infrared Microscopic Imaging and Energy Dispersive X-ray Mapping," *Analytical Methods: Advancing Methods and Applications* 7, no. 7 (2015): 2917–2927.

4. Laurah Norton, "The Twiggs County John Doe, Part 1: The Accident on Highway 16" (*The Fall Line Podcast*, April 14, 2021), www.thefalllinepodcast.com/episodes/2021/3/10/the-twiggs-county-john-doe-part-1-the-accident-on-highway-16.

5. Erin Kimmerle, Anthony Falsetti, and Ann Ross, "Immigrants, Undocumented Workers, Runaways, Transients and the Homeless: Towards Contextual Identification Among Unidentified Decedents," *Forensic Science Policy and Management* 1 (2010): 178–186.

6. Associated Press, "Two Girls Find Human Head," *Herald and Review*, Decatur, Illinois, January 31, 1993, 8.

7. www.iomcworld.com/open-access/a-preliminary-study-of-the-relationship-between-obliteration-of-cranial-sutures-and-age-at-time-of-death-2329-6577-1000163.pdf.

8. www.iomcworld.com/open-access/a-preliminary-study-of-the-relationship-between-obliteration-of-cranial-sutures-and-age-at-time-of-death-2329-6577-1000163.pdf.

9. Laurah Norton, "Dennis Doe and Christmas Doe: Dennis Doe Identified" (*The Fall Line Podcast*, July 20, 2022), www.thefalllinepodcast.com/episodes/2022/7/20/dennis-doe-and-christmas-doe-dennis-doe-identified.

10. C. A. Cunningham, "Anthropology: Skeleton; Estimating Juvenile Age," in *Wiley Encyclopedia of Forensic Science*, eds. A. Jamieson and A. Moenssens (Hoboken, NJ: Wiley-Blackwell, 2014).

11. Jonathan Raymond, "Mom Charged with Murder as Georgia Boy Whose Remains Were Found 23 Years Ago Finally Identified," 11Alive.com (11 Alive News, July 13, 2022), www.11alive.com/article/news/crime/william-dashawn-hamilton-cold-case-identified-mother-charged-murder-dekalb-county/85-c1314239-6530-4c4d-a629-0a2d2de9e8da.

12. Jonathan Raymond, "Mom Charged with Murder as Georgia Boy Whose Remains Were Found 23 Years Ago Finally Identified," 11Alive.com (11 Alive News, July 13, 2022), www.11alive.com/article/news/crime/william-dashawn-hamilton-cold-case-identified-mother-charged-murder-dekalb-county/85-c1314239-6530-4c4d-a629-0a2d2de9e8da.

13. Gita Mall, Michael Hubig, Andreas Büttner, J. Kuzník, Randolph Penning, and Matthias Graw, "Sex Determination and Estimation of Stature from the Long Bones of the Arm," *Forensic Science International* 117, no. 1–2 (2001): 23–30.

14. Kelsey Kyllonen, Terrie Simmons-Ehrhardt, and Keith L. Monson, "Stature Estimation Using Measurements of the Cranium for Populations in the United States," *Forensic Science International* 281 (2017): 184.e1–184.e9.

15. Stephen Ousley and Richard Jantz, "Ch. 15: Fordisc 3 and Statistical Methods for Estimating Sex and Ancestry," in *A Companion to Forensic Anthropology* (Hoboken, NJ: Wiley-Blackwell, 2014).

16. N. J. Sauer, "Forensic Anthropology and the Concept of Race: If Races Don't Exist, Why Are Forensic Anthropologists So Good at Identifying Them?," *Social Science & Medicine* 34, no. 2 (1992): 107–111.

17. Madeleine Hinkes, "Book Review: Atlas of Human Cranial Macromorphoscopic Traits," *Academic Forensic Pathology* (Thousand Oaks, CA: SAGE Publishing, December 2018), www.ncbi.nlm.nih.gov/pmc/articles/PMC6491539/.

18. Clyde Snow et al., "Sex and Race Determination of Crania by Calipers and Computer: A Test of the Giles and Elliot Discriminant Function in 52 Forensic Cases," Defense Technical Information Center (University of Illinois, 1979), https://apps.dtic.mil/sti/pdfs/ADA364024.pdf.

19. Jill Tucker, "Bones Found in '79 ID'd as Missing Girls; Bones Found 37 Years Ago Linked to Missing Sonoma County Girls," *San Francisco Chronicle*, February 4, 2016, E2.

20. Adam Randall and Kwear Udjar, "National Expert Gives Opinion on Mendocino County Cold Case IDs," *Ukiah Daily Journal* (Ukiah Daily Journal, August 23, 2018), www.ukiahdailyjournal.com/2016/02/05/national-expert-gives-opinion-on-mendocino-county-cold-case-ids/.

21. "Hyperostosis Frontalis Interna," NORD (National Organization for Rare Disorders), accessed 2007, https://rarediseases.org/rare-diseases/hyperostosis-frontalis-interna/.

Chapter 7

1. "African Burying Ground Memorial Park—We Stand in Honor of Those Forgotten—Portsmouth, New Hampshire," African Burying Ground Memorial Park, n.d., https://africanburyinggroundnh.org/.

Chapter 8

1. "HIPAA Rules for Dentists—Updated for 2022," *HIPAA Journal*, August 22, 2022, www.hipaajournal.com/hipaa-rules-for-dentists/.

2. Grant Robinson, "Public Help Needed in Missing and Unidentified Person Cases," wbir.com (WBIR, October 14, 2018), www.wbir.com/article/news/local/public-help-needed-to-help-missing-and-unidentified-person-cases/51-604152875.

3. "Dental Identification in a Case of Purposeful Commingling of Remains by a Toronto Serial Killer Operating in the Gay Community of Toronto, 2010–2017: The Bruce McArthur Case," Taylor Gardner, BFS; Yolanda Nerkowski, BA; Robert E. Wood, DDS, MSc, PhD. AAFS annual conference, February 21–25, 2022, Seattle.

4. Grant Robinson, "Public Help Needed in Missing and Unidentified Person Cases," wbir.com (WBIR, October 14, 2018), www.wbir.com/article/news/local/public-help-needed-to-help-missing-and-unidentified-person-cases/51-604152875.

5. "Official 9/11 Death Toll Climbs by One," CBS News (CBS Interactive, July 11, 2008), www.cbsnews.com/news/official-9-11-death-toll-climbs-by-one/.

6. Brad Mielke, Kelly Terez, and Ivan Pereira, "Forensic Investigators Work to Give 9/11 Families Peace as They ID Ground Zero Remains," ABC News (ABC News, September 12, 2022), https://abcn.ws/3B9meHx.

7. Mark Finlay, "How USAir Flight 427 Became Pennsylvania's Deadliest Air Disaster," Simple Flying, September 8, 2022, https://simpleflying.com/usair-flight-427-crash-story/.

Chapter 10

1. "Charles Holt Expo," West Virginia Public Safety Expo, n.d., www.wvsafetyexpo.com/team-member/charles-holt/.

2. Karen T. Taylor, *Forensic Art and Illustration* (Boca Raton, FL: CRC Press, 2000).

3. Sonja Gupta et al., "Forensic Facial Reconstruction: The Final Frontier," *Journal of Clinical and Diagnostic Research* 9, no. 9 (Sept. 2015): ZE26–ZE2.

4. Caroline Wilkinson, *Forensic Facial Reconstruction* (Cambridge, UK: Cambridge University Press, 2006), 39–41.

5. Sculpture by Thomas Woolner, Dickens Museum Collection, 1875.

6. M. H. Kauffman and Robert McNeil, "Death Masks and Life Masks," *British Medical Journal* 298, no. 6673 (1989): 506–507.

7. Caroline Wilkinson, *Forensic Facial Reconstruction* (Cambridge, UK: Cambridge University Press, 2006), 45.

8. "Anne Arundel County Police Use DNA Snapshot to Aid Identification of Baltimore Murder Victim, Leading to Arrest and Confession," Parabon Nano-Labs News, February 12, 2018, www.parabon-nanolabs.com/news-events/2018/02/anne-arundel-police-use-dna-snapshot-to-identify-murder-victim-leading-to-arrest-and-confession.html.

9. "Murder of Shaquana Marie Caldwell," Arundel County and Baltimore, MD, Police Departments, Murder of Shaquana Marie Caldwell—Parabon Snapshot Case Summary, n.d., https://snapshot.parabon-nanolabs.com/snapshot-case-summary—anne-arundel-county-md—shaquana-caldwell-murder.html.

10. "Murder of Shaquana Marie Caldwell," Arundel County and Baltimore, MD, Police Departments, Murder of Shaquana Marie Caldwell—Parabon Snapshot Case Summary, n.d., https://snapshot.parabon-nanolabs.com/snapshot-case-summary—anne-arundel-county-md—shaquana-caldwell-murder.html.

11. Christopher Buchanan, "She Was Found in a Georgia Cornfield in 1981. On Thursday, We Finally Learned Her Name," 11Alive.com, January 10, 2020, www.11alive.com/article/news/investigations/gone-cold/brooks-county-jane-doe-identified/85-e3aea29f-a5b3-4319-a3c5-d7d72fa621bf.

12. "Brooks County Jane Doe Killed 37 Years Ago," *Valdosta Today* (Valdosta Today, November 2018), https://valdostatoday.com/news-2/local/2018/11/brooks-county-jane-doe-killed-37-years-ago/.

13. Pat Mueller, "Victim in 1981 Brooks Co. Murder Case Identified as Fair Worker," WCTV (WCTV, September 2020), www.wctv.tv/content/news/Arrest-made-in-1981-Brooks-County-cold-murder-case-566844011.html.

14. Phillip Kish, "He Was Struck and Killed While Walking. We Don't Know His Name," 11Alive.com (11 Alive, March 15, 2019), www.11alive.com/article/news/local/he-was-struck-and-killed-while-walking-we-dont-know-his-name/85-2676beb9-0784-4ff8-a062-9843ef5c76d2.

15. Alex Whittler, "Missing Riverdale Teen Identified Three Years After Death," FOX 5 Atlanta (FOX 5 Atlanta, April 5, 2022), www.fox5atlanta.com/news/missing-riverdale-teen-identified-three-years-after-death.

16. "Update John Riverdale Doe Identified Dywimas Marquis Autman," Facebook (Clayton County Police Department, April 2022), www.facebook.com/ClaytonCountyPD/posts/380828344082386/?paipv=0&eav=AfY5VH6oCW_vlAZL45oCnjj0aDgnrTGlqgJC4GgFvwFkYdytee_Mq2uyw_Z828MEOGA&_rdr.

Chapter 12

1. Hao Fan and Jia-You Chu, "A Brief Review of Short Tandem Repeat Mutation," *Genomics, Proteomics & Bioinformatics* (U.S. National Library of Medicine, February 2007), www.ncbi.nlm.nih.gov/pmc/articles/PMC5054066.

2. "CeCe Moore Genetic Genealogist," CeCe Moore, The DNA Detective, n.d., https://cecemoore.com/.

3. Andrew Cass, "A Year After Joseph Newton Chandler's True Identity Revealed, the 'Why' Remains Unanswered," *News-Herald* (News-Herald, July 15, 2021), www.news-herald.com/2019/06/15/a-year-after-joseph-newton-chandlers-true-identity-revealed-the-why-remains-unanswered.

4. Morgan Winsor, "Body of 'Buckskin Girl' Found in Ohio in 1981 Identified as Arkansas Woman," ABC News (ABC News Network, April 2, 2018), https://abcnews.go.com/US/body-buckskin-girl-found-ohio-1981-identified-arkansas/story?id=54417156.

5. Emily Shapiro, "How the 'Golden State Killer,' a Serial Rapist, Murderer, Evaded Capture for Decades," ABC11 Raleigh-Durham, October 31, 2020, https://abc11.com/golden-state-killer-joseph-deangelo-timeline-caught/7515045/.

6. Jason Moon, "Three Bear Brook Murder Victims Identified; Citizen Sleuth, Genetic Genealogy Provide Key Clues," New Hampshire Public Radio (NHPR, February 13, 2020), www.nhpr.org/nh-news/2019-06-05/three-bear-brook-murder-victims-identified-citizen-sleuth-genetic-genealogy-provide-key-clues.

7. Alie Yang and Boaz Halaban, ABC News (ABC News Network, January 18, 2021), https://abcnews.go.com/US/terry-rasmussens-victims-unknown/story?id=69585534.

8. K. C. Downey, "Unidentified Bear Brook Victim Likely Was Born in Mid-to-Late 1970s, Has Relatives from Mississippi," WMUR (WMUR, June 30, 2022), www.wmur.com/article/terry-rasumussen-daughter-bear-brook-victim/40461037.

9. Tara Luther, "GEDmatch: A Genealogy Platform Allowing Users and Law Enforcement to Make Familial Connections," ISHI News, March 1, 2021, www.ishinews.com/gedmatch-a-genealogy-platform-allowing-users-and-law-enforcement-to-make-familial-connections.

10. Peter Aldhous, "This Genealogy Database Helped Solve Dozens of Crimes, but Its New Privacy Rules Will Restrict Access by Cops," *BuzzFeed News* (BuzzFeed News, May 19, 2019), www.buzzfeednews.com/article/peteraldhous/this-genealogy-database-helped-solve-dozens-of-crimes-but.

11. Peter Aldhous, "A Teen Allegedly Assaulted an Elderly Woman. Cops Pursued Him Like the Golden State Killer," *BuzzFeed News* (BuzzFeed News, May 15, 2019), www.buzzfeednews.com/article/peteraldhous/genetic-genealogy-parabon-gedmatch-assault.

12. Eric Levenson, "How a Utah Assault Case Upended the Cutting-Edge DNA Website That Caught the Golden State Killer," CNN (Cable News Network, June 9, 2019), www.cnn.com/2019/05/27/us/genetic-genealogy-gedmatch-privacy/index.html.

13. Eric Levenson, "How a Utah Assault Case Upended the Cutting-Edge DNA Website That Caught the Golden State Killer," CNN (Cable News Network, June 9, 2019), www.cnn.com/2019/05/27/us/genetic-genealogy-gedmatch-privacy/index.html.

14. "About Gedmatch Pro™: Gedmatch Pro™," About GEDmatch PRO™ | GEDmatch PRO™, n.d., https://pro.gedmatch.com/about.

15. Laurah Norton, "The DNA Doe Project" (*The Fall Line Podcast*, November 30, 2022), www.thefalllinepodcast.com/episodes/2022/11/29/the-dna-doe-project-part-1.

16. Erin Murphy and Jun Tong, "The Racial Composition of Forensic DNA Databases," *California Law Review*, December 31, 2020, https://californialawreview.org/print/racial-composition-forensic-dna-databases/.

17. Peggy Townsend, "Kim Tallbear: Protecting Native American DNA and Indigenous Rights," *UC Santa Cruz Magazine*, August 26, 2022, https://magazine.ucsc.edu/2022/08/kim-tallbear-protecting-native-american-dna-and-indigenous-rights/.

18. "Hispanic Heritage Month Featured Cases 1-12," Facebook (DNA Doe Project, October 31, 2022), www.facebook.com/DNADoeProject/photos/a.2036472776611497/3299319286993500/.

19. Andreas Tillmar, Siri Aili Fagerholm, Jan Staaf, Peter Sjölund, and Ricky Ansell, "Getting the Conclusive Lead with Investigative Genetic Genealogy—A Successful Case Study of a 16 Year Old Double Murder in Sweden," *Forensic Science International: Genetics* 53 (2021).

Chapter 15

1. Lee Elder, "Husband Holds onto Hope as Search Continues for Wife," *The Leaf-Chronicle*, December 31, 1992, 11.

2. N/A, "Police Continue Search for Missing Woman," *The Leaf-Chronicle*, December 29, 1992, 3.

3. N/A, "Weather Report," *The Leaf-Chronicle*, December 23, 1992, A2.

4. Lee Elder, "Police Target Kentucky in Search for Woman," January 3, 1993, 1.

5. Lee Elder, "Husband Vows to Continue Search for Missing Wife," *The Leaf-Chronicle*, January 8, 1993, 5.

6. Lee Elder, "Husband Vows to Continue Search for Missing Wife," *The Leaf-Chronicle*, January 8, 1993, 5.

7. Lee Elder, "Police Target Kentucky in Search for Woman," *The Leaf-Chronicle*, January 3, 1993, 1.

8. Lee Elder, "Husband Vows to Continue Search for Missing Wife," *The Leaf-Chronicle*, January 8, 1993, 5.

9. Lee Elder, "Husband Holds onto Hope as Search Continues for Wife," *The Leaf-Chronicle*, December 31, 1992, 11.

10. N/A, "No Grave Discovered in Search for Lund," *The Leaf-Chronicle*, April 15, 1993, 9.

11. N/A, "Missing Woman Apparently Safe," *Montgomery Advertiser* 16 (1993), 12.

Epilogue

1. Michael Levenson, "Nearly 50 Years After Murder, the 'Lady of the Dunes' Is Identified," *New York Times* (New York Times, November 3, 2022), www.nytimes.com/2022/11/03/us/provincetown-body-lady-of-the-dunes.html.

2. David Bakke, *God Knows His Name: The True Story of John Doe No. 24* (Carbondale, IL: Southern Illinois University Press, 2000).

3. David Bakke, *God Knows His Name: The True Story of John Doe No. 24* (Carbondale, IL: Southern Illinois University Press, 2000).

INDEX

3-D digital modeling, 177–178, 180–183
3-D printing, 182, 189, 241
3-D reconstruction, 76–77, 177–183, 189, 241
9/11 attacks, 26, 154–160
23andMe, 26, 207, 212, 215–216, 240, 248, 292
90 Day Fiancé (TV show), 46

AARP Magazine, 198
Abbott, Dr. Derek, 34–35
ABC Australia, 33
ABC docuseries, 208
ABC News, 159
"ACE" tattoo, 192–193
ADA News (newspaper), 149
Adam (TV show), 28
Adelaide, Australia, 32–35
Advanced Fingerprint Identification Technology (AFIT), 29
AFIP (Air Forces Institute of Pathology), 160
AFIS (Automated Fingerprint Identification System), 15, 29
AFIT (Advanced Fingerprint Identification Technology), 29
age-range estimations, xvii, 8, 14, 41, 95–97, 113, 179, 183, 191–192
Air Forces Institute of Pathology (AFIP), 160
Alabama, 252, 258–259, 276
Albee, Dr. Andrew, 165–175, 275
Alighieri, Dante, 181
"Amazon Savage," 126, 166, 168

Amelia, 166–167, 170, 174
American Dental Association, 149–151
America's Most Wanted (TV show), 28, 281
AMS dating, 169
anatomical mummy, 125–127, 138–146, 163–164, 169
ancestry estimations, xvi–xvii, 68–69, 91–113, 132–134, 183–185, 246
Ancestry.com, 207, 211–212, 215–216, 248–251, 254, 292
ANDE machine, 26
animal predation, 8, 63, 136, 204–205, 259
Anne Arundel County, Maryland, 62, 183–184
Anne Arundel County Police, 183
Arc Bio, 117
Arizona, 66, 98
Arizona State University, 66
Arkansas, 214
Astrea Forensics, 117–118, 131, 164, 193, 195, 202, 208, 216, 227–236, 245, 272, 275, 290
Atlanta, Georgia, xi–xii, 39–59, 73, 88, 97–98, 115, 123, 145, 184–185, 192, 229, 235–237, 263, 270
Atlanta Journal-Constitution (newspaper), 192
Atlanta Police Department, 185
Audiochuck, 224
Australia, 32–35, 222
Autman, Dywimas, 192–193
Automated Fingerprint Identification System (AFIS), 15, 29

"Babes in the Woods," 207, 242
"Baby Horry," xviii
Bakke, David, 294
Baltimore, Maryland, 183–184
Baltimore City Police Department,
    183–184
Barrow County, Georgia, 191
Bear Brook State Park, 214–215
Beaufort County, South Carolina, 73
Beethoven, Ludwig van, 181
Bengtson, Dr. Jen, 50–51, 89–90
Biggie Smalls, 187
birthmarks, 26–27. *See also* marks; scars
Black, Teresa Ann Bailey, 97–98
Black and Missing Foundation, 21
Blake, William, 181
Blatt, Dr. Samantha, 63–64, 67–68, 109,
    116–131, 137, 140–146, 163–167, 170,
    173–175, 178, 234, 237–243, 272
"Blinded by the White: Forensic
    Anthropology and Ancestry
    Estimation," 104
Bodies: The Exhibition (museum
    show), 141
"Body 115," 37
Bon Jovi, 201
Bonaparte, Napoleon, 181
bone samples, 141–147, 204–205, 231, 235.
    See also skeletal analysis
Bones (TV show), 63, 70
bones, broken, xv, 26, 92, 112. *See also*
    injuries
Borges, Jorge Luis, 247
Boxall, Alfred "Alf," 33–34
"Boy in the Box," xviii
Boyd, John Doe, 293–295
Branch Davidians, 154
breast implants, 25, 36. *See also* medical
    implants
Brigham Young University, 186
British Transport Police, 37
broken bones, xv, 26, 92, 112. *See also*
    injuries
Brooks County, Georgia, 188
Brown, Dr. Rodney, 149–151

Brown University, 69
Buckley, Pamela Mae, 199
"Buckskin Girl," 214
Bullard, Jeff, 270–272, 275–276
Bundy, Ted, 138, 196
Burge, Scott, 52–54, 74–78, 269
Burgess, Kyana, 42, 49–59, 73–87, 90, 127,
    130–137, 201, 252, 261–269, 272, 276
burial sites, 95, 119–120, 126, 188, 216, 258
BuzzFeed, 217

Caldwell, Shaquana, 184
California, 30–31, 37, 108, 117, 210,
    227–234
California Law Review (journal), 219
Canada, 220–222, 242
Carpenter, Mary Chapin, 294
case files
    assembly of, 22–25, 39–59, 128, 171, 193,
        198, 231
    cold cases, xi–xxi, 1–17, 20–53, 65,
        71–90, 101–125, 182, 203–247,
        264, 290
    of Ina Jane Doe, xvii–xxi, 1–17, 27,
        39–59, 63–64, 71–90, 92–113, 202,
        227–236, 245–246, 261–262
    loss of, 292–293
Centerville, Utah, 217
centimorgan (cM) matches, 213, 218–222,
    246, 249–252, 274
Charley Project, xii, 25
Charlotte, North Carolina, 98
Chicago Tribune (newspaper), 16
children
    database of, xii, 30, 98, 109, 192–193, 198
    fingerprinting, 28, 138–139
    missing, xii–xiv, 27–28, 30, 98, 109,
        192–193, 198
    stranger-danger and, 27–28
Church of Jesus Christ of Latter-Day
    Saints, 241
Clarksville, Tennessee, 256–262, 271, 286
Clarksville Leaf-Chronicle, The
    (newspaper), 256–257, 286
Clarksville Police Department, 257–259

clay busts, 42–43, 130, 178, 180–181
clay reconstructions, 42–43, 130,
     178–186, 190–191. *See also* facial
     reconstruction; forensic art
closed population event, 158
cM matches, 213, 218–222, 246, 249–252, 274
CNN, 217
CODIS, 9, 26, 207–208, 216, 220
cold cases
     investigating, xi–xxi, 1–17, 20–53, 65,
          71–90, 101–125, 182, 203–247, 264, 290
     news coverage of, xii–xv, 53, 72,
          202–203, 255–259, 269–288, 292
     number of, xii, 19–21
     publicity for, xii–xv, 53, 72, 255–259
     reviewing, 38–42
     see also unidentified decedents
Combined DNA Index System (CODIS), 9,
     26, 207–208, 216, 220
Connelly, Kaycee, 270–271, 275
Contagion (movie), 231
"contextual identification" methods, 95
Cosgriff-Hernandez, Dr.
     Meghan-Tomasita, 104
Creative Paperclay, 191
Crime Con 2022, 221
crime scene
     for Ina Jane Doe, xvii, 1–12, 27, 39, 48,
          55, 79–88, 201, 259
     investigation of, xvii, 3–12, 27, 39, 61,
          84–88
     lack of, 10, 12, 27, 39
     locations of, xvii, 3–12, 48, 61, 84–88,
          196, 238
     recovery scene and, 61, 65, 80, 94,
          154–156, 273
Crime Scene Technician (CST), 5
Cron, Thomas, 212
Cruz, Pablo Hernandez, 19
Currie, Maura, 167, 228–235, 240, 244–245

D-ABFA (Diplomate of the American
     Board of Forensic Anthropology), 64
D'Alton, David, 242
D'Alton, Derek, 242

Dardeen, Elaine, 11–13
Dardeen, Keith, 11–13
Dardeen, Peter, 11–13
Dardeen case, 12, 76–77
Dardeen family, 1–2, 11–13, 76–77
databases
     23andMe database, 26, 207, 212,
          215–216, 240, 248, 292
     AFIS database, 15, 29
     Ancestry.com, 207, 211–212, 215–216,
          248–251, 254, 292
     creating, 23–25
     DNA databases, 26, 198–227, 245–254,
          260–261, 273–274, 292
     Doe Network, xv, 23–25, 151–155, 178,
          198, 296
     DPAA databases, 65, 104
     FamilyTreeDNA, 202, 211, 215–219,
          224, 246
     FORDISC database, 92, 101–102,
          105–107, 132–134, 185
     GEDmatch, 202, 211–213, 216–221, 224,
          227, 236, 245–252, 260–261, 273–274
     IAFIS database, 29
     LAMMP database, 239, 246
     of missing children, xii, 30, 98, 109,
          192–193, 198
     NamUs database, xv, xix, 21–25, 31, 41,
          46, 49, 78, 102, 152–162, 203, 215–216,
          239, 295
     NCMEC database, xii, 30, 98, 109,
          192–193, 198
     NDIS database, 9
     POW/MIA databases, 65, 104
     searching, 15–16, 20–31, 43, 295–296
DCI (Division of Criminal
     Investigation), 6
Deadly Run (movie), 48
DeAngelo, Joseph, 10, 214, 224
decapitations
     investigations of, xvii, 2–15, 44, 48–49,
          84–85, 149, 204–205, 260, 290–292
     locations of, xvii, 2–14, 44, 149, 204
     postcrania and, 8, 13–14, 113, 131, 178
     see also Doe, Ina Jane

Defense Department, 29
Defense POW/MIA Accounting Agency
        (DPAA), 65, 104
Dekalb County, Georgia, 97
Dekalb Medical Examiner's Office, 97
"Delta Dawn," xviii
dental comparisons, 26–27, 149–175, 272
dental examinations, 6, 63–64, 136, 146–155,
        160–179, 195, 216, 227, 232–234
dental records, 4–6, 22–27, 37, 63, 96–97,
        112, 122, 135–137, 145–175, 184
dentist visit, 163–175
Department of Agriculture, 31
Department of Conservation, 6
Department of Defense, 29
Department of Justice, xix, 24
Department of the Interior, 68
Despins, Amy, 139–147
DFA (discriminant function analysis),
        101–102, 105–107
Dickens, Charles, 181
Dickens Museum, 181
Diplomate of the American Board of
        Forensic Anthropology (D-ABFA), 64
disaster scenes, 26, 154–161
Discord, 244, 247–252
discriminant function analysis (DFA),
        101–102, 105–107
dismemberment
    "Indiana arm," 203–204, 290, 296–297
    investigations of, 2–12, 44, 48–49,
        84–85, 95, 122–123, 180, 203–205,
        288, 290–292, 296–297
    locations of, 2–14, 44, 203–204, 290,
        296–297
    see also decapitations
Division of Criminal Investigation (DCI), 6
Division of State Troopers, 6
Dixie, Georgia, 188
DNA analysis, 35, 108, 117–118, 131,
        159–162, 182–183, 207–226, 291
DNA collection policies, 220
DNA databases, 26, 198–227, 245–254,
        260–261, 273–274, 292. *See also*
        specific databases

"DNA Detective," 208
DNA Doe Project, 19–20, 193, 199, 210,
        214, 218–224, 238–242, 246, 250, 295
DNA evidence, 9–10, 22, 25–27, 108
DNA extraction, 22, 51, 76, 117, 159, 205,
        208, 223, 231–234
DNA Identification Act, 9
DNA Painter, 247
DNA phenotyping, 182–183
DNA profiles, 9, 26, 35, 197–198,
        207–221, 232
DNA science, xvi, xx, 25–27, 53, 156–162,
        222, 232
DNA sequencing, 22, 117, 205, 212–213,
        231–236
DNA testing
    analysis of, 35, 108, 117–118, 131,
        159–162, 182–183, 207–226, 291
    collection policies for, 220
    cost of, xx
    exhumations and, 108, 210, 216, 225
    explanation of, 26–27, 35–36
    extraction and, 22, 51, 76, 117, 159, 205,
        208, 223, 231–234
    home DNA tests, 207, 220, 260
    investigative genetic genealogy and,
        207–226, 291
    phenotyping and, 182–183
    racial composition and, 219–222
    rapid DNA testing, 26, 156, 162
    results of, 26–27, 35–36, 51, 98, 108–109,
        131–132, 146, 156–162, 188, 207–226,
        239, 260, 291
    science of, xvi, xx, 25–27, 53,
        156–162, 232
    sequencing and, 22, 117, 205, 212–213,
        231–236
    SNP profiles and, 26, 117, 197–198,
        207–208, 216, 232
    STR DNA testing, 26, 207–208, 216, 232
DNASolves, 215
Doe, Anne Arundel Jane, 62, 183–184
Doe, Boyd John, 293–295
Doe, Christmas, xv, 40, 189
Doe, Dennis, xv, 97–98

Doe, Illinois John, 293–295
Doe, Ina Jane
    age-range estimation for, xvii, 8, 14, 41,
        95–97, 113, 179, 183, 191–192
    announcement about, 269–288
    case file of, xvii–xxi, 1–17, 27, 39–59,
        63–64, 71–90, 92–113, 202, 227–236,
        245–246, 261–262
    crime scene for, xvii, 1–12, 27, 39, 48, 55,
        79–88, 201, 259
    dental comparisons and, 26–27,
        149–175, 272
    dental examinations and, 6, 63–64,
        136, 146–155, 160–179, 195, 216, 227,
        232–234
    dental records and, 4–6, 22–27,
        37, 63, 96–97, 112, 122, 135–137,
        145–175, 184
    discovery of, 2–5
    DNA sequencing for, 231–236
    facial asymmetry and, xvii, 42–43,
        77–78, 112–113, 132–137, 173–179,
        200–201, 252, 266, 272–273
    forensic anthropology and, 63–64,
        92–113
    forensic art and, 42–43, 76–77, 137,
        173–174, 177–202, 272–273
    forensic odontology and, 4, 26, 63, 93,
        96, 149–162, 173–175
    GEDmatch for, 245–252
    hair samples from, 9, 117–118, 136, 164,
        195, 200–201, 227, 234–235
    homicide investigation and, 12–14, 260,
        271–277, 280, 289–290
    identity of, 8–9, 16–17, 252–268
    newspaper reports on, 8
    postcrania and, 8, 13–14, 113, 131, 178
    postmortem interval for, 8, 91–92, 100
    radiograph of, 165–173
    root canal of, 5, 132, 149–150, 154,
        172–173, 278
    sex estimation for, 107–113
    skeletal analysis and, 41–43, 53–55,
        63–66, 77–78, 92–113, 116–117,
        125–138

skeletal reanalysis and, 41–43, 53–55,
        64–66, 77–78, 116–117, 125–138, 203,
        272–273, 293
    tooth of, 6, 63–64, 136, 146–155,
        160–179, 195, 216, 227, 232–234
    torticollis and, xvii, 17, 42–43, 112–113,
        137, 179, 277
    VICAP for, 4–5, 10, 15
    wry neck syndrome and, xvii, 174
    X-rays of, 165–173
    see also Lund, Susan Minard
Doe, "Indiana Arm," 296–297. See also
    "Indiana arm"
Doe, Jasper County John, 241
Doe, Jefferson County John, 78–79
Doe, Julie, xv, 36, 107, 202, 210, 246
Doe, Litchfield Jane, 14–16
Doe, No. 24 John, 293–295
Doe, Riverdale John, 192–193
Doe, Twiggs County John, 94–95, 102,
    191–192
Doe Network, xv, 23–25, 151–155, 178,
    198, 296
"Doe Spotlight" drives, 221–222
Does, Jane
    DNA tests and, 208–209, 215–218
    investigations of, 19–38, 183–184, 199
    news coverage of, xii–xv, 53, 72,
        202–203, 255–259, 269–288, 292
    publicity for, xii–xv, 53, 72, 255–259
    reconstruction of, 187–192
    researching, xi, xvii–xxi, 19–38
    see also unidentified decedents
Does, John
    DNA tests and, 208–209, 215–218
    investigations of, 19–38, 78–79, 102, 155,
        166, 171, 199, 293–294
    news coverage of, xii–xv, 53, 72,
        202–203, 255–259, 269–288, 292
    publicity for, xii–xv, 53, 72, 255–259
    reconstruction of, 187–192
    researching, xi, xvii–xxi, 19–38
    see also unidentified decedents
DPAA (Defense POW/MIA Accounting
    Agency), 65, 104

Dugard, Jaycee, 197
Dunkley, George, 294
Dunne, Samantha, 275
Duvall, Shelley, 200–201

Education Week (magazine), 28
Emerson, Meredith, 48
England, 37, 54, 119, 181, 248
entomology reports, xvi, 8, 79, 126–127, 259
exhumations
  arguments for, 34
  cost of, xx
  DNA tests and, 108, 210, 216, 225
  for examination, 108, 120, 189, 210–211,
    216, 223–225
  observations of, 73
  orders for, 245, 293–295
Eyler, Larry, 241

Facebook, 42, 195, 203, 209, 214, 239, 247,
  253–254, 260, 265
FACES (Forensic Anthropology
  and Computer Enhancement
  Services), 189
facial asymmetry
  of Ina Jane Doe, xvii, 42–43, 77–78,
    112–113, 132–137, 173–179, 200–201,
    252, 266, 272–273
  torticollis and, 17, 42–43, 112–113, 137,
    179, 277
  wry neck syndrome and, xvii, 174
facial reconstruction
  3-D reconstruction, 76–77, 177–183,
    189, 241
  clay reconstruction, 42–43, 130,
    178–186, 190–191
  for Ina Jane Doe, 17, 42–43, 76–77,
    129–130, 181–190, 195–205
  portraits for, 16–17, 42–43, 177–189,
    192, 197–198, 202
  techniques for, xvi, xx, 63, 177, 181–190,
    195–206
  see also forensic art
Fall Line, The (podcast), xiv–xv, 94, 97, 102,
  117, 184, 228, 240, 261

Fallon, Alexander, 37
Falsetti, Dr. Anthony, 95
FamilyTreeDNA (FTDNA), 202, 211,
  215–219, 224, 246
FBI, 9, 15, 22, 29–31, 35, 160, 208, 281, 291
Finding Your Roots (TV show), 208
fingerprint comparisons, 9, 26–30, 156
fingerprint files, 15, 22–31, 38, 151
fingerprint technology, 15, 29
Fiore, Jasmine, 36–37
Fitzpatrick, Dr. Colleen, 35, 207, 210–214
Fitzpatrick, Dr. Leslie, 127, 138–143,
  146–147, 165–166, 172–175
Flaherty, Taylor, 109–111, 238
Florida, 19, 36, 95, 123, 145, 292
Flowers, Ashley, 224
Flowers in the Attic (book), 140
FOIA (Freedom of Information Act),
  xiv–xvii, 4, 15, 57, 145, 198, 292
FORDISC (Forensic Discriminant)
  database, 92, 101–102, 105–107,
  132–134, 185
forensic anthropology, 22–24, 61–70,
  91–113, 120, 137, 154–155, 189. *See
  also* skeletal analysis
Forensic Anthropology and Computer
  Enhancement Services (FACES), 189
Forensic Anthropology Identification and
  Recovery (FAIR) Lab, xvi
forensic art
  3-D digital modeling, 177–178, 180–183
  3-D reconstruction, 76–77, 177–183,
    189, 241
  clay busts, 42–43, 130, 178, 180–181
  clay reconstructions, 42–43, 130,
    178–186, 190–191
  digital images, 166, 177, 180–183, 192, 202
  facial reconstruction, 17, 42–43, 76–77,
    129–130, 181–190, 195–205
  portraits, 16–17, 42–43, 177–189, 192,
    197–198, 202
  process for, 22–23, 42–43, 54, 98–102,
    129–130, 137, 173–174, 177–202, 227,
    238–241, 260, 272–273
  renderings, 16–17, 42–43, 178, 202

Forensic Art and Illustration (book), 180

Forensic Discriminant (FORDISC)
database, 92, 101–102, 105–107,
132–134, 185

forensic genealogy, 208–209, 238, 270–273.
See also investigative genetic
genealogy

forensic odontology, 4, 26, 63, 93, 96,
149–162, 173–175. *See also* dental
comparisons

forensic reconstruction, xvi, xx, 63, 177,
181–190, 195–206

forensics
anthropology and, 22–24, 61–70,
91–113, 120, 137, 154–155, 189
art and, 16–17, 22–23, 42–43, 54, 76–77,
98–100, 102, 129–130, 137, 173–174,
177–202, 227, 238–241, 260, 272–273
early forensics, 9
genealogy and, 208–209, 238, 270–273
odontology and, 4, 26, 63, 93, 96,
149–162, 173–175
reconstruction techniques, xvi, xx, 63,
177, 181–190, 195–206
skeletal analysis and, xiv–xxi, 22–27,
38, 41–55, 61–78, 91–113, 116–120,
125–138, 154–155, 183, 189, 195, 203,
271–272, 293

Forestville, California, 108

Fort Campbell, 256, 258, 278, 280

Franklin County, Illinois, 1–4, 6, 13, 15

Franklin County Sheriff's Department, 6

Freedom of Information Act (FOIA),
xiv–xvii, 4, 15, 57, 145, 198, 292

Freund, James Paul, 199

FTDNA (FamilyTreeDNA), 202, 211,
215–219, 224, 246

Gates, Henry Louis Jr., 208

Gatliff, Betty Pat, 186, 197

GBI (Georgia Bureau of Investigation), 74,
94, 102, 185–189, 191

GCLAITH (Grupo Científico
Latino-Americano de Trabajo Sobre
Identificación Humana), 222

GEDmatch, 202, 211–213, 216–221, 224,
227, 236, 245–252, 260–261, 273–274

gender identification, 20–21, 36, 91–93,
97–101, 107–111, 238–239, 242, 246.
See also sex estimation

Genetic Detective, The (TV show), 208

genetics, 10, 20–22, 150, 207–226, 230

Georgia, xi–xii, 39–59, 73–74, 88, 94–102,
115, 123, 184–192, 229, 235–237,
263, 270

Georgia Bureau of Investigation (GBI), 74,
94, 102, 185–189, 191

Georgia State University, 270

Glen Burnie, Maryland, 183

Golden State Killer, 10, 207, 211, 214, 224

Goldman, Ron, 196

Goliath, Dr. Jesse, 101, 104–107

Google, 80

Google Alert, xv, 276

Google Docs, 293, 297

Google Drive, 44, 88, 122

Google Earth, 44

Google Scholar, xii

Goots, Alex, 109

Gould, D. Rae, 69

Grady Memorial Hospital, 184

Grafton, Sue, 210–211

Graham, Kerry, 108

gravesites, 61–69, 95, 119–120, 126, 188,
216, 258

Green, Donna, 184–185

Green, Raymond, 184–185

Greytak, Dr. Ellen, 182–184

Grupo Científico Latino-Americano de
Trabajo Sobre Identificación Humana
(GCLAITH), 222

hair samples, 9, 117–118, 136, 164, 195,
200–201, 227, 234–235

Hallmark, Josh, 125, 138

Hamilton, William DaShawn, 97–98

Hammack, Shirlene "Cheryl," 189

Hanrahan, Chelsea, 248, 275

Happy Face Killer, 123

Hargrove, Brooke, xiii, 50, 55, 189, 240

Harris, Kaylene Jo "Katy," 12
Hassanamisco Band of Nipmucs of
    Massachusetts, 69
Health Science Centers, 22
Heath, Becky, 214
Help Find The Missing Act, 152
HFI (hyperostosis frontalis interna), 113,
    134–136
Highland, Indiana, 254
Hilton, Gary, 48
Holt, Charles, 178
Home Depot, 190
homicides
    experience with, 11, 53
    Ina Jane Doe and, 12–14, 260, 271–277,
        280, 289
    investigation of, 8–9, 11–13, 20–21,
        36–37, 51–53, 223, 271–277, 280, 289
    missing people and, 8–9, 20–21, 223
    unidentified decedents and, 8–9,
        20–21, 223
Honeychurch, Marlyse, 215
Hopkinsville, Kentucky, 258
Hubbard Center for Genome Studies,
    131–132, 205, 275, 290
Huntington Beach, California, 30
Hurricane Katrina, 154
hyperostosis frontalis interna (HFI), 113,
    134–136

IAFIS (Integrated Automated Fingerprint
    Identification System), 29
Idaho, 67, 241
Idaho State University, 63, 67, 109, 118
identification methods
    gender and, 20–21, 36, 91–93, 97–101,
        107–111, 238–239, 242, 246
    Ida Jane Doe identity, 8–9, 16–17, 252–268
    photo identification, 22–28, 35, 41,
        88–89, 111, 179–191, 198–201
    racial categories and, 21, 99–106, 219–222
    transgender identification, 36, 107–111,
        238–239, 242, 246
    types of, xv–xvi, xx, 15, 26–29, 95
    see also specific methods

IGG, 10, 20, 207–226, 291. See also
    investigative genetic genealogy
I'll Be Gone in the Dark (book), 214
Illinois, xvii, 1–15, 41–56, 71–90, 117,
    122–123, 137, 149, 178, 193–195,
    200–203, 227–228, 234, 245, 249,
    259–271, 277–280, 288–296
Illinois Division of Criminal
    Investigation, 2
Illinois State Police, 2, 6, 15, 53, 295
implants, 25–26, 36–37, 112, 168
Ina, Illinois, 1–14, 71–90
Indiana, 203–205, 254, 256, 259, 281, 290,
    296–297
"Indiana arm," 203–204, 290, 296–297
injuries, xv, 26, 62–63, 112–113, 134–135,
    170, 184, 282–283. See also marks;
    scars
insect activity, xvi, 8, 79, 126–127, 259
Instagram, 72, 120, 229
Integrated Automated Fingerprint
    Identification System (IAFIS), 29
International Symposium on Human
    Identification (ISHI), 222
investigative genetic genealogy (IGG)
    DNA analysis and, 35, 108, 117–118, 131,
        159–162, 182–183, 207–226, 291
    explanation of, 10, 20
    forensic genealogy and, 208–209, 238,
        270–273
    funding for, 215, 223–225
    gender and, 20–21, 36, 91–93, 97–101,
        107–111, 238–239, 242, 246
    importance of, 10, 20
Isa, Dr. Mari, 109
ISHI (International Symposium on
    Human Identification), 222
isotopic testing, xvi, 127, 137, 140, 146, 163

Jacksonville, Illinois, 293
"Japanese Gardens Girl," 292–293
Jefferson County, Illinois, xvii, 1–15,
    41–56, 74–87, 117, 123, 137, 149, 178,
    193–195, 200–203, 227–228, 234, 245,
    249, 260–271, 277–280, 288–296

Jefferson County Sheriff's Office, 6, 53, 74, 195, 203, 227–228, 261, 271
Jenkins, Ryan, 37
"Jestyn," 33–34

Keats, John, 181
Kentucky, 2, 13, 23, 49, 258
Kerr, Isabella, 180–181
Keyes, Israel, 125, 138
Keyes, Kelly, 30–31
Kimmerle, Dr. Erin H., 95
Kincaid, Dr. Kelly Harkins, 117, 223, 228–230, 290, 296
King, Marcia, 214
King's Cross Underground, 37
Klepinger, Dr. Linda, 95–97, 99–100, 107, 112–113, 135–136, 179, 277
KMOV News, 13
Koppelman, Carl, 193, 196–202, 227, 260
Kuiper, Andrea, 30–31

LA Times (newspaper), 30–31, 196
Lady Chatterley's Lover (book), 140
"Lady of the Dunes," xviii, 291–292
Lake County, Indiana, 254
Lake Lou Yaeger, 15
LAMMP: LGBT+ Accountability for Missing and Murdered Persons, 239, 246
Latin American Scientific Working Group on Human Identification, 222
Lavoie, Rebecca, 125
Lawson, Kelly, 184–197
Lawson, Marla, 185–192, 196
Lewis, William "Bill" Joseph, 241
LGBTQ+ community, 239
"Lime Lady, The," 199
Litchfield, Illinois, 14–15
Little, Samuel, 48
Lompoc, California, 210
London, England, 37
Los Angeles, California, 37, 228
Louisiana, 189
Loveless, Joseph Henry, 241
Lowery, Bob Jr., 109
Lund, Angel, 256

Lund, Crystal, 255–256, 285–287, 290, 296
Lund, Paul, 254–262, 278–284
Lund, Paul Jr., 256
Lund, Susan Minard
  announcement about, 269–288
  background of, 253–288
  children of, 252, 255–256, 260–262, 276–280, 284–287, 290, 296
  family of, 252–272, 275–290, 296
  homicide investigation of, 289–290
  husband of, 254–262, 278–284
  identifying, 252–268
  see also Doe, Ina Jane

Marion, Illinois, 2
marks/scars, xv, 25–27, 76, 112, 131–135, 164–165, 169, 205. See also tattoos
Marshall, Elizabeth, 275
Mary Queen of Scots, 181
Maryland, 62, 183–184
mass disasters, 26, 154–161
Massachusetts, 69, 125, 138, 229, 237–239, 261, 291
Massachusetts State Police, 291
Matchem-Thomas, Lynn, 16
Matthews, Todd, 23–25, 151–152, 155–158, 178
McArthur, Bruce, 155–156
McCandless, Katherine, 139
McCarthy, Andrea, 275
McGruff the Crime Dog, 28
McNamara, Michelle, 214
McWaters, Sarah, 215
medical devices, 36–37
medical implants, 25–26, 36–37, 112, 168
medical records, 26, 37–38, 112, 137–138, 157, 165–166, 181. See also dental records
Megan Wants a Millionaire (TV show), 37
Miami-Dade County, Florida, 292
Michael, Dr. Amy, xvi–xviii, 22, 38, 41–90, 96, 99, 102, 109, 115–147, 150–157, 163–175, 179, 195–205, 223–227, 230, 234–246, 252, 260–266, 269–273, 276–278, 283, 289–297

Michigan State University, 109
military fingerprints, 29
military intelligence, 34, 256
military mystery, 33–34
military records, 29, 173–174
Millbrook, Dannette, xii–xiv
Millbrook, Jeannette, xii–xiv
Minard, Ann Marie, 254–255, 260–267,
    270–271, 276–283, 288–290, 296
Minard, Charles (Chuck), 255, 264,
    270–271, 276, 281
Minard, Mary, 281
Minard, Pam, 254–256, 260–267, 270–272,
    275–289
Minard, Susan, 253–255. *See also* Lund,
    Susan Minard
Minecraft, 45, 247
missing-persons cases
    age-range estimations for, xvii, 8,
      14, 41, 95–97, 113, 179, 183,
      191–192
    cM matches and, 213, 218–222, 246,
      249–252, 274
    DNA testing and, 212–213
    homicides and, 8–9, 20–21, 223
    investigation of, 8–30, 43, 78–88,
      103–108, 122–128, 151–158, 172, 184,
      189, 223, 238–243, 253–262
    number of, xviii–xx, 20–22
    researching, xiv–xx, 10–30, 43,
      78–88, 103–108, 122–128, 151–158,
      192–197, 238–243, 253–262,
      273, 287
    sex estimation for, xvii, 20–21, 91–113,
      134, 182–183, 238–243, 272
    see also unidentified decedents
Mississippi, 192–193, 215
Mississippi State University, 101, 104
Missouri, 2, 13, 16, 47, 50–51, 54, 58–59,
    71, 89–90
Moore, CeCe, 207–212, 215
most recent common ancestor (MRCA),
    250, 274–275
Mount Vernon, Illinois, 11, 71–72, 122,
    149, 195, 202, 261–263, 269

MRCA group, 250, 274–275
MSU Forensic Anthropology Lab
    (MSU-FAL), 109
Muldavin, Guy, 291–292
mummification, 66, 125–127, 138–146,
    163–171
Murphy, Erin, 220
Myrtle Beach, South Carolina, 119

NAGPRA (Native American Graves Pro-
    tection and Repatriation Act), 68–69
NamUs database, xv, xix, 21–25, 31, 41, 46,
    49, 78, 102, 152–162, 203, 215–216,
    239, 295
National Center for Missing and Exploited
    Children (NCMEC), xii, 30, 98, 109,
    192–193, 198
National Crime Information Center
    (NCIC), 24, 79, 88
National DNA Index System (NDIS), 9
National Forest (National Park), 48
National Institute of Justice (NIJ), 22,
    66–67, 208
National Missing and Unidentified
    Persons System (NamUs), xv, xix,
    21–25, 31, 41, 46, 49, 78, 102, 152–162,
    203, 215–216, 239, 295
National September 11 Memorial &
    Museum, 159
Native American and Indigenous Studies
    Initiative, 69
Native American Graves Protection
    and Repatriation Act (NAGPRA),
    68–69
NBC, 28, 67
NBC News, 67
NCIC (National Crime Information
    Center), 24, 79, 88
NCMEC database, xii, 30, 98, 109,
    192–193, 198
NDIS database, 9
Netflix, 46
New Hampshire, xviii, 45–46, 65, 115–147,
    163–175, 227, 295
New Hampshire State Police, 65

New York Office of the Chief Medical Examiner (NYC OCME), 159
New York Times (newspaper), 291–292
News Herald (newspaper), 213
Newsome, George, 188
Newspapers.com, 116, 251
Newton, Joseph Chandler, 212
Next Generation Identification (NGI), 22, 29
Nichols, Robert Ivan, 213–214
NIJ (National Institute of Justice), 22, 66–67, 208
Ninety Six, South Carolina, 237
North Carolina, 22, 98
Nyden, Donald, 199

odontology, 4, 26, 63, 93, 96, 149–162, 173–175. *See also* dental comparisons; dental records
Ohio, 214
On the Hunt with John Walsh (TV show), 28
One Strange Thing (podcast), 228–229
open population event, 158
Orange, Massachusetts, 125, 237–239
Orange County, California, 30–31, 228
Orange County Sheriff's Office, 30
"Orange Socks," xviii
Othram Inc., 215, 291

panoramic X-rays, 126, 138, 153, 166–167, 170–174
Pantagraph (newspaper), 14
Parabon NanoLabs, 182–183, 189, 208
Parker, Charles, 2
Pasqual, Sebastian, 19
PBS, 208
Pectol, Doug, 258
Pembroke, Florida, 95
Pembroke, New Hampshire, 165–166
Pennsylvania, 159, 161
Peoria, Illinois, 294–295
person of interest (POI), 122–123
Philip, Dr. Sneha, 158–159
photo identification, 22–28, 35, 41, 88–89, 111, 179–191, 198–201

PMI (postmortem interval), 8, 40, 91–92, 100
POI (person of interest), 122–123
Poltak, Dr. Steffen, 121, 200
population event, 158
Portsmouth, New Hampshire, 116–119
postcrania
explanation of, 8
identity and, 13–14
Ina Jane Doe and, 8, 13–14, 113, 131, 178
postmortem interval (PMI)
explanation of, 8
for Ina Jane Doe, 8, 91–92, 100
understanding, 8, 40, 91–92
POW/MIA Accounting Agency, 65, 104
Press, Dr. Margaret, 207, 210–214, 219, 224, 242
Primitive Camp area, 5, 80–83
Pro Publica (news site), 68–69
Project EDAN: Everyone Deserves a Name, 178

Quantico, 53, 178
"Queered Science: Interdisciplinary Approaches to Gender-Inclusive Research," 109

racial categories, 21, 99–106, 219–222
racial composition, 219–222
"Racial Composition of Forensic DNA Databases, The," 219–220
radiocarbon, 66–67, 93, 137–140, 146, 163
radiographs, 152–160, 165–173
Rae-Venter, Dr. Barbara, 207, 211–212, 214–215
"Railroad Killer," 12
rapid DNA testing, 26, 156, 162
Rasmussen, Terry, 215
reconstruction techniques, xvi, xx, 63, 177, 181–190, 195–206. *See also* facial reconstruction
recovery scene, 61, 65, 80, 94, 154–156. *See also* crime scene
Reddit, xii, 42, 50, 85, 150, 242, 262
Redgrave, Anthony, 109–110, 237–252, 260–261, 265, 270–275

Redgrave, Lee, 237–252, 260–261
Redgrave Research Forensic Services, 125,
    138, 202, 227, 234–254, 260–262, 265,
    270–275
"Redhead Murders," 48–49
Rend Lake, 1–4, 11, 80–83
Rend Lake Resort, 2, 80
Research Triangle Institute (RTI), 22
Reséndiz, Ángel Maturino, 12
Return of the Living Dead (movie), 141–142
Ritter, Nancy, xix
Riverdale, Georgia, 192
Rogers, Curtis, 217
Rogerson, Mary Jane, 180–181
RootsWeb, 209
Ross, Dr. Ann H., 95
RTI (Research Triangle Institute), 22
Rubáiyát of Omar Khayyám (book), 33–34
Rule, Ann, xii
Ruxton, Buck, 180

St. Louis Dispatch (newspaper), 15
St. Louis, Missouri, 16, 50–51, 54, 58–59
San Francisco Chronicle (newspaper), 108
Santa Cruz, California, 117, 227–234
Saved by the Bell (TV show), 73
Scanlon, Dr. Richard, 155–162
scars, xv, 25–27, 76, 112, 131–135, 164–165,
    169, 205
Schechter, Harold, 48
Seabright Beach, California, 229
Sells, Tommy Lynn, 12
September 11 (9/11) attacks, 26, 154–160
serial killers, 12, 47–49, 122–125, 155–156,
    214–215, 224, 241–242
serial-number matching, 25–26, 36–37, 154
sex estimation, xvii, 20–21, 91–113, 134,
    182–183, 238–243, 272. *See also*
    gender identification
short tandem repeat (STR) tests, 26,
    207–208, 216, 232
Simpson, Nicole Brown, 196
Simpson, O. J., 196
single nucleotide polymorphism (SNP)
    profiles, 26, 117, 197, 207–208, 216, 232

skeletal analysis
    bone samples, 141–147, 204–205, 231, 235
    broken bones, xv, 26, 92, 112
    forensics and, xiv–xxi, 22–27, 38,
        41–55, 61–78, 91–113, 116–120,
        125–138, 154–155, 183, 189, 195, 203,
        272–273, 293
    Ina Jane Doe and, 41–43, 53–55, 63–66,
        77–78, 92–113, 116–117, 125–138
    method of, 91–113
    reanalysis of, 41–54, 64–66, 77–78,
        116–117, 125–138, 203, 272–273, 293
    skeletal asymmetry and, xvii, 42–43
    skeletal remains and, xiv–xxi, 1–16,
        44–52, 61–69, 84–171, 180–188,
        195–225, 232–241
skeletal asymmetry, xvii, 42–43. *See also*
    facial asymmetry
skeletal reanalysis, 41–54, 64–66, 77–78,
    116–117, 125–138, 203, 272–273, 293
skeletal remains, xiv–xxi, 1–16, 44–52,
    61–69, 84–171, 180–188, 195–225,
    232–241
Smithsonian (magazine), 32, 35, 62
Smithsonian Institute, 62, 65, 79
Snapshot Advanced DNA Analysis
    Service, 182–184
SNP profiles, 26, 117, 197–198, 207–208,
    216, 232
social media
    Facebook, 42, 195, 209, 214, 239, 247,
        253–254, 260, 265
    Instagram, 72, 120, 229
    Reddit, xii, 42, 50, 85, 150, 242, 262
    TikTok, 224, 296
    Twitch, 224, 270
    Twitter, 291
    Unidentified Wiki, 25, 30, 292
    Websleuths, 42, 197–198, 209, 262
    YouTube, 104, 224, 232, 270
"Somerton Man, The," xviii, 32–35, 181,
    210, 222
South Carolina, 73, 119, 237, 263, 295
Southeast Missouri State University
    (SEMO), 89–90

Spokane, Washington, 199
State Police Case Action Report, 4
Stevik, Lyle, xviii, 19, 199
Stigsen, Pam, 275
STR DNA testing, 26, 207–208, 216, 232
stranger-danger era, 27–28
Strontium Isotopes analysis, 169
Stubblefield, Dr. Phoebe R., 104
Suncook Dental, 165–174, 275

tattoos, xv, 25–27, 58, 89, 192–193, 237, 240
Taylor, Barbara Ann Hackman, 23
Taylor, Karen, 180–181, 186, 197–198
TBI (Tennessee Bureau of
    Investigations), 258
TDTF (Trans Doe Task Force), 109–111,
    237–239, 242, 246
Tennessee, 13, 26, 49, 101, 152–155,
    252–265, 271–284, 289–291
Tennessee Bureau of Investigations
    (TBI), 258
"Tent Girl," 23
Terry, Ruth Marie, 291–292
Texas, 22, 74, 122–123, 154, 229
Texas Tech University, 109
Thomas, Curtis, 16
Thomas, Lynn, 16
Thomaston, Georgia, 189
Thomson, Jessica Harkness, 34–35
Thomson, Robin, 34–35
Tigard, Tamara Lee, 199
TikTok, 224, 296
Tilton Mummy, 126–127, 138–146,
    163–164, 169
Tong, Jun H., 220
tooth examination, 6, 63–64, 136,
    146–155, 160–179, 195, 216, 227,
    232–234. See also dental comparisons
torticollis, xvii, 17, 42–43, 112–113, 137,
    179, 277. See also wry neck syndrome
Tradewinds Shopping Center, 256
Trans Doe Task Force (TDTF), 109–111,
    237–239, 242, 246
transgender identification, 36, 107–111,
    238–239, 242, 246

Trimble, Francine, 108
Troy, Ohio, 214
Tupac, 187
Twiggs County, Georgia, 94–95, 102,
    191–192
Twitch, 224, 270
Twitter, 291

UID cases, xvi, 19–21. See also unidenti-
    fied decedents
Ukiah Daily Journal (newspaper), 109
unidentified decedents (UID)
    age-range estimations for, xvii, 8, 14, 41,
        95–97, 113, 179, 183, 191–192
    cM matches and, 213, 218–222, 246,
        249–252, 274
    DNA testing and, 212–213
    explanation of, xvi, 19–21
    gender of, 20–21, 36, 91–93, 97–101,
        107–111, 238–239
    homicides and, 8–9, 20–21, 223
    investigation of, 20–38, 90, 103–108,
        212–213, 218–222
    number of, xviii–xx, 20–22
    race of, 20–21
    racial categories and, 21, 99–106
    sex estimation of, xvii, 20–21, 91–113,
        134, 182–183, 238–243, 272
    see also cold cases; missing-persons
        cases
Unidentified Wiki, 25, 30, 292
Uniform Anatomical Gift Act, 125, 140
University of Adelaide, 34
University of California, Berkeley, 68
University of Florida, 104
University of Nevada Las Vegas (UNLV),
    109, 111
University of New Hampshire (UNH),
    xvi, 50–52, 87, 127, 138, 205, 248, 272,
    275, 290
University of North Dakota, 67
University of North Texas, 22
University of Tennessee, 101
Unsolved Mysteries (TV show), xi–xii, 30
Utah, 186, 217

Vancouver, Canada, 242
Vancouver Police, 242
Vanderburgh County, Indiana,
    204–205
Vaughn, Marie, 215
Veltstra, Viktor, 239–248, 260, 275
Verdugo, Dr. Cristina, 230–235
VH1, 37
Violent Criminal Apprehension
    Program (VICAP), 4–5, 9–10, 15,
    24, 88
Virginia, 30–31, 262

Waco, Texas, 154
Walker, Carla, 207
Wallace, Bobby, 74, 260, 269, 280, 289
Walsh, Adam, 28
Walsh, John, 28
Warder, Robin, xii
Washington, 19, 199
Waterman, Audrey, 42, 50–52, 56–59,
    73–87, 90
WATO probability, 274–275
Wayne Fitzgerrell State Park, xvii, 1–5, 55,
    79–83, 201, 259

Wayne Fitzgerrell State Recreation
    Center, 80
Webb, Charles "Carl," 35, 181
Websleuths, 42, 197–198, 209, 262
West Virginia, 19, 240
What Are the Odds (WATO) tool, 274–275
Whittington, Illinois, 1, 4
Wilson bands, 118, 164
Winn Dixie, 256
Wood, Dr. Jim, 108
World Trade Center, 158–159
World War II, 33, 213
Worters, Bryan, 241
wry neck syndrome, xvii, 174. *See also*
    torticollis

X-ray comparisons, 26, 38, 125–126,
    137–138, 151–160, 165–174

Yahoo, 209
YouTube, 104, 224, 232, 270
YouTuber MrBallen, 224

Zoom, 55, 117, 137, 140, 147, 167, 200, 208,
    245–248, 261